BRADY

PARAMEDIC
EXAMINATION
REVIEW
MANUAL

DAVID P. EDWARDS BA, EMT-P

MARK WEINGARTNER RN, EMT-P

Brady
A Prentice Hall Division
Englewood Cliffs, New Jersey 07632

Library of Congress Cataloging-in-Publication Data

Edwards, David P.
   Paramedic examination review manual/David P. Edwards, Mark
  Weingartner
    p.m.
   Includes bibliographical references and index.
   ISBN 0-89303-805-9
   1. Emergency medicine—Examinations, questions, etc.
  I. Weingartner, Mark. II. Title.
   [DNLM: 1. Emergency Medical Technicians—examination questions.
  2. Emergency Medicine—examination questions. WB 18 E26p]
  RC86.9.E39 1991
  616.02 '5 '076—dc20
  DNLM/DLC
  for Library of Congress   90–15164
                                   CIP

Editorial/production supervision and
  interior design: Fred Dahl and Rose Kernan
Cover design: Karen Stephens
Prepress manufacturing buyer: Mary McCartney
Manufacturing Buyer: Edward O'Dougherty
Acquisitions Editor: Natalie Anderson

©1991 by Prentice-Hall, Inc.
A Simon & Schuster Company
Englewood Cliffs, New Jersey 07632

Printed in the United States of America

10 9 8 7 6 5 4 3 2 1

ISBN 089303-805-9

Prentice-Hall International (UK) limited, *London*
Prentice-Hall of Australia Pty. Limited, *Sydney*
Prentice-Hall Canada Inc., *Toronto*
Prentice-Hall Hispanoamericana, S.A., *Mexico*
Prentice-Hall of India Private Limited, *New Delhi*
Prentice-Hall of Japan, Inc., *Tokyo*
Simon & Schuster Asia Pte. Ltd., *Singapore*
Editora Prentice-Hall do Brasil, Ltds., *Rio de Janeiro*

Contents

Preface

When it's time to take paramedic board exams, the usual method of review involves corraling a considerable collection of study materials. This probably includes an ACLS text, PHTLS text, maybe a PALS textbook, the latest paramedic class textbook, a PDR or other pharmacologic reference, some old tests and notes, or even a copy of the DOT National Standard Curriculum for Paramedics, The purpose of this book is to allow paramedics access to review materials in a single text that conform closely to the National Standard Curriculum and incorporates the essence of other resources considered to be "standard of care."

The idea for summarizing the essentials of the paramedic curriculum to facilitate studying for EMS exams arose out of meetings of the Field Paramedic Committee, a small group of experienced field medics assembled by the Missouri Bureau of EMS (facilitated by Jason White) and charged with exploring ideas for shaping the future of EMS in Missouri. While discussing a side issue, Mark Weingartner expressed the opinion that a document should be produced that gives guidance to medics retaking their board examinations. The authors, Edwards and Weingartner, have between them 30 years of field experience as paramedics and have tried to approach the subject with an economy of material, while still covering subjects that are fair game for examiners.

The authors would like to thank the following people for their outstanding job in reviewing the text manuscript: Greg Mullen, EMT-P, Swedish Medical Center, Englewood, Colorado; Ted Tully, EMT-P, Westchester City EMS; William R. Roush, MD, Akron City Hospital; Bryan Bledsoe, D.O., EMT-P, Scott & White Hospital, Texas A&M University College of Medicine; and Keith Meely, EMT-P, Oregon Health Sciences University.

Acknowledgments

We appreciate the help of many in the preparation of this manuscript from our employers and co-workers who endured our obsession with writing, to the many paramedics (and paramedic students) facing exams who agreed to use our material in their preparation and review. A special thank you is extended to Jason White.

Most of all, this book is indebted to Mary (David's wife) and Marie (Mark's wife). The wife of a paramedic is protective of her family's time together. However, both Mary and Marie gave of their time to cajole, inspire, and encourage when writing was an arduous and time-consuming task that took both of us from family and friends.

How to Take a Test

Nearly as important as your choice of study materials is the way that you prepare for an examination.

1. Begin your study several weeks before the exam, if possible, and approach the subjects in an organized and realistic manner. Don't wait until the last minute. Know when to refuse social pleasantries (or even overtime) when you really need to study.

2. When studying, organize your resources so that you do not have to jump from area to area. (Study drugs, for example, at the same time.)

3. Beware of old administrators who think they have a copy of the test or a similar test that can help you. Put stock in your knowledge instead.

4. Don't cram the evening before. If possible, don't study at all the night before the exam (at most, do a light review). The answers you need should be in your long-term memory, not the short-term unless you plan on short-changing your patients.

5. Get plenty of sleep the night before the test.

6. It may be helpful to study with someone else in your final review sessions. They may know answers you don't and you can stimulate each other in finding resources and answers.

Then, as test day dawns:

1. Dress comfortably. Board exams are not a fashion show.
2. If unfamiliar with the examination site, locate it in advance. You don't need any of those kind of hassles on test day.
3. Get up early or leave in plenty of time to allow for bad traffic, car trouble, and so on. Try to follow your usual daily routine the day of the test.
4. Take only the materials you are told to, or the materials mentioned in the official exam notice.
5. Don't eat high-sugar foods before the test (you may experience a let-down at some crucial point). Take a cue from long-distance runners and do some carbo-loading the night before, then have a light reasonable high-protein meal approximately two hours before taking the test.
6. See if you can reschedule the exam if you are seriously ill.

When you are comfortably arranged in your seat at zero hour, with a sharp #2 pencil in claw:

1. Consider limiting your intake of coffee before and during test time. Caffeine is like the short-term high of sugar—it may leave you stranded.
2. Have some idea of the time limitations for each question. If you know there are 160 questions to complete in a four-hour time limit, you know you have an average of two minutes per question. At the end of hour one, you should be near or past question #40, while at the end of hour three you should be near or past question #120.
3. Find out if you are penalized for wrong answers. If you are not, guess at the correct answer when stumped. The most frequent correct answer on multiple choice tests is usually "b." If you have decided to guess and have absolutely no clue as to the answer, guess "b."
4. Find out if you may use a scratch pad during the test. If so, keep one handy to figure dosages and make calculations (and to keep track of the questions you need to go back to). If you are allowed a calculator, keep it handy.
5. Listen to the instructions and do not start until instructed to do so.

After the proctor has read the instructions and handed out the test:

1. Scan the test. Look at the format and spot difficult areas that might require more time.

2. Read each question and all responses thoroughly before answering. Don't just pick the first one that seems correct—there may be a better or more precise answer. Be sure you understand what the question is asking. Pay particular attention to key words, such as "least", "most", "best", "describe" and the like.

3. If you have trouble on a question (or even a section), leave it and come back later. This will allow you to finish more questions before spending time on the tough ones. After answering the other questions, you may have more insight into the best way to approach the question. At times, a late question in the test gives away the answer to an early question.

When you are finished with the test:

1. Go back and check your answers if you have time, looking for obvious mistakes.

2. Scan your answer sheet for extra marks, multiple answers, and so on. The machines that usually grade standardized exams interpret extra marks, poorly erased answers and smudges as real answers. This may reduce your score.

3. If you skipped questions during the test, be sure you started again in the right place. If you get off by one question, you can incorrectly mark a whole section.

Obviously some people have an easier time than others performing on written evaluations. Following these simple suggestions (and using this book) will increase your chances of accurately reflecting your knowledge base on your exam score.

Roles and Responsibilities

The EMT-Paramedic is a health care professional who must understand his/her legal and ethical responsibilities, demonstrate a high level of professionalism, and strive for a standard of care that places the patient above all else.

Roles and Responsibilities

Ethics Derived from the Greek word meaning "character", ethics are the principles and standards of conduct governing the EMT-P. Though ethics deal with the rightness or wrongness of conduct, they do not address morality.

Professionalism In the field of emergency prehospital care, professionalism involves acquiring a specialized body of skills and knowledge and conforming to specific standards of conduct and performance within that area.

Roles of the EMT-P At the scene of an emergency, the EMT-P must:

1. Recognize and treat life-threatening emergencies.
2. Send for (and coordinate with) other supportive agencies (as needed).

3. Establish rapport with patients.
4. Communicate data to the appropriate medical command authority.

When transporting to an appropriate medical facility, the EMT-P must:

1. Continue prioritized treatment and stabilization.
2. Maintain appropriate communication with medical command.

Upon arrival at the destination medical facility, the EMT-P must:

1. Effect an orderly transfer of patient(s) to the care of receiving personnel.
2. Provide receiving personnel with relevant patient records and history.
3. Document the call, accurately and in detail (including pertinent negatives). Remember, if it isn't written, it didn't happen!
4. Disinfect appropriate equipment and resupply.

Credentials

Registration/Certification Registration/certification is the process by which an agency/association grants recognition to an individual who has met pre-determined qualifications specified by that agency/association. (This is a traditional way of assuring minimum competency in the medical arena.)

Licensure This is the process by which a governmental agency grants permission to an individual to engage in a specific occupation upon recognition that the applicant has demonstrated the minimal degree of competency necessary to ensure the public of reasonable protection.

Reciprocity Reciprocity is the recognition by one agency of minimum proficiency levels in respecting the certification of another agency. It may involve a mutual exchange of privileges or licenses by the agencies.

Continuing Education Continuing education is an on-going educational process designed to:

1. Maintain skill levels attained at licensure or certification.

2. Keep personnel aware of current trends, techniques, and changing standards in patient care.

3. Encourage further professional development.

4. Protect the community-at-large against erosion of skills and knowledge.

Summary

Paramedics play a key role in emergency health care delivery. They are expected to:

1. Analyze chaotic scenes (and send for appropriate supportive agencies).

2. Recognize, prioritize, and treat life-threatening injuries and illnesses (utilizing advanced emergency medical procedures).

3. Carefully package and transport victims to appropriate facilities.

4. Transfer care to other health care professionals and appropriately document the event.

Participation in state and national EMS organizations, refresher courses, special seminars, further study and continuing education help EMT-P's maintain their skills, certifications, and licenses.

SELF-TEST

Chapter 1

1. Define ethics.

    ANSWER: Ethics deals with the rightness or wrongness of conduct.

2. Define professionalism.

    ANSWER: Professionalism involves acquiring specialized skills and knowledge that conform to specific standards of conduct and performance within that area.

3. What is the role of the EMT-P at the scene of an emergency?

    ANSWER: To recognize and treat life-threatening emergencies, send for supportive agencies as needed, establish a rapport with patients, and communicate data to the appropriate medical authority.

EMS Systems

This chapter reviews the EMS System, its basic components, and their relationships. An emphasis must be made on the importance of commitment, cooperation, and communication between participatory members and agencies.

EMS System The EMS system's purpose is to provide rapid prehospital evaluation, advanced treatment, and timely transport to appropriate medical facilities of acutely ill and injured citizens. The effective extension of hospital care into the field can only be accomplished by an informed committed community, properly trained and managed prehospital care agencies (including the police department), aggressive supportive hospital emergency departments, and the support and understanding of area physicians.

System Access System access is the way in which the Emergency Medical System is activated. Calls are received from private citizens, law enforcement agencies, medical facilities, schools, automatic notification systems, and other prehospital care providers. Most communities now have 911 direct-dialing systems that utilize specialized technology to ensure rapid and appropriate response to calls for emergency assistance.

Field Stabilization This is definitive medical intervention designed to stabilize patients for safe transport from the prehospital environment to the hospital environment. Some medical patients receive extensive field treatment, while some trauma patients receive only a rapid cursory evaluation before immediate transport to the hospital.

Medical Control Medical control is a broad concept referring to a physician's direction of advanced prehospital care. It may also involve the development of patient care protocols, standing orders (where legal), Medical Command Authority and on-line physician (or physician designee) direction of patient care.

Medical Director The medical director is a licensed physician who provides direction and assumes medical responsibility for prehospital care providers. Though the medical director's responsibilities vary from state to state, he/she generally is the authority who approves patient care protocols, standing orders, prescription medications and controlled substances carried, and may provide some portion of continuing education training, run reviews, and personnel evaluation.

Protocols Protocol describes patient management guidelines which apply to a proscribed set of circumstances and provide accepted standards of treatment. Protocols often cover a wide variety of commonly encountered EMS situations.

Standing Orders Standing orders are specific patient care procedures that are pre-approved for use when:

1. The delay necessary to establish contact and provide a proper report to the proper medical control would be detrimental to patient outcome.
2. Attempts to contact medical control have been unsuccessful and the patient needs immediate definitive care.
3. Circumstances unique to a EMS delivery system make standing orders the only viable stopgap to deal with emergency medical/trauma situations.

Constructive Audits These audits are run reviews intended to isolate weaknesses and strengths in the procedures of an EMS system and the performance of its personnel. Constructive audits are not intended as a disciplinary tool, but provide a way to ensure quality control and consistent levels of performance.

Continuing Education Continuing education is training that incorporates a review of original training and new information to help maintain levels of proficiency. Continuing education should provide:

1. Review of core curriculum (DOT National Standard Curriculum).
2. Updated drug information and dosages.
3. Introduction to new devices and procedures.
4. Supervised practice of basic and advanced skills.

Community Education This form of education is an on-going effort to advance community awareness in the area of advanced prehospital emergency care. Some benefits of aggressive community education are:

1. Widespread understanding of proper (rapid) system access (usually 911).
2. Earlier system access by high-risk cardiac patients (due to increased public awareness of the early warning signs of impending heart attack).
3. A higher level of basic life support skills within the general population.
4. Adequate financial support of EMS system components.
5. More accurate, more positive press coverage.
6. Enhanced citizen cooperation (and less complaints).

Major Incident/Disaster Planning This form of planning incorporates a realistic assessment of community assets and liabilities in planning a system-wide response to disaster (or major system overload). Remember that a disaster can be any situation where the demand for emergency care outstrips available resources.

Summary

In the end, the quality and performance of an EMS system depends most directly on the personnel responsible for patient care. If they are well-trained, if they demonstrate common sense and perform in a professional manner, and if they put the interests of the patient above all else, the system will function successfully.

SELF-TEST

Chapter 2

1. What functions should an EMS system provide?

   ANSWER: It should provide rapid prehospital evaluation, advanced treatment and timely transport to appropriate medical facilities of acutely ill and injured citizens.

2. A broad concept refering to physician direction of advanced prehospital care is called _____ _____ .

   ANSWER: Medical control

3. Who is a "medical director?"

   ANSWER: A licensed physician who provides direction and assumes medical responsibility for prehospital care providers.

4. What are "protocols?"

   ANSWER: Patient management guidelines that apply to a proscribed set of circumstances and provide accepted standards of treatment.

5. Specific patient care procedures that are pre-approved by a physician medical director for use in the field are called _____

   ANSWER: Standing orders

Medical/Legal Considerations

This chapter reviews patient rights and protections as well as the protections and obligations of the EMT-P. Though the intricacies of legal definitions vary from state to state, the following explanations represent a faithful attempt to convey the essence of these concepts. All EMT-Ps should thoroughly understand these terms and their implication to "hands-on" patient care.

Terminology

Medical Practice Act This act defines the minimum qualifications and skills of health care professionals and details their method of certification.

Good Samaritan Act Where applicable, this act protects those who render emergency assistance at the scene of an emergency from legal action, providing that they acted unselfishly and within the boundaries of their training.

State EMS Legislation Enabling Legislation dealing specifically with statutes relating to the administering of emergency medical care and usually defines levels of personnel certification and training, equipment requirements, medical and quality control, communications, protocols and standing orders, and other administrative technicalities.

Negligence (Neglect/Omission/Medical Liability) This is considered failure to provide a standard level of care. Four elements *must* be proven in order to establish negligence:

1. There existed a clear "duty to act."
2. There was a failure to respond to this "duty to act."
3. The patient suffered injury or damages.
4. The patient's damages were a result of the "failure to act."

Consent Consent is an agreement to accept care (*or* failure to refuse care). There are several accepted forms of consent:

1. Informed Consent—The patient is told (in such a way that he/she understands) the nature and extent of what procedures are to be performed and agrees to accept treatment.
2. Expressed Consent—When the patient gives verbal or written permission for treatment.
3. Implied Consent—When the patient's condition warrants immediate treatment, but he/she is unable to request it.

Consent can be obtained from:

1. The patient.
2. A parent or legal guardian.
3. The state, if the patient is a ward of the state.

Abandonment This is the process of ending the provider/patient relationship without ensuring that the patient receives equal services (such as, providing care and then discontinuing that care without the patient's permission). Abandonment can also mean inappropriate relinquishment of care of the patient to a lesser level of provider.

Assault Assault means creating the fear of bodily harm without permission.

Battery Battery is the physical touching of a patient without consent.

False Imprisonment Intentional and unjustified detention (and/or transportation) of a mentally competent patient without his/her consent is considered false imprisonment.

Obligatory Reporting Statues Most states have laws that require emergency medical personnel to report reasonable suspicion of the following:

1. Child abuse or neglect.
2. Abuse or neglect of the elderly.
3. Rape.
4. Gunshot wounds.
5. Animal Bites.

Privilege/Responsibility Statutes Many states have laws that deal with special circumstances the emergency care provider may encounter such as:

1. Living wills.
2. DNR (do not resuscitate) orders.
3. Limits on restraint and degree of force.
4. Access to restricted areas.
5. Scene control (who's in charge?).
6. Obtaining blood samples for suspected ETOH (alcohol) levels.

Libel Injuring a person's name or reputation by false and malicious writings is considered libel.

Slander Injuring a person's name or reputation by false and malicious spoken words is considered slander.

Reducing Risk of Litigation/Liability The likelihood of legal action can be dramatically reduced by:

1. Clear and accurate documentation of actions and events.
2. Taking the trouble to clearly obtain consent.
3. Establishing and utilizing workable protocols.

4. Maintaining confidentiality (and limiting oral reporting to appropriate personnel).

5. Describing behavior and surroundings in lieu of subjective speculation.

6. Avoiding labels and slang terms, unless used in quotes from patient, family and/or bystanders.

7. Maintaining medical liability insurance and understanding the specific limits and protections of its coverage.

8. Holding the patient's interests above all else.

Summary

The legal profession has discovered EMS. We knew it was coming, we knew life would get difficult, and so it has become. Our best protection is quality professional patient care and careful comprehensive documentation of that care.

SELF-TEST

Chapter 3

(Answers to some of these questions may vary from state to state.)

1. What is the function of a "Medical Practices Act?"

   ANSWER: It defines the minimum qualifications and skills of health care professionals and details their method of certification.

2. A law that protects those who render emergency assistance at the scene of an emergency from legal action—providing that they acted within the boundaries of their training—is called a "_____ _____ _____."

   ANSWER: Good Samaritan Law

3. What are the four elements necessary to prove "negligence?"

   ANSWER: a. There existed a clear "duty to act."

   b. There was a failure to respond to this "duty to act."

   c. The patient suffered injury or damages.

   d. The patient's damages were a result of this "failure to act."

4. What kind of consent exists when a patient understands the nature and extent of procedures that are to be performed and agrees to accept treatment?

   ANSWER: "Informed consent."

5. What is "expressed consent?"

   ANSWER: When a patient gives verbal or written permission for treatment.

6. What kind of consent exists when a patient's condition warrants immediate treatment, but the patient is unable to request it or agree to it.

   ANSWER: "Implied consent."

7. Who can give consent for treatment?

   ANSWER: a. The patient (if of legal age to consent or emancipated).

   b. A parent or legal guardian (sometimes, the extended family).

   c. The state, if the patient is a ward of the state.

8. Ending the provider/patient relationship without ensuring that the patient receives equal services—and doing so without the patient's permission—is considered _____ .

   ANSWER: abandonment

9. Creating the fear of bodily harm without permission is called _____ .

   ANSWER: assault

10. The physical touching of a patient without consent is considered _____ .

    ANSWER: battery

11. The intentional detention or transportation of a mentally competent patient without that patient's consent is considered _____ .

    ANSWER: false imprisonment

12. Injuring a person's name or reputation by false and malicious writings is termed _____ .

    ANSWER: libel

13. What is slander?

    ANSWER: Injuring a person's name or reputation by false and malicious spoken words.

EMS Communications

A study of any EMS system would reveal the absolute importance of reliable communications. From the use of 911 to the transmission of ECGs from the field to the hospital, our dependence upon varying degrees of communications technology requires a firm understanding of system components.

This chapter deals with the technical aspects of communications equipment (in the context of public safety radio), rules governing radio transmissions, communication through written or spoken words, and communication (written and verbal) of patient information.

Terminology

Base Stations Base stations may be limited in effectiveness by geography and terrain. Both the transmitter and the receiver are usually in the same physical location and may be controlled by remote console or by an attached speaker and microphone. It's power output of 45–275 watts is determined by the FCC and is printed on the radio station license. A base station may transmit on only one channel at a time in multiple channel systems.

Mobile Transmitter/Receivers (Two-way Radios) Usually vehicular-mounted, the power output of 20–50 watts (well below base station) of these single or multiple (8–12) channel units have an effective transmission range of about 10–15 miles. Flat land or water expanse will increase this range while tall buildings, mountains or thick forestation will decrease range.

Portable Transmitter/Receivers (Walkie-Talkies) Hand-carried transmitter/ receivers with a power output of 1–5 watts (and, therefore, limited range). It may be single or multiple (up to 14 or more) channel units and a "power boost" (and range increase) is possible through the use of repeaters.

Repeater/Base Stations These may be fixed or mobile, and extend transmission range by intercepting low-power signals (such as portables) and retransmitting at a higher power on another frequency. (Essentially a miniature base station.) Repeaters, if vehicular mounted, can retransmit low-power portables at mobile radio power levels. This also allows portables to "hear" each other communicate, and minimizes instances of "walking" on each other (mutual cut-off by simultaneous transmission).

Remote Consoles Utilized when unavoidable, or when advantageous to locate dispatching center away from the base station, a remote console extends control of the base station to a remote location by means of microwave relay, dedicated phone lines, underground cables, and so on.

Satellite Receivers Utilized when mobile and portable radios do not have the range to reliably reach their base station, satellite receivers can be strategically placed to ensure that low-power units are always within range of the communications system. They are connected to repeater(s) by microwave relay, dedicated phone lines, and so on.

Encoders and Decoders Resembling telephone dials or push button telephone pads, *encoders* send pulses or tones over the air to *decoders,* which recognize their unique codes and activate audio circuits in receivers.

Radio Frequencies These frequencies are designated by cycles per second or megahertz per second.

1. Hertz (Hz) = cycles per second.
2. Kilohertz (KHz) = 1,000 cycles per second.

3. Megahertz (MHz) = 1,000,000 cycles per second.
4. Gigahertz (GHz) = 1,000,000,000 cycles per second.

VHF VHF stands for *very high frequency* and is equal to 30–175 MHz.

1. VHF "low band" = 30–50 MHz. Has ranges up to 2,000 miles, but is somewhat unpredictable since changes in ionospheric conditions often cause "skips" (patchy losses in communication).
2. VHF "high band" = 150–170 MHz. Almost free of "skips", but has shorter range.

UHF UHF is ultra high frequency which is equal to 300–3,000 MHz. Most medical communications occur in the 450–470 MHz range where transmissions are entirely free of skip interference and have minimal signal distortion. UHF has a shorter ranger than VHF and better penetration in dense urban areas. Ten UHF frequencies (soon to be expanded) are allocated and licensed by the FCC for EMS use (two for dispatch and eight for paramedic-to-medical control).

FM/AM Radio equipment used for EMS communications is usually FM (frequency modulated), which is less likely to suffer interference than AM (amplitude modulated) systems.

Biotelemetry of ECGs ECG voltage changes are converted to audio tones and transmitted to hospital receivers which convert the audio signal back to a reproducable ECG.

Interference Telemetry interference may be caused by the following:

1. Loose ECG electrodes.
2. 60-cycle interference (electrical).
3. Patient movement (muscle tremor).
4. Variations in transmitter power.

Simplex Radio System This radio system has one frequency only, but is "non-repeating."

Duplex Radio System This system involves simultaneous two-way communications, much like a telephone conversation (requires two frequencies).

Multiplex Radio System This system combines signals (ECG and voice) for transmission simultaneously on one channel.

Proper Radio Use Proper radio use can be utilized if you adhere to the following guidelines:

1. Transmissions should be clear, concise, and professional.
2. Speak slowly and clearly, pronouncing each word distinctly.
3. *Be brief* and know what you are going to say *before* pressing the transmit button.
4. Use a normal tone of voice which is free of emotion.
5. *Don't waste air time* with long drawn-out phrases or descriptions.
6. If your report must be of considerable length, pause periodically to confirm that the receiving agency is copying your transmission.
7. Avoid ten-codes, especially when they seem awkward or are likely to be misunderstood. Use plain English whenever in doubt.
8. Protect patient privacy whenever possible.
9. Avoid slang and *do not* use profanity.
10. *Repeat physician orders* (and other significant instructions).
11. When completing a transmission, obtain confirmation that your message was received.

Radio Format Proper radio format should include the following:

1. Identify unit's name and call number (and/or name of EMT-P).
2. Brief description of scene (in a residence, on a highway, and so forth).
3. Patient's age, sex, and approximate weight (if appropriate).
4. Chief complaint and associated symptoms.
5. Brief history of present illness/injury.
6. Pertinent past medical history, medications (and over-the-counter meds), and allergies. (Identify patient's physician if appropriate.)
7. Physical exam findings:
   a. Level of consciousness (LOC).
   b. Vital signs (VS).
   c. Neuro exam.
   d. Appearance and degree of distress.

   e. ECG findings (if appropriate).

   f. Trauma Score and/or Glasgow Coma Scale.

   g. Other pertinent observations. INCLUDE PERTINENT NEGA-TIVES!

8. Description of treatment (Tx) already initiated.

9. Estimated time of arrival (ETA) at receiving facility.

10. Request orders as needed (and repeat if received).

Written Communications (EMS Forms) Written documentation is essential to:

1. Provide written evidence of patient's condition before intervention (and stay with patient record at the receiving hospital).

2. Serve as legal record of prehospital patient care.

3. Document refusals of care and/or transport (don't forget witnesses!).

4. Serve as source documents for audits, quality control, data collection, and billing (and should, therefore, be legible and complete).

Summary

EMS communications encompass a wide variety of equipment technologies, standardized procedures and informational "digest-and-transfer skills." A basic understanding of these components and their appropriate utilization increases the likelihood of quality patient care.

SELF-TEST

Chapter 4

1. Which radio frequency has a longer range, VHF or UHF?
   ANSWER: VHF

2. Which radio frequency is most often used for medical communication, and why?
   ANSWER: UHF has a shorter range than VHF, but has better penetration in dense urban areas and/or areas with obstacles to radio waves.

3. How does ECG biotelemetry work:

   ANSWER: ECG signals are converted to audio tones and transmitted to a hospital receiver which receives and converts the audio tones back into an ECG.

4. Encoders send pulses or tones over the air to decoders. What do the decoders do?

   ANSWER: Decoders recognize their unique codes and activate audio circuits in their receiver. This allows their receiver to receive the transmissions meant for it without having to monitor all traffic on that channel.

5. Finish this sentence: If it wasn't written, it wasn't _____!

   ANSWER: done

6. What does a multiplex radio system do?

   ANSWER: It combines ECG and voice for transmission on one channel.

Rescue

Rescue is defined as the removal (or freeing) of subjects from danger, harm, or entrapment and has been a widely used term in our profession. Every fire department has some type of "rescue" truck; every lifeguard is trained in "rescue" breathing. We have rope rescue, search-and-rescue, mountain rescue, water rescue, confined space rescue, dive rescue, high-angle rescue, cave rescue, air rescue, boat rescue, hostage rescue, farm rescue, vehicle rescue, medical rescue, and so on. You name it, we've got a rescue designation to slap along with it.

This chapter briefly reviews the principles involved with rescue in general. The specialized nature of rescue education demands methodical "hands-on" training, therefore, our treatment of rescue is conceptual only. We will examine the following components:

Safety	Emergency Care
Assessment	Disentanglement
Gaining Access	Preparation for Removal
	Removal

Safety

The most important aspect of any rescue operation is the safety of the rescuer and patient and this must be considered at all times (especially before the rescuer attempts the rescue). Many rescuers have been lost because of poor pre-rescue planning and an absence of adequate safety precautions.

Personal Safety Sometimes seen as "impractical" by some paramedics, most or all of these items should be available for utilization at rescue scenes to ensure personal safety:

1. Protective head gear;
2. Protective coat, pants, or overalls;
3. Gloves (the kind you need depends upon the nature of the rescue);
4. Eye protection;
5. Protective shoes or boots;
6. Self-contained breathing apparatus.

Patient Safety Often we have seen rescuers in full bunker gear working on and around a confined patient with heavy tools, while patient protection from broken glass, jagged metal, and extrication hazards is meager or nonexistent. A well-prepared rescue team should have most or all of these items available for patient protection at a rescue scene:

1. Protective blankets;
2. Protective shields;
3. Breathing aids;
4. Fire protection;
5. Climatic protection from:
   a. Hypothermia;
   b. Hyperthermia;
   c. Wind, rain, sun, and so on.

Hazards All rescue scenes contain hazards that must be evaluated prior to rescue operations. These might include:

1. Hazardous materials:
   a. Chemicals;
   b. Caustic substances;
   c. Volatile liquids;
   d. Gases;
   e. Radiation.
2. Fire potential:
   a. Gas or volatile liquid spill;
   b. Electrical hazards;
   c. "Sparking" hazards.
3. Environmental hazards:
   a. Ice, snow, avalanche, and other extremes of cold;
   b. Hot environment and high humidity (such as heat waves and fire scenes);
   c. Severe storms (lightning, tornadoes, hurricanes, wind, and flooding).
4. Other scene hazards:
   a. Electrical hazards (downed wires);
   b. Sharp objects (jagged metal in cars, glass, and so on);
   c. Vehicle stability (is cribbing required?);
   d. Traffic (re-route, if necessary);
   e. Crowd and bystander control;
   f. Compartment collapse (shore up if necessary—provide an escape path).

Pre-planning Pre-planning is essential to provide adequate rescue scene risk management. This requires careful review and assessment of:

1. Ability to summon appropriate help to ensure scene safety.
   a. Local communication capability;
   b. Range of resources available to aid rescue response;
   c. Additional personnel available to aid rescue response.
2. Crowd or bystander control (includes recruitment for assigned tasks with specific instructions).
3. Local major incident plan(s).

Assessment

Assessment refers to the "sizing up" of a situation to determine the specific needs for that rescue scene. Several elements are involved.

Response Response includes the:

1. Exact location;
2. Number of victims;
3. Type of situation;
4. Possible hazards;
5. Weather conditions.

Other Factors Other factors include:

1. Location:
   a. Near a school or other densely populated area?
   b. Road condition?
   c. The need for other types of response vehicles?
2. The time of day:
   a. Is there a concern for rush-hour traffic?
   b. Darkness?
   c. Are there high concentrations of people in the area during the response time period?

Resources Resources (determined by the type of situation) cover:

1. Whether the responding units can handle the situation at hand:
   a. Call for a major incident response;
   b. Ask for the specific type of resource.
2. Hazard control:
   a. Call for the appropriate response;
   b. Control the scene.
3. Victim assessment:
   a. Quick scan for the number of victims;
   b. Quick scan for critical injuries.

4. Other special resources.

5. Other ALS or types of transport units.

Gaining Access

Once steps have been taken to assure scene safety and respond the appropriate support units, gaining access to patients takes priority. Rapid access to critical patients is essential, BUT STILL MUST BE DONE SAFELY.

1. *Alternatives* to usual routes or methods should be explored (if necessary).
2. *Resources* on the scene should be assessed to if they are adequate for the task at hand.
3. *Recognition* of the need for special rescuers/tools/techniques must be made if the paramedic is unable to gain adequate (or safe) access to patients—including the sense to stand back and let specially trained personnel do the job.

Emergency Care

The primary purpose for paramedic response to a rescue scene is to render appropriate prehospital emergency care, once safe access to the patient has been accomplished.

Assessment Assessment includes:

1. *Primary survey* (A,B,C,D,E):
    a. **A**irway (open, patent) *and* cervical spine (immobilize if indicated);
    b. **B**reathing (present, rate, quality—immediate chest exam if distressed);
    c. **C**irculation (cartoid/radial pulses, rate, quality, capillary refill, skin color/temperature, JVD, scan for severe external bleeding);
    d. **D**isability (AVPU—level of consciousness);
    e. **E**xpose (chest, neck, sites of severe bleeding).

2. *Decision!*
   a. LOAD and GO (rapid extrication if necessary)! Consider Trauma Center or other appropriate destination.
      OR
   b. Continue with assessment.
3. *Vital signs* and *secondary survey* (head to toe).

Management Management includes:

1. Recognition of critical injuries and immediate intervention (may require basic/advanced life support while still entrapped);
2. Appropriate care on the scene;
3. Appropriate packaging of patient prior to transport;
4. Continuation of basic/advanced life support enroute to hospital.

Disentanglement

Disentanglement, if required, is the most technical component of rescue operations and requires a great deal of specialized training. Quite simply, it involves separating patients from hazardous confining surroundings. Some examples of disentanglement would include the following:

1. Auto extrication;
2. Plane, train, bus, and subway extrication;
3. Extrication from cave-ins;
4. Extrication from mountainous terrain (wrecks, rock-climbing accidents);
5. Underwater rescue.

Preparation for, and Removal

The final phase of rescue, and sometimes the most physically demanding or difficult, it involves the stable removal of patients from the rescue scene to reliable and appropriate transportation to an appropriate facility.

Coordination of Removal Coordination of removal involves:

1. Patient packaging:
   a. Wounds bandaged;
   b. Fractures splinted;
   c. IVs secure and untangled;
   d. Patient securely strapped;
   e. All appropriate basic and advanced life support performed before removal (if possible).
2. Coordination of manpower and equipment for smooth removal.
3. Is the exit pathway secure?

Removal Once the method of preparation has been accomplished and the patients can be removed from confinement, considerations for other equipment related to patient care need to be made.

1. Patient transport to ambulance or helicopter:
   a. Wheeled stretcher;
   b. Flat or break-down stretcher or spineboard;
   c. Other (stokes basket, stair-chair, and so on).
2. Patient care equipment:
   a. Oxygen and advanced airway equipment;
   b. PASG (pneumatic anti-shock garment);
   c. IV fluids and medications;
   d. Cardiac monitor/defibrillator.

Transport Patient care is continued during transport, while the patient's status is updated and any special needs anticipated are communicated to the receiving facility.

Summary

Rescue is the nuts-and-bolts essential job that many in the prehospital emergency care arena consider "the continuing challenge." Those that have become experts in rescue stress the overriding importance of safety, preplanning, adaptation, common sense, proper equipment and constant training. Knowing your own limitations, knowing who to call and knowing that they will respond are the keys to successful rescue operations.

SELF-TEST

Chapter 5

1. _____ is the most important aspect of a rescue operation?

   ANSWER: Safety (of both the rescuer and the patient).

2. List some items that a rescue team might use for patient protection.

   ANSWER: Blankets, tarps, breathing aids, fire suppression equipment, and so on.

3. List the six major components involved in rescue (as many as you can).

   ANSWER: a. Safety.

   b. Assessment.

   c. Gaining access.

   d. Emergency care.

   e. Disentanglement.

   f. Preparation for, and removal of victim.

Major Incident/Disaster Response

A major incident/disaster can exist in any situation that places a stress on local EMS resources—it will usually involve more patients than can be handled by responding units. It can have multiple sites (such as, tornadoes) and be community-wide. This chapter is meant to briefly review the components of a successful "major incident response." Your local "disaster plan" should address the specifics of command and individual agency responsibilities.

Components of Disaster Response

When to Declare a "Major Incident" Of course, this is a judgement call, but, for many regions, an event that requires more than two ambulances would qualify (as would a situation involving hazardous materials or requiring special resources not normally requested).

Pre-Planning In order to properly deal with a disaster area EMS agencies and hospitals need to cooperate in joint efforts. Each entity needs to hold practice drills to ensure effectiveness and familiarize personnel with their disaster plan. Rescuers must be able to access special resources (such as, air evacuation, disaster services, public health agencies, hazardous material teams, special rescue teams, and heavy equipment).

Communications A vital factor in response to any major incident is an adequate communications system—one that allows responding agencies to talk with each other. A separate frequency should be assigned to a major incident if possible, and command personnel should stay physically together (at a command post) after their arrival at the incident scene.

EMS Command Upon arrival, a predetermined individual (EMT or paramedic) should assume the role of EMS COMMAND. He/she will determine if a major incident exists, activate the response plan, request appropriate EMS assistance and coordinate the overall scene from a medical standpoint. Treatment areas should usually (not always) be established away from the immediate incident scene. All communications from scene to medical control should go through EMS COMMAND.

Triage A TRIAGE OFFICER should perform a rapid assessment of each victim, geared towards identifying *and tagging* those who will require immediate treatment and transport and those whose treatment/transport can be delayed. In a major incident, survival of the largest number of victims is the objective, so priorities of treatment must be based on the severity (and survivability) of injuries. Critically injured victims with little chance of survival (and who require a large commitment of personnel and resources) may, out of necessity, have treatment withheld, where normally, treatment would be aggressive.

Staging The decision on where to stage units should be made jointly between the EMS COMMAND, FIRE COMMAND, and POLICE COMMAND (or appropriate law enforcement authority). The staging area for EMS units should allow easy access, be relatively safe and allow the units to rapidly leave the scene. Units are called up as needed by EMS COMMAND.

Transfer of EMS Command It may be appropriate to transfer EMS COMMAND from the first arriving EMS unit to a late arriving unit or predetermined EMS authority. Specialized disaster vests with EMS COMMAND, TRIAGE, STAGING, and/or EMS COMMUNICATIONS are helpful, and if command is shifted, so are the vests.

Patient Information It is the TRIAGE OFFICER'S responsibility to quickly determine the total number of patients and their severity. This information should go immediately to EMS COMMAND, who will make a determination as to the need for additional assistance and notify area hospitals what (and how many) to expect.

Depending upon the situation (although not desirable), the EMS COMMAND and the TRIAGE OFFICER may be committed to providing a good deal of patient care, thus it is important to pre-plan for major incidents, aware of the responsibilities that must be assumed to provide the most appropriate care for the most number of patients. Agencies involved in the response *must communicate and coordinate* with each other, or a longer, less efficient incident/disaster scene will prevail.

Incident Command System The Incident Command System, utilized by most fire departments, is an excellent tool for functioning within the broader scope of a disaster plan. It can be used on the smallest of incidents, and yet expand as an emergency event expands. *It does not take the place of a disaster plan,* which of necessity goes beyond scene control and requires cooperation from many sectors of the community in extensive pre-planning, mobilization of many additional resources and cementing mutual aid relationships.

Summary

The wrong time to plan for a major incident/disaster is while it occurs. With common sense, foresight, inter-agency cooperation and training, and frequent review by all personnel of their own role in disaster response, you can be reasonably certain of managing the unmanageable responsibility.

SELF-TEST

Chapter 6

1. Define a major incident.

   ANSWER: Generally, this is an incident that outstrips available resources. This might involve hazardous materials, require specialized resources or present more patients than can be handled by responding units.

2. What is the role of EMS COMMAND?

ANSWER: EMS COMMAND determines if a major incident exists, activates the response plan, requests appropriate EMS assistance, and coordinates the overall scene from a medical standpoint.

3. What is the role of the TRIAGE OFFICER?

ANSWER: The TRIAGE OFFICER performs a rapid assessment of all victims to identify (and tag) those who require immediate attention and those whose care can be delayed.

4. What is "staging?"

ANSWER: The process of routing all incoming units to a specified location, in order that they be called into the scene as needed.

5. What is the most important aspect of developing a disaster plan.

ANSWER: Pre-planning.

Stress

Paramedics, as much as any career or professional group, are likely to encounter situations and emotions that cause stress. In fact, stress is a performance edge for some paramedics, while it hinders the performance of others. In this chapter we offer a brief overview of stress, its causes and our reactions to it while focusing on job-related stresses faced by paramedics (such as death and dying) and how they can be managed.

Introduction to Stress

Stress The definition of stress is a response of the body to demands that are made upon it. Further, stress may produce a need to adapt and try to re-establish normalcy. Stress is always present, but varies greatly in degree.

Stressors Stressors are any agent or situation that causes stress (can be emotional or physical).

Causes of Psychological Stress The causes of psychological stress are:

1. Loss of valued objects;
2. Bodily injury (or threat of injury);

3. Illness, poor nutrition;
4. Frustration of drives (such as sexual drive);
5. Inability to cope effectively.

Three Stages of Stress The three stages of stress are:

1. *Alarm reaction*—The initial response to a stressor:
   a. Occurs at first exposure to stressor;
   b. Resistance is diminished, physiologic and emotional response is great.
2. *Stage of resistance*—The bodies ability to adapt to a stressor:
   a. Individuals begin to adapt;
   b. Physiologic parameters return to normal;
   c. Resistance rises above normal.
3. *Stages of exhaustion*—Energy is depleted due to prolonged stress:
   a. Follows long, continued exposure to same stressor;
   b. Adaptation energy is exhausted;
   c. Signs of alarm reaction reappear, but are now irreversible.

Reactions to Stress

Defense Mechanisms

1. Adaptive functions of the personality that assist us in adjusting to stressful situations that confront us. This is a healthful mechanism unless it is used to the degree where reality becomes distorted.
2. Most defense mechanisms are unconscious and automatic, while some are consciously employed. All are utilized in an attempt to seek relief.

Common Defense Mechanisms

1. *Repression*—Involuntary relegation of unacceptable ideas or impulses into the unconscious:
   a. Unconscious forgetting;
   b. Repressed conflicts (unchanged in quality and intensity) constantly seek expression.

2. *Regression*—The return to an earlier level of emotional adjustment.

3. *Projection*—Attributing to another person or object those thoughts, feelings, motives, or desires which are really one's own unacceptable traits. It may present an aggression toward others, but is actually anger with self.

4. *Rationalization*—The process of ascribing acceptable or worthwhile motives to feelings, thoughts, or behavior which really have other unrecognized motives:

   a. Commonly employed as a defense mechanism;

   b. Usually an unconscious, retrospective process;

   c. A way of "explaining" our behavior—often self-deceiving.

5. *Compensation*—A conscious or unconscious attempt to overcome real or imagined shortcomings by developing individual skills or traits to compensate for those deficiencies.

6. *Reaction formation*—Directing overt behavior or attitudes in the opposite direction of an individual's underlying unacceptable impulses.

7. *Sublimation*—The diversion of instinctive but unacceptable drives into socially acceptable channels.

8. *Denial*—The unconscious disavowal of thoughts, feelings, wishes, or needs which are consciously unacceptable (this is closely related to rationalization).

9. *Substitution*—The replacement of an unattainable or unacceptable activity by one which is attainable or acceptable, or the redirection of an emotion from the original object to a more acceptable substitute object.

10. *Isolation*—The separation of an unacceptable impulse, act or idea from its memory origin, thereby removing the associate emotional charge—conscious retention of the memory, but not the feeling that accompanied it.

Anxiety Anxiety is an emotional state caused by stress that is a key ingredient in the coping process. It alerts a person to impending danger, maintains all potential resources (body and mind) in readiness for emergencies, helps us cope by narrowing and focusing our field of attention, and enables us to increase tolerance for stress by developing effective coping mechanisms and defenses. Sometimes, anxiety fails to stimulate coping behavior and, instead, stimulates reaction to perceived threats

that is out of proportion to actual danger. It plays a negative role in coping behavior when it interferes with thought processes and performance.

Physical Effects Subjects feeling anxiety may experience a variety of
physical effects such as:

1. Heart palpitations, rapid or difficult breathing, and dry mouth;
2. Chest pain (or tightness);
3. Anorexia, nausea, vomiting, abdominal cramps, flatulence, or
    butterflies;
4. Flushing, diaphoresis, and body temperature fluctuation;
5. Urgency and frequency in urination along with decreased sexual
    drive/performance;
6. Aching muscles, joints, backache, and headache.

Unconscious Effects *Unconscious effects* might include:

1. Increased blood pressure and heart rate;
2. Increased blood glucose;
3. Shunting of blood to muscles;
4. Pupil dilation;
5. Increase in epinephrine production.

Reactions to Stress *Reactions to anxiety/stress* include:

1. Patient and family:
    a. Anger towards God, themselves, or anyone around (including you);
    b. Guilt (whether or not it is based on fact);
    c. Indecisiveness (don't give too many alternatives when anxiety level
        is high.
2. Paramedic:
    1. Impatience;
    2. Fear;
    3. Anger;
    4. Important to maintain professional attitude despite these emotions;
        remain non-judgmental.

Job Stressors Job Stressors for Paramedics (hazards of the trade) include:

1. Multiple roles and responsibilities (often widely diverse);
2. Dealing with angry or confused citizens;
3. Unfinished tasks;
4. Meeting continuous timelines;
5. Absence of challenge and "burnout;"
6. Necessary restrictions on "scope of practice;"
7. Lack of recognition for performance (lack of esteem);
8. Lack of upward career mobility;
9. Dealing with death, critical and dying patients and their families.

Stress Management Stress Management (tools of the trade) include:

1. Learn to recognize the early warning signs of anxiety.
2. Identify stressful situations:
   a. Do you really see what's happening?
   b. Are you blaming yourself unjustly?
   c. Sort events into categories of importance, urgency, and degree of actual threat.
3. Take advantage of your means of support:
   a. Talk to someone else (perhaps a peer or partner) about the stress;
   b. Group discussions of difficult situations (that affect the group);
   c. Critical incident stress debriefing.
4. Get enough sleep and rest (very important)!
5. Pursue positive activities with others and consciously balance work with recreation.
6. Learn to accept what cannot be changed if it's beyond your control.
7. Learn to consciously use coping mechanisms:
   a. Evaluate your defense mechanisms. Adopt those most likely to reduce your level of stress.
   b. Consider physical exertion as a means of stress control.
   c. Don't waste your energy—choose activities carefully.

Death and Dying Your attitudes and perceptions (about death) color your treatment of patient and family. Be aware of the stages of healthy grief process and how it affects behavior:

1. Denial (and possibly isolation);
2. Anger;
3. Bargaining;
4. Depression;
5. Acceptance (disengagement).

Educate yourself to the needs of patient/family/close friends in these high-stress situations. Don't lie to a dying patient that asks you if he's dying. Touch these patients and keep communicating—they may need to talk about dying. If the patient is DOA, the family becomes the "patient." Do what you can, but recognize your limitations. *You may need to go through the same grief stages!* Don't be afraid to use the word "dead" (instead of "passed away" or "expired"). It conveys a realistic nature of what has happened and the family may well need to hear it.

Summary

The paramedic is affected by calls that involve death and dying. He has a responsibility to patients and their families to understand their grief and how it affects behavior. He has an obligation to be truthful and supportive in these situations. Further, he has an obligation to himself to acknowledge his own feelings (at an appropriate time) about death and dying which will be based on past experiences, personal attitudes, and his personal involvement with the current situation.

SELF-TEST

Chapter 7

1. Define "stress."
   ANSWER: A response of the body to demands that are made upon it.
2. A _____ is any agent or situation that causes stress.
   ANSWER: Stressor.

3. List the three stages of stress.

ANSWER: a. Alarm reaction.

b. Resistance.

c. Exhaustion.

4. Why do we use "defense mechanisms?"

ANSWER: To assist us in adjusting to stressful situation in an effort to seek relief.

5. Anxiety can play both positive and negative roles in the coping process. Name one of the positive roles.

ANSWER(S): a. Alerts us to impending danger.

b. Maintains all potential resources (body and mind) in readiness for emergencies.

6. What are the five classic stages of a normal grief process:

ANSWER: a. Denial.

b. Anger.

c. Bargaining.

d. Depression.

e. Acceptance.

_____

Medical Terminology

Paramedics must be able to decipher a myriad of medical terms in the course of their jobs, often without the benefit of detailed background information in related medical arenas. An understanding of medical abbreviations, prefixes and suffixes provides a way to break a term down into its logical components, and thus reveal it's meaning. In this chapter, we have defined many of the abbreviations, prefixes, and suffixes common to the medical field. Though by no means complete, an overview of the subject is presented and should provide adequate review.

Abbreviations

aa of each.

abd abdomen.

ac before meals.

ad lib as much as desired.

aq water.

AMA against medical advice or American Medical Association.

AMI acute myocardial infarction.

ant   anterior.

AP   front-to-back (anteroposterior).

A + P   auscultation and percussion.

A&P   anatomy and physiology.

art   artery.

ASA   aspirin.

APC   aspirin-phenacetin-caffeine.

approx   approximately.

BBB   bundle branch block:
  RBBB   right bundle branch block.
  LBBB   left bundle branch block.

BF   black female.

bid   twice daily.

BM   black male, bowel movement.

BP   blood pressure.

BSA   body surface area.

BUN   blood urea nitrogen.

C   centigrade.

c or **/w**   with.

CA   cancer.

CAD   coronary artery disease.

cap(s)   capsules.

CBC   complete blood count.

cc   cubic centimeter.

CC   chief complaint.

CCU   coronary care unit.

CHF   congestive heart failure.

c/o   complains of.

CO$_2$ carbon dioxide.

cont   continue.

COPD   chronic obstructive pulmonary disease.

CPR   cardiopulmonary resuscitation.

CVA   cerebrovascular accident.

CVP   central venous pressure.

dc   discontinue.

DC   discharge from hospital.

DNA   does not apply.

DNR   do not resuscitate.

DNS   did not show.

DOA   dead on arrival.

DOE   dyspnea on exertion.

Dr   doctor.

Dx   diagnosis.

EEG   electroencephalogram.

ED   emergency department.

ER   emergency room.

EKG or **ECG**   electrocardiogram.

ETOH   alcohol.

Ex   examination.

F   Fahrenheit.

Fx   fracture.

GB   gall bladder.

GI   gastrointestinal.

g or **gm**   gram.

gr   grain.

GU   genitourinary.

h or **hr**   hour.

H or **(H)**   hypodermic.

H&P   history and physical.

H&H   hemoglobin and hematocrit.

Hb or **Hgb**   hemoglobin.

Hct   hematocrit.

Hg   mercury.

Hx   history.

IC   intracardiac.

ICU   intensive care unit.

IM   intramuscular.

IV   intravenous.

L   liter, left.

LLQ   left lower quadrant (of abdomen).

lmp   last menstrual period.

LOC   level of consciousness, loss of consciousness.

LUQ   left upper quadrant (of abdomen).

MAE   moves all extremeties.

mEq   millequivalent.

mg   milligram.

MI   myocardial infarction.

MICU   mobile intensive care unit, medical intensive care unit.

ml   milliliter.

MS   morphine sulphate, multiple sclerosis.

NaHCO$_3$ sodium bicarbonate.

neg   negative.

NPO   nothing by mouth.

NTG   nitroglycerin.

O$_2$ oxygen.

OB   obstetrics.

OD   overdose.

OR   operating room.

p   after.

pc   after meals.

PCU   Progressive Care Unit.

PE   physical exam.

PI   present illness.

po   by mouth.

pt   patient.

PT   physical therapy.

PERL   pupils equal and react to light.

q   every.

qh   every hour.

qid   four times a day.

gt   drop.

gtt   drops.

RBC   red blood cells.

RHD   rheumatic heart disease.

RO or **R/O**   rule out.

RLQ   right lower quadrant (of abdomen).

ROM   range of motion.

RUL   right upper lobe (of lung).

RUQ   right upper quadrant (of abdomen).

Rx   treatment.

s or **w/o**   without.

sc or **SC**   subcutaneous.

SICU   surgical intensive care unit.

SL   sublingual.

SOB   short of breath.

sol   solution.

ss   half.

stat   immediately.

subQ   subcutaneously.

sym   symptoms.

tab   tablet.

T   temperature.

T or **Tbsp**   tablespoon.

tid   three times a day.

TPR   temperature-pulse-respiration.

tsp   teaspoon.

u   unit.

UA   urinalysis.

UCHD   usual childhood diseases.

URI   upper respiratory infection.

USP   *United States Pharmacopeia.*

UTI   urinary tract infection.

VD   veneral disease.

VO   verbal order.

vol   volume.

VS   vital signs.

/w   with.

WBC   white blood cells.

WD   well developed.

WF   white female.

WM   white male.

WNL   within normal limits.

wt   weight.

yo   year old.

+   positive.

−   negative.

+/−   postive or negative.

/   per.

<   less than.

>   more than.

≈   approximately equal.

±   plus or minus.

    increase.

    decrease.

*   birth.

    death.

    male.

    female.

×   times, power.

Prefixes

a- or **an-**   (without) such as, **a**pnea—without breath; **an**emia—lack of blood.

ab-   (away from) such as, **ab**normal—away from the normal.

abdomi(n)- (abdomen) such as, **abdomi**nal—pertaining to abdomen.

acr- (extremity) such as, **acr**omegaly—enlargement of extremity.

ad- (to/toward) such as, **ad**hesion—stuck to/remaining in close proximity to.

aden- (gland) such as, **aden**itis—inflammation of gland.

angio- (blood vessel) such as, **angio**gram—study of vessels.

ante- (before, forward) such as, **ante**natal—occurring or formed before birth.

anti- (against) such as, **anti**pyretic—against fever.

arter- (artery) such as, **arter**iogram—study of arteries.

arthro- (joint) such as, **arthro**scopy—inspection of joint.

auto- (self) such as, **auto**-transfusion—transfusion using the body's own blood.

bi- (two) such as, **bi**lateral—both sides.

bio- (life) such as, **bio**logy—study of life.

blast- (germ or cell) such as, **blast**oma—a true tumor of cells.

brady- (slow) such as, **brady**cardia—slow heart rate.

cardi- (heart) such as, **cardi**ography—recording of the movements of the heart.

cerebr- (brain) such as, **cerebr**al—pertaining to brain.

cerv- (neck) such as, **cerv**ical—pertaining to neck.

cephal- (head) such as, **cephal**opathy—any disease of the head.

chole- (bile) such as, **chole**lithiasis—stones in the gall bladder.

chondr- (cartilage) such as, costo**chondr**al—junction of ribs and cartilage.

circum- (around, about) such as, **circum**oral—around the mouth.

contra- (against/opposite) such as, **contra**stimulant—against stimulating.

cost- (rib) such as, **cost**al margin—margin of lower limits of ribs.

cyan- (blue) such as, **cyan**osis—bluish discoloration.

cyst- (bladder, sac) such as, **cyst**itis—inflammation of urinary bladder.

cyt- (cell) such as, **cyt**ology—study of cells.

derma- (skin) such as, **derma**titis—inflammation of the skin.

di- (twice, double) such as, **di**plopia—double vision.

dia- (through, completely) such as, **dia**gnosis—knowing completely.

dys- (with difficulty) such as, **dys**pnea—difficulty breathing.

ecto- (out from) such as, **ecto**pic—out of place.

edem- (swelling) such as, **edem**a—swelling.

electr- (electricity) such as, **electr**oencephalogram—electric record of brain activity.

endo- (within) such as, **endo**metrium—within the uterus.

enter- (intestines) such as, **enter**itis—inflammation of the intestines.

epi- (upon) such as, **epi**dermis—on the skin.

erythro- (red) such as, **erythro**cyte—red blood cells.

exo- (outside) such as, **exo**genous—produced outside the body.

febr- (fever) such as, a**febr**ile—without fever.

gastr- (stomach) such as, **gastr**itis—inflammation of the stomach.

glyco- (sugar) such as, **glyco**uria sugar in the urine.

gynec- (women) such as, **gynec**ology—study of diseases of women.

hem- or **hemat-** (blood) such as, **hem**oglobin—coloring matter of red cells.

hemi- (half) such as, **hemi**plegia—paralysis of one side of the body.

hepat- (liver) such as, **hepat**itis—inflammation of the liver.

hydr(o)- (water) such as, **hydr**ophobia—fear of water.

hyper- (over, excessive) such as, **hyper**glycemia—excessive sugar in the blood.

hypo- (under, deficient) such as, **hypo**tension—low blood pressure.

hyster- (uterus) such as, **hyster**ectomy—surgical removal of the uterus.

infra- (below) such as, **infra**scapular—below the scapular bone.

inter- (between) such as, **inter**costal—between the ribs.

intra- (within) such as, **intra**cellular—within the cells.

iso- (equal) such as, **iso**tonic—having equal tension.

later(o)- (side) such as, **later**al—pertaining to side.

leuk- (anything white) such as, **leuk**ocyte—white blood cells.

macro- (large) such as, **macro**blast—abnormally large cell.

mal- (bad abdominal disorder) such as, **mal**aise—general discomfort, unease.

mening(o)- (meninges) such as, **mening**itis—inflammation of the meninges.

micro- (small) such as, **micro**plasia—dwarfism.

mono- (one) such as, **mono**cular—one eye.

my- (muscle) such as, **my**eloma—muscle tumor.

nas(o)- (nose) such as, **nas**opharynx—pertaining to nose and pharynx.

neo- (new) such as, **neo**plasm—new growth.

nephr- (kidney) such as, **nephr**ectomy—surgical removal of kidney.

neur(o)- (nerve) such as, **neur**ogenic—caused by nerve.

olig- (little) such as, **olig**uria—decreased urine output.

oophor- (ovary) such as, **oophor**ectomy—surgical removal of ovary.

opthal- (eye) such as, **opthal**mic drops—drops for the eye.

orchi- (testicle) such as, **orchi**tis—inflammation of testicle.

ortho- (straight) such as, **ortho**pnea—unable to breathe supine.

os- (mouth) such as, cervical **os**—mouth of cervix.

osteo- (bone) such as, **osteo**peritis—inflammation of bone and surrounding tissue.

ot- (ear) such as, **ot**itis medea—inflammation of the middle ear.

para- (by the side of) such as, **para**medic—along side of a physician.

per- (through) such as, **per**foration—a breaking through.

phago- (to eat) such as, **phago**cyte—cells that eat debris.

pharyng- (throat) such as, **pharyng**itis—inflammation of the pharynx.

peri- (surrounding) such as, **peri**osteum—covering of bone.

phleb- (vein) such as, **phleb**itis—inflammation of vein.

pneum- (air or lung) such as, **pneum**othorax—air in the chest cavity.

poly- (many, excessive) such as, **poly**trauma—multiple trauma.

post- (after, behind) such as, **post**partum—after childbirth.

pre- (before) such as, **pre**diastolic—before diastole.

pro- (before, in front of) such as, **pro**gnosis—forecast as to extent of disease.

pseudo- (false) such as, **pseudo**anemia—condition of paleness without true anemia.

psych- (mind) such as, **psych**iatry—treatment of mental diseases.

pulmon- (lung) such as, **pulmon**ary thrombosis—clot in lung.

pyo- (pus) such as, **pyo**rrhea—discharge of pus.

pyel- (pelvis or kidney) such as, **pyel**itis—inflammation of kidney.

quadr- (four) such as, **quadr**ilateral—four sides.

retro- (backward) such as, **retro**flexion.

rhin- (nose) such as, **rhin**itis—inflammation of nose.

sclero- (hard) such as, **sclero**sis—hardening.

semi- (half) such as, **semi**lunar—half-moon, or crescent-shaped.

sub- (under, moderately) such as, **sub**acute—moderately sharp.

super-, **supra-** (above) such as, **supra**ventricular—above the ventricles.

sym- (with, together) such as, **sym**physis—grow together.

tachy- (fast) such as, **tachy**cardia—fast pulse.

thorac(o)- (chest) such as, **thorac**otomy—cutting into chest.

topo- (surface) such as, **topo**graphy—record of surface.

trans- (across) such as, **trans**fusion—pour across.

tri- (three) such as, **tri**cuspid—having three cusps.

uni- (one) such as, **uni**lateral—one-sided.

vaso- (vessel) such as, **vaso**constriction—constriction of vessels.

Suffixes

-algia (pain) such as, neur**algia**—pain along a nerve.

-asthenia (weakness) such as, myos**thenia**—muscle weakness.

-blast (germ of immature cell) such as, myeo**blast**—bone marrow cell.

-cele (tumor, hernia) such as, extero**cele**—hernia of the intestine.

-centesis (puncturing) such as, thoro**centesis**—puncturing and drainage of pleural space.

-cyte (cell) such as, leuko**cyte**—white cell.

-ectomy (cutout/remove) such as, tonsill**ectomy**—surgical removal of the tonsils.

-emia (blood) such as, an**emia**—lack of blood.

-esthesia (sensation) such as, an**esthesia**—without sensation.

-genic (causing) such as, carcino**genic**—cancer causing.

-gram or **-graph** (record) such as, electrocardio**gram**—record of heart's electrical activity.

-itis (inflammation) such as, tonsill**itis**—inflammation of the tonsils.

-megaly (enlargement) such as, cardio**megaly**—enlargement of heart.

-ology (science of) such as, bi**ology**—science or study of life.

-oma (tumor, swelling) such as, carcin**oma**—cancerous tumor.

-osis (condition) such as, psych**osis**—condition of the mind.

-ostomy (opening) such as, trache**ostomy**—opening in the trachea.

-otomy (cutting into) such as, cricothyroid**otomy**—cutting into the crico-thyroid cartilage.

-paresis (weakness) such as, hemi**paresis**—one-sided weakness.

-pathy (disease) such as, cardiac myo**pathy**—disease of the heart muscle.

-phagia (eating) such as, poly**phagia**—excessive eating.

-phasia (speech) such as, a**phasia**—loss of speech ability.

-phobia (fear) such as, hydro**phobia**—fear of water.

-plasty (repair of; tying of) such as, nephro**plasty**—suturing of a kidney.

-plegia (paralysis) such as, hemi**plegia**—one-sided paralysis.

-pnea (breathing) such as, a**pnea**—without breathing.

-rhythmia (rhythm) such as, ar**rhythmia**—variation from normal rhythm.

-rrhagia (bursting forth) such as, hemo**rrhage**—flowing of blood.

-rrhea (flowing) such as, dia**rrhea**—discharge of feces.

-trophia (nourishment) such as, a**trophy**—wasting.

-scopy (exam) such as, broncho**scopy**—inspection of bronchus.

-uria (urine) such as, pol**yuria**—excessive secretion of urine.

Summary

This review of medical terminology should equip you to logically decipher basic medical terms and handle most anything thrown at you on state boards or final exams. Spelling is important, so be careful.

Patient Assessment

Responsibility for recognizing and correcting life-threatening conditions lies with the paramedic, thus the development of rapid accurate patient assessment skills is crucial to a paramedic's effectiveness.

Accepted principles of emergency prehospital care mandate that life-threatening conditions be treated first. Often, this means simultaneous assessment and treatment. With medical patients, definitive care is started in the field (defibrillation for ventricular fibrillation, glucose for insulin shock), while with significant trauma patients, field treatment is directed toward maintaining oxygenation and perfusion and controlling bleeding while rapidly transporting the victim to an appropriate facility that can provide definitive care (usually the operating room).

A review of accepted patient assessment procedures is presented in this chapter. Few paramedics perform the assessments in quite the same order as recommended in textbooks, yet the principles and priorities of patient assessment remain the same—and will be addressed in most paramedic exams. This chapter assumes that *scene safety* and the paramedic's *personal safety* have already been assured. These two factors must always be confirmed before patient assessment/treatment begins.

Primary Survey

The primary survey is designed to uncover life-threatening problems, and if they exist, the appropriate treatment must be initiated before continuing with assessment. For our purposes, we will follow the A-B-C-D-E mnemonic:

A = Airway/C-Spine
B = Breathing
C = Circulation
D = Disability
E = Expose and Examine

Airway/C-Spine This is one combined step, because maintaining a good airway position is directly related to protecting the cervical spine until further assessment. Ask yourself these important questions:

1. Is the airway open?
   YES—maintain manually in neutral position while continuing assessment.
   NO—open the airway with an appropriate procedure.
2. Can cervical spine injury be ruled out?
   YES—Use head-tilt chin-lift to open the airway.
   NO—Consider modified jaw thrust to open the airway.

Breathing Ask yourself these questions:

1. Is the patient breathing?
   a. Is the chest rising and falling?
   b. Is there audible or palpable air exchange?
   YES—continue with assessment.
       a. Rate (rapid, normal, slow)?
       b. Rhythm (regular, irregular)?
       c. Depth (shallow, normal, deep, equal chest movement bilaterally)?
       d. Noisy (rales, ronchi, wheezing, snoring, stridor)?

      e. Labored (slight, moderate, severe, accessory muscles in use)?

      f. Skin color (flushed, normal, pale, ashen, cyanotic)?

NO—ventilate twice, check for a pulse and continue with assessment. (If obstructed, follow AHA standards for obstructed airway.)

2. Do I need to assist ventilations?

    YES—a. If rate is < 10 or > 28.

        b. If tidal volume or expansion seems inadequate;

        c. If flail chest or pneumothorax is present;

        d. In the presence of suspected significant head injury.
Methods and adjuncts available:

        a. Mouth-to-mouth;

        b. Mouth-to-mask;

        c. Bag-valve-mask;

        d. Demand valve (with care);

        e. EOA (esophageal obturator airway);

        f. EGTA (esophageal gastric tube airway);

        g. PTL (pharyngeal tracheal lumen airway);

        h. Endotracheal intubation;

        i. Transtracheal ventilation (cricothyrotomy, jet insufflation).

NO—continue assessment.

Circulation Perfusion (delivering adequate amounts of oxygenated blood to body tissues) status is extremely important. Ask yourself these questions:

1. Is there a pulse? (Check the carotid.)

    YES—a. Rate (fast, slow, normal);

        b. Rhythm (regular, irregular);

        c. Character (strong, weak, thready);

        d. Location:

          1. Carotid (BP > 60 systolic);

          2. Femoral (BP > 70 systolic);

          3. Radial (BP > 80 systolic, absence may indicate shock).

NO—find correct hand placement and begin cardiac compressions.

2. What is the capillary refill? (Check when removing fingers from the carotid artery pulse check.)

   a. Normal = less than 2 seconds (suggests adequate perfusion);

   b. Delayed = 2–4 seconds (suggests decreased perfusion and/or shock);

   c. Absent = more than 4 seconds (suggests poor perfusion and profound shock).

3. What is the skin color? (Can also be done while checking for pulse.)

   a. Flushed or normal (suggests adequate perfusion);

   b. Pale (inconclusive—may be normal or decreased perfusion);

   c. Ashen, cyanotic or mottled (suggests poor tissue perfusion and/or profound shock).

4. Is there any obvious severe bleeding? (Quick visual scan—any pools?)

   YES—apply direct pressure and control;

   NO—continue assessment.

Disability (Mini-Neuro Exam)—Refers to measuring the responsiveness of a patient to his environment, both to determine the seriousness of the present condition and to establish a baseline level of consciousness against which future changes can be measured. Use the mnemonic A-V-P-U:

A = Alert.

V = Responds to verbal stimuli.

P = Responds to painful stimuli.

U = Unresponsive (unconscious and will not respond to painful stimuli).

Expose and Examine If the condition is serious, expose the entire body for examination. Hidden injury sites and hidden bleeding can be catastrophic. Of course, some factors that will limit the amount of actual exposure are:

1. Environment (cold weather, rain, and so on);

2. Bystanders (versus need for examination);

3. Critical trauma (exposure of the chest is mandatory in the primary survey);

4. Common sense (remove whatever is necessary to rule out or confirm a condition or injury).

Vital Signs

Vital signs, combined with the results of the primary survey, supply enough information to make a decision regarding immediate transport versus continued patient assessment. The baseline vital signs are:

1. Pulse (rate, rhythm, character);
2. Respirations (rate, effort, adequacy of ventilation);
3. Blood pressure (measurement by auscultation or palpation);
4. Skin color and temperature;
5. Pupils (equality, size, shape, reaction to light).

Decision

Immediate rapid transport or continued assessment? Some indications for rapid transport you might discover during the primary survey would be:

1. Shock.
2. Inadequate respirations—causes might include:
    a. Open chest wound (sucking);
    b. Large flail chest;
    c. Tension pneumothorax;
    d. Major blunt chest injury;
    e. Airway obstruction (unrelieved by mechanical methods).
3. Head injury with any of the following:
    a. Unconsciousness;
    b. Unequal pupils;
    c. Decreasing level of consciousness.
4. Traumatic "Code Blue" (cardiopulmonary arrest).
5. Severe uncontrolled bleeding.

Secondary Survey

The secondary survey is an orderly head-to-toe examination designed to assess the entire patient and provide more information about problems revealed in the primary survey. You are specifically checking for:

1. Pain;
2. Tenderness;
3. Edema;
4. Deformities/fractures;
5. Bleeding;
6. Soft tissue damage (lacerations/contusions/abrasions);
7. Other abnormalities.

using the assessment tools of:

1. Inspection (LOOKING);
2. Auscultation (LISTENING);
3. Palpation (FEELING);
4. Percussion;
5. Smell.

There are situations (with critical patients) when you may never reach the secondary survey, as all your energies will be involved in correcting problems encountered in the primary survey, while rapidly transporting the patient. *Should you encounter any of the following conditions while performing the secondary survey:*

1. Development of shock, respiratory difficulty, or decreasing level of consciousness;
2. Tender distended abdomen;
3. Bilateral femur fractures;
4. Unstable pelvis.

upgrade the patient to critical status, apply the PASG and transport immediately. (The use of PASG is controversial and not universally accepted)
    An appropriate secondary survey includes assessment of the:

1. Head;
2. Neck;
3. Thorax;
4. Abdomen;

5. Extremities;
6. Neurological exam;
7. Back.

Head

1. Skin and scalp (deformities/depressions, lacerations, hematomas);
2. Eyes (pupils re-checked—size, shape, equality, reaction to light);
3. Ears (blood and/or CSF);
4. Nose (blood and/or CSF);
5. Mouth (broken teeth, bleeding, speech);
6. Bones (structural integrity):
   a. Facial;
   b. Mandible/maxillary;
   c. Cranium.

Neck

1. Skin (color, capillary refill, dryness);
2. Soft tissue (subcutaneous emphysema, contusions, edema);
3. Trachea (mid-line/deviated, use of accessory muscles);
4. Vessels (carotid pulse, JVD-jugular vein distension, flat or distended);
5. Cervical spine (obvious deformities, pain/tenderness).

Thorax

1. Skin (abrasions, contusions, lacerations, punctures);
2. Chest wall (intact, fractures, splinting, expansion during ventilaton);
3. Lungs (breath sounds all fields, hyperresonance, pulmonary edema/rales, wheezes, ronchi, stridor, rate or respirations, labored/normal);
4. Heart:
   a. Auscultation;
   b. Palpation;
   c. ECG (if indicated).

Abdomen

1. Skin (abrasions, contusions, lacerations, punctures, edema, tightness);
2. Muscles ("guarding", bulges/distension, rigidity);
3. Retroperitoneal space (tenderness/pain, rigidity);
4. Lumbar spine (obvious deformity, pain/tenderness);
5. Pelvis (stable/unstable, pain/tenderness, "grating", deformity);
6. Genitalia (lacerations, edema, pain/tenderness, blood in urine).

Extremities

1. Skin (lacerations, abrasions, contusions, temperature/color);
2. Muscles (cramping/spasms, function, edema);
3. Soft tissues (edema, lacerations, punctures);
4. Vessels (pulses distal to injury, presence of peripheral pulses—both upper and lower extremities);
5. Bones (fractures/dislocations, deformity, pain/tenderness);
6. Function/sensation (movement/feeling, range of motion, parasthesia, paralysis).

Neurological Exam

1. Level of consciousness (repeat AVPU—look for changes). Is patient alert to person, time and place? Determine GLASGOW COMA SCALE when time permits, and determine TRAUMA SCORE for trauma victims.
2. Seizure activity or posturing?
3. Motor function intact?
4. Sensory function intact?
5. Pupils (re-assessed for size, shape, equality, reaction to light).

History

A patient/scene history must often be obtained from several sources. These might include:

1. Patient;

2. Relatives;

3. Paramedic's own observations;

4. Bystanders;

5. Law enforcement/fire/rescue/ambulance personnel;

6. Medic alert tags.

A good history must include:

1. Chief complaint (verbal or non-verbal);

2. Mechanisms of injury (if applicable);

3. Present illness or injury;

4. Past history—take an A-M-P-L-E history:

    A = Allergies to medications;

    M = Medications (both prescription *and* non-prescription);

    P = Past medical history;

    L = Last oral intake;

    E = Events leading up to emergency.

Reassessment

Even though assessment is thorough, the patient must be constantly re-assessed at regular intervals. Should a patient suddenly deteriorate, return to the primary survey and reassess. Some of the items to monitor would include:

1. Airway/C-spine control;

2. Adequacy of ventilations (chest rise, breath sounds);

3. Oxygenation (flow rates, delivery, skin color, capillary refill);

4. Level of consciousness (especially any changes);

5. Vital signs (note any changes);

6. Circulatory status (especially distal to injuries);

7. ECG;

8. IV fluids (rates, patency of lines, signs of infiltration);

9. PASG (pressures, placement, signs of pulmonary edema);

10. Adequacy of immobilization.

Summary

The skill of patient assessment is founded upon good training, extensive practice and common sense. The recognition and correction of life-threatening conditions identified in the primary survey is absolutely essential for field paramedics and adequacy of care is directly related to assessment skills. Knowing when to take time and care, knowing when to cut short and transport with minimal on-scene intervention this is the key to effective advanced prehospital care.

SELF-TEST

Chapter 9

1. What is the goal of the primary survey?

   ANSWER: To rapidly identify and treat life-threatening problems.

2. Define the A-B-C-D-E mneumonic for the primary survey.

   ANSWER: A = Airway.

   B = Breathing.

   C = Circulation.

   D = Disability.

   E = Expose and Examine.

3. Define the A-V-P-U mneumonic for the neurological exam.

   ANSWER: A = Alert.

   V = Verbal (responds to verbal stimuli).

   P = Painful (responds to painful stimuli).

   U = Unresponsive.

4. What situations require rapid transporation instead of continued assessment? (Name some examples.)

   ANSWER: a. Severe respiratory distress.

   b. Shock.

   c. Decreased level of consciousness.

5. Define the A-M-P-L-E mnemonic for obtaining history.

   ANSWER: A = Allergies to medications.

   M = Medications (prescription and over-the-counter).

   P = Past medical history.

   L = Last meal (or oral intake).

   E = Events leading up to emergency.

6. What is the goal of the secondary survey?

   ANSWER: An orderly head-to-toe examination designed to assess the entire patient and provide more information about problems revealed in the primary survey.

Airway Management

Maintaining an open airway is the top priority in emergency airway management. All other considerations are secondary. Lack of adequate airway and ventilation is *the* major cause of non-survival and/or neurological, cardiac, and pulmonary complications of both medical and trauma prehospital disease processes. It is probably the most important skill performed in the prehospital arena, and probably the most easily neglected. Airway control while protecting the C-spine, the timely application of oxygen, early and appropriate assistance of ventilations, assuring adequate pulmonary volumes, maintaining airtight mask/facial seals, adequate preoxygenation before changing airway adjuncts or suctioning, auscultation of the chest and constant reassessment of airway and ventilatory status—these are the standards by which the paramedic's performance is judged.

Fick Principal This principal states that adequate oxygenation depends upon:

1. Oxygenation of the red blood cells (RBCs).
2. Delivering this oxygen (via the RBCs) to the tissues.

Anatomy of the Upper Airway

Nasopharynx The nasopharynx cleans, warms and humidifies air as it enters the upper airway.

Oropharynx The oropharynx is the common entrance for both food and air. The digestive process begins here as food is broken down by the teeth and digestive enzymes.

Vallecula This is the area/indentation between the tongue and the epiglottis that should receive the tip of the curved blade during oral endotracheal intubation.

Epiglottis The epiglottis is the soft flap of tissue that quickly reacts to cover the opening of the trachea and prevent aspiration of solids/liquids into the lungs.

Larynx The larynx is also called the "voice box", where sound is produced as air passes across the vocal cords. It consists of:

1. Thyroid cartilage.
2. Cricothyroid cartilage—site utilized during cricothyroidotomy.
3. Vocal cords—these should be visualized during oral endotracheal intubation.

Anatomy of the Lower Airway

Trachea The trachea is 4–5 inches in length. It consists of C-shaped cartilaginous rings and is a direct passageway to the lungs. The walls of the trachea are lined with cilia (little hairs that help filter air and move secretions) and mucous-producing cells.

Carina The carina is where the trachea bifurcates (splits) into the right and left mainstem bronchi.

Bronchi (right and left) These are the air passages below the trachea that narrow progressively and lead eventually to the lungs. They are followed by the:

FIGURE 10.1.

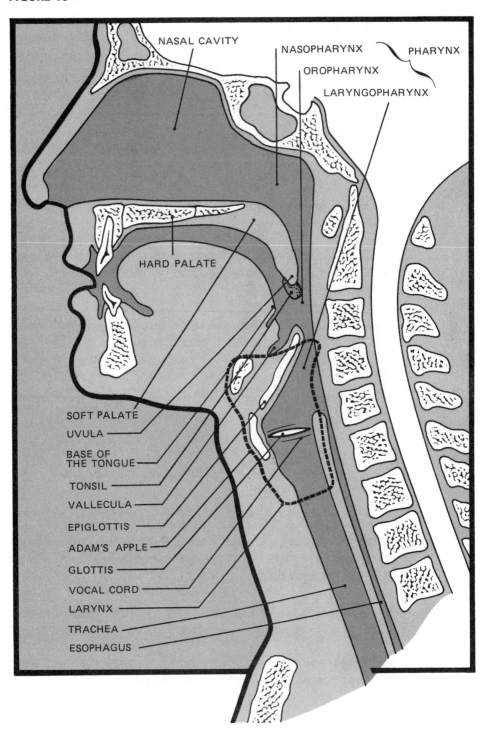

NASAL CAVITY

NASOPHARYNX   PHARYNX

OROPHARYNX

LARYNGOPHARYNX

HARD PALATE

SOFT PALATE
UVULA
BASE OF
THE TONGUE
TONSIL
VALLECULA
EPIGLOTTIS
ADAM'S APPLE
GLOTTIS
VOCAL CORD
LARYNX
TRACHEA
ESOPHAGUS

1. Secondary bronchi—Narrower continuations of the mainstem bronchi.
2. Bronchioles—Numerous smaller air passages that branch from the secondary bronchi.
3. Respiratory bronchioles—Comprised only of connective muscular tissue, these passages can narrow and even occlude during bronchospasm.
4. Alveolar ducts—Connect the bronchioles to the alveoli.

Alveoli These are small thin-walled air sacs where O_2/CO_2 gas exchange (respiration) takes place. They are surrounded by a network of microscopic capillaries that originate in the pulmonary artery.

Lungs These are the organs of respiration, consisting of the respiratory bronchioles and the alveoli. The right lung has three lobes, the left lung has two, and an extensive blood supply is provided by both the pulmonary and bronchial arteries and veins.

Visceral Pleura This is the smooth membrane that covers the outside of both lungs.

Parietal Pleura This is the smooth membrane that covers the inside of the chest cavity.

FIGURE 10.2.

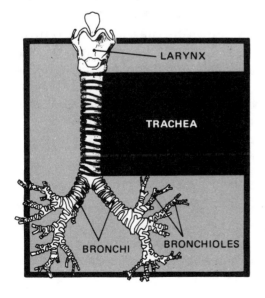

FIGURE 10.3.

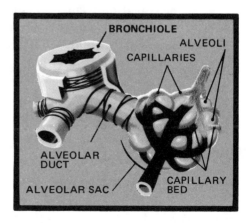

Pleural Space A "potential" space between the visceral and parietal pleura (a vacuum with lubricating fluid)—it may become a real space when one or both of the pleura are damaged to the point that air, blood or both can enter, destroying the vacuum that helps the lungs cling to the chest wall.

Mechanics of Respiration and Ventilation

Respiration Respiration is the exchange of gases between a living organism and its environment.

Pulmonary Ventilation This is the process that moves air into and out of the lungs.

Respiratory Cycle:

1. Inspiration—The diapragm (the major muscle in respiration) contracts, moving downward, while the intercostal muscles contract, moving the ribs outward and upward. The elastic lungs, because of the suction present between the visceral and parietal pleura, follow the diapragm downward and the chest wall outward, expanding and dramatically increasing in volume. This creates a low-pressure area inside the lungs. Air from outside the body (now a high-pressure area) flows into the lungs and alveoli (in an attempt to equalize pressures), bringing oxygen to exchange for carbon dioxide (respiration).
2. Expiration—The diapragm and intercostal muscles relax, returning to their previous neutral positions. As the lung volume decreases dramatically, air that had filled the lung is compressed (creating a high-pressure area). The air in the lungs flows to the outside (now a low-pressure area) in a further attempt to equalize pressures, and in the process carbon dioxide from the lungs is eliminated.

Pulmonary Circulation

Unoxygenated blood (low in oxygen and high in carbon dioxide) from the systemic venous system returns to the right heart and is pumped from the right ventricle via the pulmonary artery to the lungs, where microscopic capillaries surround the alveoli and exchange carbon dioxide for oxygen across the alveolar membrane. The freshly oxygenated blood (now high in oxygen and low in carbon dioxide) returns via the pulmonary vein to the left heart and is pumped from the left ventricle into the systemic arterial system.

Gas Exchange in the Lungs

The exchange of carbon dioxide and oxygen at the alveolar level is reflected by measurements of gas molecules in the blood (blood gases).

Torr (Toricellia Unit) A measurement of pressure. One torr is the pressure required to support one millimeter of mercury (mmHg) at 0 degrees Centigrade. This value is expressed in millimeters of mercury (mmHg). 1 torr = 1 mmHg.

Partial Pressure A concentration of gas in a mixture measured in torrs.

PO$_2$ (PaO$_2$) This is partial pressure of oxygen. Normal values are:

PO$_2$ in alveoli = 140 torr (room air);
PO$_2$ in arterial blood = 80–100 torr (freshly oxygenated); and
PO$_2$ in venous blood = 46 torr (returning to heart).

PCO$_2$ (PaCO$_2$) Partial pressure of carbon dioxide. Normal values are:

PCO$_2$ in alveoli = nearly zero;
PCO$_2$ in arterial blood = 35–40 torr (freshly oxygenated); and
PCO$_2$ in venous blood = 46 torr (returning to the heart).

Diffusion This is when gases move from an area of high concentration to an area of lower concentration.

Regulation of Respiration

Though control of respirations can be voluntarily overridden for short periods, primary control of respiration is involuntary and rests in the brainstem. In response to chemical, physical and nervous reflexes, it sends nerve impulses to the diaphragm and intercostal muscles to contract and initiate inspiration.

1. Microscopic stretch regulators (in the lungs and pleura) sense the expansion of the lungs and send impulses back to the brainstem that end inspiration, allowing the passive phase of exhalation to begin.
2. Central chemoreceptors in the medulla and peripheral chemoreceptors in the carotids and aortic arch are stimulated by certain blood gas concentrations, such as:
   a. Increases in PCO_2 (carbon dioxide—PRIMARY stimulus to breath);
   b. Decreases in PO_2 (oxygen); and
   c. Decreases in pH (signaling increasing blood acidity).
3. Carbon dioxide concentrations provide the primary stimulus to breathe in normal healthy individuals:
   a. High CO_2 concentrations increase respiratory activity;
   b. Low CO_2 concentrations decrease respiratory activity.
4. Hypoxic drive is present when respirations are stimulated by low concentrations of oxygen (instead of high CO_2). It is most often present in those who have had long-term chronic obstructive pulmonary disease (COPD)—and thus have chronically high levels of CO_2 in their blood. The body learns to ignore the high PCO_2 levels and instead depends upon low PO_2 levels for stimulus to breathe. When administering high levels of supplemental oxygen to these patients, you must monitor the respiratory rate carefully, because the high PO_2 levels you create may fool the body into respiratory arrest, requiring you to support ventilations.

Normal Respiratory Functions

Respiratory Rate This is the number of respirations (inspiration + expiration) in one minute. Normal respiratory rates (at rest) are:

Adults = 10–16 breaths per minute;

Children = approximately 24 breaths per minute; and

Infants = approximately 40–60 breaths per minute.

Some factors that may increase the respiratory rate are:

1. Hemorrhage;
2. Head injury;
3. Hypoxia;
4. Fever/infection/metabolic imbalance;
5. Anxiety, hysteria;
6. Activity; and
7. Some drugs. (Example: aspirin overdose or amphetamines.)

Some factors that may decrease the respiratory rate are:

1. Sleep/unconsciousness;
2. Head injury;
3. High oxygen levels in patients with hypoxic drive (example: Long-term COPD patients);
4. Some drugs (example: morphine, CNS depressants).

Lung Capacity The average lung capacity is 6 liters in the adult male.

Tidal Volume This is the volume of gas inhaled or exhaled during a single respiratory cycle (500 cc).

Dead Space This is the air that remains in the air passageways, unavailable for gas exchange (150 cc).

Alveolar Air The amount of air that normally reaches the alveoli for gas exchange (350 cc).

Minute Volume The amount of air moved in and out of the respiratory system in one minute. (TIDAL VOLUME × RESPIRATORY RATE = MINUTE VOLUME.)

Vital Capacity The amount of air that can be forcefully exhaled from the respiratory tract in one exhalation.

Factors Altering Carbon Dioxide Levels in the Blood

Arterial carbon dioxide levels (PCO_2) represent a balance between carbon dioxide produced during metabolism and carbon dioxide eliminated during respiration.

Increased PCO_2 This condition may be due to fever, muscular exertion, shivering, aneurobic metabolism (resulting in acidosis) or any other metabolic process that results in an excess of acid in the blood or an interference in the natural elimination process of carbon dioxide.

Note: Most importantly, increased PCO_2 will result from hypoventilation.

Some causes may be:

1. Airway obstruction;
2. Chest trauma;
3. Impact apnea (from blow to the head);
4. Some drugs (example: morphine, CNS depressants); and
5. COPD/asthma.

Decreased PCO_2 This condition is usually due to hyperventilation from anxiety, hysteria, brain injury, diabetic ketoacidosis, and so on.

Note: Hyperventilation *may* be the body's attempt to compensate for ineffective ventilations, perhaps due to:

1. Trauma;
2. Pulmonary edema; and
3. Pulmonary embolism.

Factors Altering Oxygen Levels in the Blood

Arterial oxygen levels in the blood (PO_2) represent a balance between the oxygen concentration inspired, circulatory function (transport medium for the oxygen), the respiratory rate, and respiratory function.

Increased PO_2 This may be due to supplemental oxygen and/or high ventilation rates.

Decreased PO$_2$ This may be due to a variety of causes such as:

1. Airway obstruction/asphyxia;
2. Circulatory collapse (malfunction of the transport medium);
3. Pulmonary edema;
4. Alveolar collapse (example: freshwater near-drowning victims);
5. Pulmonary embolism;
6. COPD/asthma;
7. Some drugs (CNS depressants and so forth);
8. Chest trauma (reducing effective ventilations); and
9. Neurological trauma.

Common Airway Problems

Obstruction Causes for obstruction include:

1. Tongue—The most common cause of airway obstruction, the tongue, will relax into the back of the throat, occluding the posterior pharynx.
2. Foreign Bodies:
   a. Food aspiration;
   b. Trauma (broken teeth, vomitus, clotted blood, fractured bones);
   c. Loose teeth or dentures;
   d. Other objects (example: child attempts to eat or swallow balloon).
3. Cord or laryngeal trauma (causes edema or blockage of trachea).
4. Laryngospasm (cord edema/spasm, toxic fumes, intubation attempts).

Aspiration This is the inhalation of blood, fluid, vomitus, and so on.

Inadequate Ventilation Some contributing factors of inadequate ventilation would include:

1. Rate (*hyper*ventilation or *hypo*ventilation).
2. Depth (shallow or deep).

3. Trauma:
   a. Flail chest;
   b. Tension pneumothorax;
   c. Pneumothorax/hemothorax; and
   d. "Splinting" due to chest wall trauma.
4. Disease:
   a. COPD/asthma;
   b. Pulmonary edema;
   c. Pulmonary embolus;
   d. Heart disease/AMI; and
   e. Pneumonia.

Airway Assessment

Chest The evaluation of the chest is a critical component of airway assessment. A complete evaluation would include:

1. Inspection:
   a. Watch for rise and fall of the chest wall;
   b. Look for equal and adequate expansion;
   c. Scan for punctures, lacerations, abrasions, bruising, fractures or flail segments;
   d. Note any nasal flaring or use of accessory muscles in ventilatory efforts (retraction of intercostals, supraclaviculars, and so on);
   e. Look for jugular vein distension (JVD);
   f. Check the position of the trachea (mid-line or shifted); and
   g. Evaluate the skin color.
2. Auscultation:
   a. Listen for air exchange at the mouth and nose;
   b. Check lung fields (using stethoscope):
      1. Bilateral anterior and lateral chest walls;
      2. If accessible, bilateral posterior chest wall (superior and inferior).
3. Palpation:
   a. Feel for air exchange at the mouth and nose, using the back of your hand, the hairs in your ear, or your cheek.

    b. Evaluate the chest wall, feeling specifically for:

       1. Punctures/open wounds (especially "sucking chest" wound);

       2. Deformities/fractures/flail segments;

       3. Equal chest rise;

       4. Pain/tenderness; and

       5. Crepitus/subcutaneous emphysema.

    c. Thump for hyperresonance or dullness (if in distress).

    d. When ventilating manually, also check for:

       1. Lung compliance (resistance to filling);

       2. Air leaks; and

       3. Rate of bag-valve emptying/filling.

Neck The neck can provide a wealth of information during airway assessment. Evaluation would include:

1. Inspection:
   a. Look for jugular vein distension (JVD);
   b. Look for bruising, abrasions, lacerations, and deformities;
   c. Look for position of trachea (mid-line or shifted);
   d. Note the skin color;
   e. Check capillary refill. (< 2 sec. = normal, 2–4 = delayed, > 4 = absent).
2. Auscultation:
   a. If in distress, listen for stridor and other sounds;
   b. If in distress, listen for air movement.
3. Palpation:
   a. Feel for subcutaneous emphysema or edema;
   b. Feel for position of trachea (mid-line or shifted); and
   c. Feel for skin temperature.

Airway Management

Maintaining an open airway is the top priority in emergency airway management. All other considerations are secondary. Airway management decisions involve a blend of judgment, common sense, assessment skills, available equipment, and individual skill levels. *Whenever suspected or unknown, the possibility of cervical spine damage should affect the selection of appropriate airway management equipment and techniques.*

Manual Methods (appropriate for initial management)

1. Head tilt-chin lift (contraindicated if spinal injury suspected);
2. Jaw lift;
3. Jaw thrust;
4. Chin lift.

Mechanical Methods (appropriate for continued management)

Nasal Airway (nasopharyngeal) A soft flexible flanged curved tube is inserted through the nares to provide an air passage past the tongue.

Advantages:

1. Rapid insertion;
2. Bypasses the tongue;
3. Well-tolerated (less chance of stimulating vomitus) in the patient who still has a gag reflex or is returning to consciousness.

Disadvantages:

1. Won't always go beyond the tongue;
2. Tough to suction through;
3. Does not protect the trachea from aspiration.

Method Insert the tube gently through nare until only the flange is visible. If resistance is encountered, do not force. Use other nare or discontinue use.

Oral Airway (oropharyngeal) A semi-rigid or rigid curved device (usually hollow) with a flange or a block on one end that is inserted orally to maintain an air passage past the tongue.

Advantages:

1. Bypasses the tongue;
2. Holds the tongue down and forward;

FIGURE 10.4. Nasopharyngeal Airway   **FIGURE 10.5.** Oropharyngeal Airway

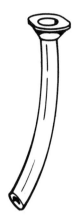   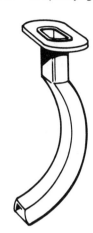

3. Facilitates suctioning;
4. Acts as a bite block to protect the tongue and/or an endotracheal tube.

Disadvantages:

1. Does not protect the trachea from aspiration;
2. May cause obstruction if improperly inserted;
3. Usually not tolerated in the presence of a gag reflex—may stimulate vomitus when the level of consciousness improves;
4. Sometimes difficult to insert.

Method Size properly before insertion (should reach from the corner of the mouth to the tip of the earlobe). Insertion may be:

1. Straight (with a tongue blade holding back the tongue);
2. Reverse (inserted to soft palate, then rotated 180 degrees—this holds the tongue back during insertion);
3. Side (inserted sideways to soft palate, then rotated 90 degrees).

Esophageal Obturator Airway (EOA) This is a flexible tube blindly inserted into the esophagus to inhibit vomiting, maintain an airway, and provide a method for supplemental ventilation. The closed distal end of the 15-inch tube has an inflatable cuff; the open proximal end has a standard mask adapter; and the proximal third of the tube has a series of per-

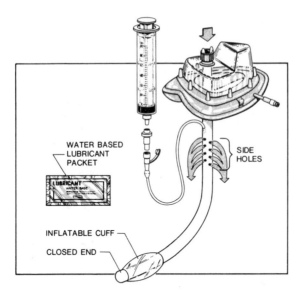

WATER BASED
LUBRICANT
PACKET

SIDE
HOLES

INFLATABLE CUFF

CLOSED END

FIGURE 10.6. Esophageal Obturator Airway

forations through which air and oxygen may enter the airway in area of the oropharynx. A detachable face mask with oxygen inlet snaps onto the proximal end of the tube and accepts a standard bag-valve or demand-valve positive pressure source. Before insertion the following equipment should be at hand:

35 cc syringe   bag-valve or demand-valve
lubricant   adequate suction
oxygen source with tubing   stethoscope
oral airway   gloves
EOA/mask

Advantages:

1. Rapid insertion;
2. Inhibits vomiting and reduces the danger of aspiration;
3. High concentrations of oxygen may be delivered;
4. May be inserted with head/neck in neutral position;
5. May be inserted blindly (without visualization);
6. May be utilized by EMTs (less training than with ET tubes);

7. Endotracheal intubation may be accomplished with an EOA still in place.

Disadvantages:

1. Patient must be unresponsive with no gag reflex;
2. Must be removed when gag reflex returns;
3. Air-tight seal must be maintained with mask;
4. Potential for damage to the esophagus;
5. Appropriate only for short-term use;
6. May intubate the trachea by mistake—effectively creating a complete airway obstruction.

Contraindications:

1. Esophageal disease;
2. Recent ingestion of caustic materials;
3. Presence of gag reflex;
4. Height—under 5 feet or over 7 feet;
5. Weight—under 100 pounds (age is not a reliable criteria).

Method Test inflatible cuff (leave syringe attached), snap mask onto tube and lightly lubricate distal tube end. Vigorously preoxygenate patient and then, with head in a neutral position (immobilized by second rescuer if possible):

1. Grasp tongue and lower jaw and pull forward;
2. Advance tube into the esophagus until mask is firmly against the face;
3. Establish a good mask seal and ventilate orally while auscultating bilateral lung fields and epigastrum;
4. If tube is positioned properly, inflate distal cuff with about 35 ccs of air by syringe—judge by firmness of pilot tube, *not* the volume of air pushed through syringe;
5. Ventilate with an appropriate source and check for chest rise;
6. Recheck lung fields and epigastrum;
7. Continue ventilation with supplemental high-flow oxygen.

Removal Done in prehospital setting only if the patient regains consciousness or if a strong gag reflex returns. Have suction working and ready, then:

1. Turn patient on side;
2. Remove mask from proximal tube end;
3. Deflate cuff;
4. Quickly and carefully remove tube (patient will almost always vomit);
5. Reassess respiratory status and oxygenate.

Esophageal Gastric Tube Airway (EGTA) Another form of EOA, this airway allows for optional stomach lavage/decompression by passing a nasogastric (NG) tube through the lumen of the EOA into the esophagus. Instead of ventilating through perforations in the tube, air/oxygen is delivered through the mask into the naso/oropharynx. The contents of the stomach are still prevented from compromising the airway by an inflatable cuff. Equipment needed for insertion is the same as with the EOA, with the optional addition of a nasogastric tube.

FIGURE 10.7. Esophageal Gastric Tube Airway

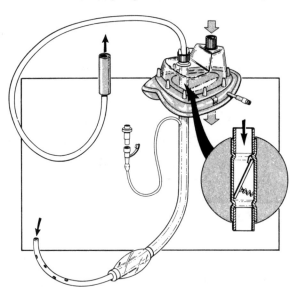

Advantages:

1. Same as with EOA;
2. May decompress and/or lavage stomach, reducing the likelihood of vomiting and decreasing pressure on the diaphragm.

Disadvantages, Contraindications, Method and Removal: Same as for EOA. If an NG tube is used, it should be measured from the tip of the nose to the earlobe to the xiphoid process.

Pharyngeo-Tracheal Lumen Airway (PTL) Considered essentially a "no-fault" EGTA, the PTL combines the advantages of an EOA and ET with the inability of improper tube placement. If blind insertion results in tracheal intubation, the airway acts as an endotracheal tube. If blind insertion results in esophageal placement, the airway acts as an EGTA (minus the need for maintaining a mask seal). The PTL is basically an endotracheal tube attached to a short tube with a large balloon cuff that occludes the oropharynx and makes an effective internal seal. When the longer tube is placed in the esophagus (probably > 90% of the time), ventilations are accomplished through the short tube via standard adapter.

FIGURE 10.8. PTL Airway

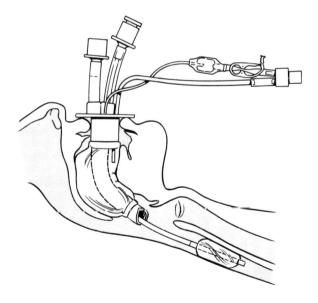

When the longer tube is placed in the esophagus (< 10% of the time), ventilations are accomplished through the long tube via a standard adapter. The oropharyngeal balloon can be deflated to allow endotracheal intubation (while the distal balloon cuff on the long tube stays inflated to prevent regurgitation).

Advantages:

1. Cannot be improperly placed;
2. Eliminates the need for an external face mask seal;
3. Can always be placed with head in neutral position;
4. Same as for the EOA (when placed in esophagus);
5. Same as for ET tube (when placed in trachea);
6. Requires minimal training (and can generally be placed by first responders and EMTs);
7. Facilitates suctioning/gastric lavage/decompression.

Disadvantages:

1. Patient must be unresponsive with no gag reflex;
2. Must be removed when gag reflex returns;
3. Appropriate only for short-term use;
4. Possibility (though slight) of cuff malfunction.

Contraindications: Same as for an EOA.

Method Vigorously preoxygenate patient if you have the means. You have the option of neutral head/neck position (mandatory in trauma, with second rescuer immobolizing manually) or hyperextension (when this position is not contraindicated). If your goal is esophageal placement, keep the patient in neutral position (immobolized by second rescuer if trauma is suspected):

1. Grasp the tongue and lower jaw and pull forward.
2. Advance tube until the teeth block is firmly against the teeth. Do not force. If resistance is encountered, redirect the tube or pull out and start over.
3. Blow forcefully into the main inflation valve (marked #1) with a sustained breath (until you can pass no more air). An alternative is to

hold the bag-valve firmly against the inflation valve and inflate as much as you can (the valve may "squeal" when optimal pressure is reached).

4. Ventilate orally through the green tube (marked #2). If the chest rises, auscultate bilateral lung fields and epigastrum. (ESOPHAGEAL PLACEMENT)

5. If the chest does not rise, pull stylet from long tube (marked #3) and ventilate orally. Auscultate bilateral lung fields and epigastrum. (TRACHEAL PLACEMENT)

6. Attach positive pressure device (with oxygen source) and continue ventilations.

Removal Done in the prehospital setting only if the patient regains consciousness or a strong gag reflex returns. Have suction working and ready, then:

1. Turn patient on side.

2. Remove the cap from the inflation valve (marked #1). This will allow both balloon cuffs to deflate.

3. Quickly and carefully remove tube (patient will almost always vomit).

4. Reassess respiratory status and oxygenate.

Endotracheal (ET) Intubation (oral) When properly placed, this is considered the most effective airway/ventilation control for the prehospital patient. It provides direct access to the lungs, protects against aspiration and can be used as an alternative site for drug administration when intravenous access is unavailable. The ET-tube is a flexible curved tube with a balloon cuff on one end and a standard adapter for ventilation devices on the other. It comes in many sizes, and the length of the tube is proportioned to its internal diameter. Special equipment is usually required for insertion including:

laryngoscope w/batteries	stylet (optional)
curved or straight blade	endotracheal tube
syringe (usually 10cc)	stethoscope
lubricant	tape
suction	magill forceps (optional)

FIGURE 10.9. Endotracheal Tube

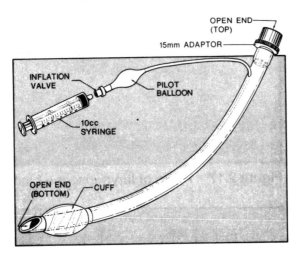

Advantages:

1. Complete control of airway;
2. Prevents aspiration;
3. Best airway for delivering positive pressure;
4. May be used as alternate route for some medications (Narcan, Atropine, Valium, Epinephrine, Lidocaine);
5. Prevents gastric distension;
6. Facilitates tracheal suctioning;
7. Allows high-volumes of high oxygen concentrations;
8. May be inserted while an esophageal or PTL airway is still in place.

Disadvantages:

1. Advanced training and frequent practice is required to maintain skill;
2. Proper placement requires direct visualization of the vocal cords;
3. Tissue damage can occur during placement;
4. No oxygenation is possible during placement process;
5. Laryngospasm may occur during placement attempts;
6. Must be removed upon return of significant gag reflex.

Contraindications:

1. Hyperextension in the trauma patient—oral intubation must be done with constant manual in-line neutral stabilization;
2. Prolonged insertion attempts (increases hypoxia).

Method (should be accomplished within 15–20 seconds):

1. Pre-ventilate with high-flow oxygen.
2. Estimate the proper size of ET-tube (average adult = 8 mm.) and prepare all equipment.
3. Place head in "sniffing position" (slight extension). Trauma victims must remain in neutral position with manual in-line stabilization during entire procedure.
4. Stop ventilation, insert laryngoscope into right side of the mouth, sweeping the tongue to the left.
5. Do not "crank back on the teeth", but lift the tongue and mandible "up and out" gently until the epiglottis, larynx, and vocal cords can be visualized (downward pressure on the larynx by another person sometimes brings the cords into better view).

FIGURE 10.10. View of Larynx with Laryngoscope

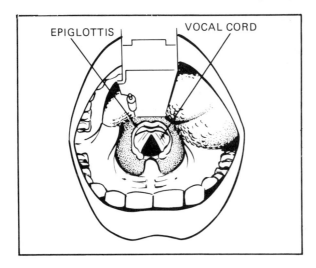

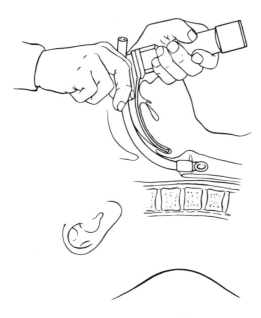

FIGURE 10.11.

6. Keeping the vocal cords in view, carefully pass the endotracheal tube through the opening in the cords. After the distal cuff disappears past the cords, pass another 1/2"–1" and stop. Do not let go of the tube!

7. Remove the laryngoscope/blade, inflate the balloon cuff with 6–10 cc air (if you watched the tube go past the cords) and ventilate.

8. Watch for chest rise, auscultate bilateral lung sounds and the epigastrum.

9. Secure tube position with tape (or other securing device) and continue ventilation.

10. If one of these situations apply, return to ventilation by BVM and make another intubation attempt after re-oxygenation:

    a. The vocal cords cannot be visualized.

    b. Tube placement cannot be confirmed and the chest does not rise.

    c. The patient's color deteriorates upon further ventilation.

11. If evaluation of tube placement confirms breath sounds on the right side only, withdraw the tube slowly until sounds are heard on the left.

Removal Usually not indicated in the field unless spontaneous respirations return and the patient fights the tube. To remove:

1. Ready suction (be ready to turn the patient on their side);
2. Deflate the balloon cuff completely;
3. Withdraw tube on inspiration;
4. Assess respiratory status;
5. Re-oxygenate patient.

Nasotracheal Intubation If a patient is still breathing spontaneously, yet intubation is judged desirable, blind nasotracheal intubation may be a viable alternative. It is accomplished with the head in a neutral in-line position (an important factor when confronted with trauma victims). If a nasotracheal tube is not available, use an endotracheal tube one size smaller than you would have used in an oral intubation. Equipment necessary for insertion includes:

syringe (usually 6–12 cc)	endotracheal or nasotracheal tube
lubricant	
suction	positive pressure source w/oxygen
	stethoscope

Advantages:

1. Same as for endotracheal intubation;
2. Does not require hyperextension of the head (trauma victims);
3. May be utilized when spontaneous respirations are present.

Disadvantages:

1. May cause damage to tissues;
2. May cause laryngospasm during placement attempts;
3. Accidental intubation of the esophagus is possible;
4. Oxygenation is not possible during intubation attempts.

Contraindications:

1. Extensive facial trauma that affects the nasopharynx;
2. Prolonged intubation attempts that increase hypoxia.

Method:

1. Lubricate the tube and largest (or chosen) nostril.
2. With head in neutral position, insert tube through nostril, advancing only during exhalation. Keep your ear to the tube opening.
3. When the exhalation heard/felt through the tube gets noticeably louder, the cords are near. If the victim gags, stop, then slide the tube through the cords on the next exhalation.
4. The tube should "mist up" immediately upon correct insertion and exhalations should be easily felt coming from the end of the tube.
5. Confirm placement by chest rise, auscultation of bilateral lungs sounds and epigastrum.
6. Secure with tape and continue ventilation.

Removal Same as for endotracheal intubation.

Cricothyrotomy (NOT A DOT-REQUIRED SKILL) This method is used in cases of complete airway obstruction when less invasive procedures have failed. It involves cutting an opening in the cricothyroid membrane and enlarging the opening to pass a pediatric endotracheal tube (approximately 4.0 mm) into the trachea. A less complicated (but less effective) variation would be to puncture the cricothyroid membrane with a large

FIGURE 10.12.

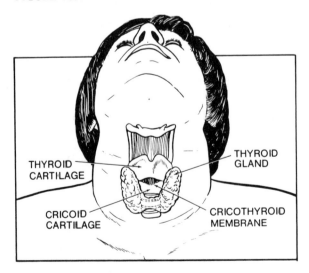

THYROID CARTILAGE

THYROID GLAND

CRICOID CARTILAGE

CRICOTHYROID MEMBRANE

gauge over-the-needle catheter (10, 12, or 14 gauge), remove the needle and allow passive air exchange through the catheter. Various styles of special kits are also available for cricothyrotomy.

Transtracheal Jet Insufflation (TTJI) If the patient with complete airway obstruction (unrelieved) is not breathing once the airway has been opened with a NEEDLE CRICOTHYROIDOTOMY, ventilation can be accomplished in the following way:

1. Connect a length of oxygen supply tubing to a 40–50 psi oxygen source. (the portable oxygen tanks and wall-mount oxygen currently used in the field fall into this category).
2. Near the distal end, bend the tubing and cut a hole in one side with a pair of scissors or knife.
3. Force the distal end of the tubing over the hub of the catheter that has been inserted into the trachea through the cricothyroid membrane (a quick application of tape securing this joint is advisable).
4. Turn the oxygen flow up to 15 liters (or highest setting) and cover the hole in the supply tubing with a thumb for one second to inflate the lungs, while uncovering the hole for four seconds for deflation.
5. Maintain this cycle until reaching the hospital. This emergency ventilation method may be good for 30–45 minutes—even with hyperinflation of the chest and CO_2 retention.

Note: A simple TTJI kit can be "homemade" and stored in a reclosable sandwich bag.

Ventilation

Mouth-to-Mouth
Advantages:

1. Provides immediate ventilation with potentially high volumes of air;
2. No special equipment is required;
3. Lung compliance is easily felt;
4. It can be done anywhere, in many different positions and environments.

Disadvantages:

1. Cannot provide supplemental oxygen;
2. Mouth-to-mouth seal must be maintained during ventilations;
3. Risk of exposure to communicable diseases.
4. Tiring to rescuer after a period of time.

Mouth-to-Pocket Mask
Advantages:

1. Easy to use and easy to carry;
2. Uses the lung power of the rescuer to provide high volumes;
3. With supplemental oxygen, a range of 50–80% concentration can be achieved;
4. Attachable one-way valve protects rescuer from possible contaminants;
5. May be used in conjunction with bag-valve when one becomes available;
6. Lung compliance is easily felt.

Disadvantages:

1. Mask-to-mouth seal must be maintained;
2. Tiring to rescuer after a period of time.

FIGURE 10.13. Pocket Mask

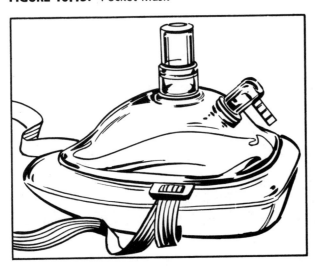

FIGURE 10.14. Bag-Valve-Mask with Reservoir

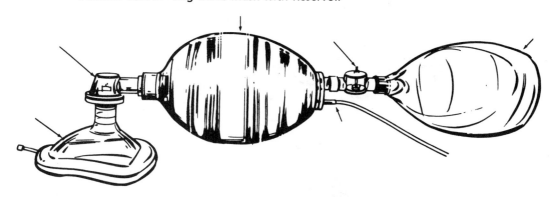

Bag-Valve-Mask (BVM) (effectiveness of BVM varies with model used)
Advantages:

1. Has a 21–100% range of oxygen concentration possible—depending upon type of supplemental oxygen reservoir, liter flow, and so on;
2. Provides positive pressure ventilations;
3. Protects rescuer from possible contaminants;
4. Lung compliance still can be felt;
5. May be connected to any standard 15 mm adapter (EOA, EGTA, PTL, ET).

Disadvantages:

1. Requires practice to maintain skill level (can be difficult for some);
2. Mask-to-mouth seal must be obtained;
3. Provides limited tidal volumes;
4. Requires two people to operate in some situations (in the presence of alveolar collapse or increased pulmonary resistance);
5. May require the simultaneous use of an oropharyngeal or nasopharyngeal airway.

Demand Valve
Advantages:

1. Provides 100% oxygen concentration and positive pressure;
2. May be used to assist the breathing of conscious patients (the negative pressure created in the mask when breathing attempt begins trig-

FIGURE 10.15. Demand Valve

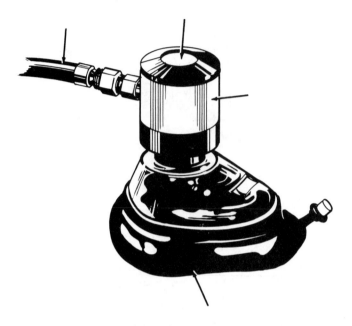

gers the demand valve to open and provide 100% oxygen until the negative pressure subsides);

3. May be manually triggered to ventilate non-breathing victims;

4. When used in conjunction with an ET-tube, one rescuer may perform CPR at near-two rescuer standards (one hand for ventilations, one hand for compressions);

5. May be attached to any standard 15 mm adapter (EOA, EGTA, PTL, ET).

Disadvantages:

1. Compliance of the lungs is not easily felt;

2. Contraindicated for pediatric and geriatric patients;

3. Potential exists for lung damage (due to ventilation pressures);

4. Greater danger of gastric distension (when used without ET-tube);

5. Because it's oxygen-powered, when the oxygen is gone—it quits working.

Suction

Adequate suction is a critical component of airway maintenance. It is used to remove fluids and some solid particles from the airway that restrict the effectiveness of ventilations, pose an aspiration hazard and obstruct the view of anatomical structures. Materials most often suctioned from the airway include:

1. Vomitus;
2. Blood;
3. Saliva;
4. Food;
5. OXYGEN!

Tracheal Suction Suction through an endotracheal tube or nasopharyngeal airway may be performed with a whistle-tip catheter (small enough to fit within the lumen of the tube). Insert the catheter completely, then suction as the catheter is withdrawn. If possible, keep suction time within 10 seconds, then quickly re-oxygenate.

Pharyngeal Suction Suction of the mouth and hypopharynx may be performed with a large bore rigid suction device (such as a tonsil-tip catheter), or even with the suction tubing itself. Insert the catheter into the hypopharynx (beside the oral airway, if present), activate suction and withdraw slowly. If it is safe to turn the patient's head (or body as a whole), this may help pool the material on one side and facilitate suctioning. Again, keep suction time under 10 seconds if possible.

Note: Though most authoritative sources recommend that:

1. The patient be well oxygenated before beginning suction.
2. Suction be discontinued after 10 seconds.

Experienced field paramedics know that until adequate suction has cleared the airway, further ventilation and oxygenation are futile.

Summary

Recognition and management of airway insufficiency is the top priority for prehospital care providers. Until this is effectively treated, and oxygen is available for transport by the circulatory system, other treatment for life-threatening emergencies is useless. Once adequately treated, the chances of survival for the seriously ill or injured patient in the prehospital phase is significantly increased. This is the most important skill that paramedics can master, and one by which they will best be judged.

SELF-TEST

Chapter 10

1. Small thin-walled air sacs where O_2/CO_2 gas exchange (respiration) takes place are called the _____ .

   ANSWER: alveoli

2. Name the major muscle of respiration?

   ANSWER: the diaphragm

3. What are the only major veins in the body that carry oxygenated blood?

   ANSWER: pulmonary veins

4. Define diffusion.

   ANSWER: When gases move from an area of high concentration to an area of lower concentration.

5. Primary (involuntary) control of respiration is located in the

   _____ .

   ANSWER: brainstem

6. Which blood gas concentration is the primary stimulus to breathe?

   ANSWER: A high level of carbon dioxide

7. The stimulation of respirations by low concentrations of oxygen instead of high concentration of carbon dioxide is called _____

   _____ .

   ANSWER: hypoxic drive

8. Name at least three factors that may increase the respiratory rate.

   ANSWER: a. hemorrhage   d. anxiety, hysteria

                 b. head injury   e. activity

                 c. hypoxia   f. pneumothorax

g. pulmonary embolism
h. fever, infection
i. pulmonary edema
j. drugs (am-
   phetamines, ASA
   overdose)

k. metabolic im-
   balance (acidosis)
l. chest trauma (flail
   chest, sucking chest
   wound, myocardial
   contusion, tension
   pneumothorax, and
   so on

9. Name at least two factors that may decrease the respiratory rate.

ANSWER: a. sleep

b. unconsciousness

c. head injury

d. drugs (morphine, CNS depressants)

10. The volume of gas inhaled or exhaled during a single respiratory cycle is called the _____ _____ .

ANSWER: tidal volume

11. The amount of air moved in and out of the respiratory system in one minute is called the _____ _____ .

ANSWER: minute volume

12. What is the most common cause of airway obstruction?

ANSWER: the tongue

13. Name at least two causes of increased PCO_2 and/or decreased PO_2.

ANSWER: a. airway obstruction

b. chest trauma

c. impact apnea

d. pulmonary edema

e. drugs (morphine, CNS depressants)

f. COPD, asthma

g. significantly decreased resp. rate

h. pulmonary embolism

14. Name at least two methods of opening the airway.

ANSWER: a. head-tilt, chin-lift

b. jaw lift

c. chin lift

d. jaw thrust

15. The _____ _____ keeps the tongue from blocking the airway and is better tolerated in the presence of a gag reflex than the oropharyngeal airway.

    ANSWER: nasopharyngeal airway

16. Name at least two contraindications of the esophageal obturator airway.

    ANSWER: a. known esophageal disease

    b. recent ingestion of caustic materials

    c. return or presence of gag reflex

    d. under 5 feet tall or over 7 feet tall

    e. under 100 pounds

17. Why is the PTL airway (pharyngeo-tracheal lumen airway) considered a "no-fault" airway?

    ANSWER: Whether blindly inserted into the esophagus or trachea—the PTL airway can still effectively ventilate the patient.

18. _____ _____ is the most effective method of ventilation and airway control in the prehospital patient?

    ANSWER: Endotracheal intubation

19. Is oral endotracheal intubation contraindicated in the trauma patient?

    ANSWER: No. If the head and neck are manually maintained in neutral position during intubation, it is a viable alternative.

20. What kind of patient is a good choice for nasal endotracheal intubation:

    ANSWER: An unconscious patient who is still breathing.

21. The demand valve provides 100% oxygen under positive pressure. Are there any patients who should not receive ventilation by demand valve?

    ANSWER: Yes. The demand valve should not be used for pediatric and geriatric patients (because of the pressures involved).

22. How long should tracheal suction be maintained?

    ANSWER: Ideally, less than 10 seconds.

Shock, Fluids, and Electrolytes

Profound shock is an extreme emergency, one that paramedics must recognize and manage immediately. Initial management can be as simple as airway positioning, elevation of extremities, bleeding control or oxygen administration, but *may* require the PASG (pneumatic anti-shock garment), intravenous fluid administration, assisted ventilations, and, most important in traumatic shock, *rapid transportation to the appropriate medical facility.*

An understanding of cellular metabolism, acid-base balance, and fluids and electrolytes is crucial to understanding shock, therefore, a brief review of these subjects is included.

Shock

Shock Shock is most often defined as *inadequate tissue perfusion,* or the lack of cellular oxygenation (and nutrition). *Normal* tissue perfusion requires four components—*IF ANY OF THESE COMPONENTS ARE ABSENT, SHOCK CAN OCCUR!*

1. *Adequate Pump* (cardiac output).
2. *Adequate Fluid Volume* (blood, ICF, ECF).

3. *Intact Vascular System* (capable of dilation/constriction, and transportation).

4. *Adequate Ventilation* (volume, rate, with O_2/CO_2 exchange possible).

Adequate Pump An efficient, effective heart muscle is necessary to pump blood through the vascular system against *systemic vascular resistance* (SVR). Cardiac output is governed by baroreceptors located within the aorta. Stimulation of these baroreceptors causes sympathetic nervous system stimulation which leads to:

1. An increase in the force of cardiac contractions;

2. An increase in the heart rate;

3. Arterial constriction (and thus increased SVR) necessary to maintain perfusion.

Adequate Volume An adequate circulating blood volume (and red blood cells) is necessary for oxygen to be transported in sufficient amounts to the cells of the body and its organs. This volume is also necessary to maintain SVR (systemic vascular resistance—afterload) and cardiac preload.

Intact Vasculature A closed contained system, capable of dilation and constriction, is necessary to convey oxygen-enriched blood to all organs and body parts and return oxygen-depleted blood (and CO_2) to the heart and lungs.

Adequate Ventilation Proper rate and depth of ventilations is necessary to provide oxygen for exchange with CO_2 in the lungs (respiration). There must be unimpeded access for this exchange to take place (no pulmonary edema).

Classifications of Shock

Hypovolemic Shock This is shock caused by significant decrease in blood or plasma volume (severe bleeding).

Cardiogenic Shock This is shock caused by failure of the heart muscle (myocardial infarction, cardiac myopathy).

Neurogenic Shock This is shock caused by a relative enlargement of the vascular system, usually due to nerve paralysis (spinal cord injury).

Psychogenic Shock This is a mild form of shock caused by temporary reduction of blood supply to the brain, usually due to vaso-vagal stimulation that temporarily dilates the blood vessels (simple fainting).

Septic Shock This is shock caused by toxins released during overwhelming bacterial infections. These create dilation of the blood vessels and loss of plasma through the vessel walls, and thus a decrease in circulating volume.

Metabolic Shock This is shock caused by fluid loss from vomiting, diarrhea, urination, or because of severe acid-base disruptions (severe diabetes, severe untreated illness).

Anaphylactic Shock This is shock triggered by the body's violent allergic reaction to a substance (after being sensitized by previous contact). Histamines are released, fluid may escape into the tissues (causing a decrease in volume) and lungs (pulmonary edema), shock symptoms develop rapidly, and severe edema may appear in upper airway.

Pertinent Definitions

Compensated Shock This form of shock occurs when an increase in heart rate, strength of contractions, and peripheral resistance are sufficient to maintain tissue perfusion at adequate levels. (Blood pressure may be normal—perhaps even elevated, though blood volume and/or blood oxygen is below normal.)

Uncompensated Shock This form of shock occurs when the body is unable to maintain adequate tissue perfusion to the vital organs. (Falling blood pressure is a *late* sign of uncompensated shock. The lack of sufficient oxygen to the cells eventually triggers anaerobic metabolism and widespread cellular damage—beginning with the brain, heart muscle and lungs— and extending to other organs as time progresses.)

Aerobic Metabolism This is normal cellular metabolism utilizing oxygen to combine with nutrients to produce energy (and easily discardable waste products).

Anaerobic Metabolism This is abnormal cellular metabolism triggered when oxygen is not available, that excretes ketones and lactic acid as byproducts of energy production.

Fluids and Electrolytes

Intracellular Fluid (ICF) This is the fluid inside of the cell membrane (40% of total body weight).

Extracellular Fluid (ECF) This is the fluid outside of the cell membrane (20% of total body weight) further composed of:

1. *Interstitial Fluid*—Water bathing the cells (includes cerebrospinal fluid [CSF] and introcular fluid); and
2. *Intravascular Fluid* (plasma)—Water within the blood vessels (carries red blood cells (RBCs), white blood cells (WBCs) and essential nutrients)

Electrolytes Electrolytes are solutes whose molecules dissociate into charged components (ions) when placed in water. In physiologic solutions, the total number of *cations* always equals the total number of *anions*. The *milliequivalent* (mEq) is the unit of measurement for electrolytes.

Cations These are positively charged ions.

1. *Sodium* (Na+)—The chief extracellular cation, and a primary factor in water distribution throughout the body. Remember—WATER FOLLOWS SODIUM!
2. *Potassium* (K+)—The chief intracellular cation, and a prime mediator of electrical impulses in nerves and muscles (including the heart).
3. *Calcium* (Ca++)—Versatile cation that aids bone development, blood clotting, and neuromuscular activity.

Anions These are negatively charged ions.

1. *Chloride* (Cl−)—Anion found primarily in extracellular fluid that tends to follow sodium and has an affinity for bicarbonate.
2. *Bicarbonate* (HCO_3−)—The chief buffer in the body, responsible for maintaining acid-base balance.

Milliequivalent (mEq) The chemical combining power of the ion, based upon the number of available ionic charges in an electrolyte solution. (1 mEq of any cation can react completely with 1 mEq of any anion.)

Nonelectrolytes These are solutes with no electrical charge. The milligram (mg) is the unit of measurement for nonelectrolytes (urea, glucose).

Osmosis The process by which water moves from an area of lower concentration to an area of higher concentration (across a semipermeable membrane) in an attempt to equalize the solute concentrations of each.

Diffusion This occurs when solute molecules move across semipermeable membranes (they move much more slowly than water).

Hypertonic Solution A solution with a higher concentration of solute molecules than is inside the cells (50% dextrose, 7.5% saline).

Isotonic Solution A solution having a concentration of solute molecules equivalent to that inside the cells (normal saline, lactated ringers).

Hypotonic Solution A solution with a solute concentration *lower* than that of the cells (1/2 normal saline, 5% dextrose).

Blood The circulating fluid of the vascular system, blood contains red blood cells (and hemoglobin), white blood cells and platelets suspended in plasma (proteins, inorganic salts, nutrients, waste materials, and gases in solution).

Whole Blood This is blood as it exists normally in the vascular system, drawn and kept from clotting, then refrigerated (good for 2–3 weeks). This is the best choice for patients suffering from acute blood loss, if available, typed and crossmatched.

Colloids These are solutions containing protein. They stay in the vascular space longer and help maintain volume (albumin).

Crystalloids These are solutions that do *not* contain protein. When using as stopgap for hemorrhagic shock, it takes 3 times the volume of crystalloid to replace blood lost to be effective—and its stay in the vascular space is short (2/3 lost to interstitial space in one hour). No more than 3 liters should be infused during volume expansion efforts (lactated ringers, normal saline).

Glucose This is simply sugar. It provides an immediate expansion in volume but rapidly leaves the vascular space. It can be used as an adjunct to provide energy for brain metabolism and to counter diabetic states (D5W, D50W).

Plasma Plasma is a temporary volume expander processed from whole blood that does not need to be typed (unless fresh-frozen) or crossmatched. Fresh-frozen plasma contains active clotting factors. Normally, plasma is the transport medium for blood components.

Dextran Dextran is a temporary volume expander (plasma substitute) made of a glucose polymer that tends to stay in the vascular space because of its large size.

Packed Red Blood Cells This is a concentrated volume of red blood cells that improve the oxygen-carrying capacity of the blood (without adding much volume).

Acid-Base Balance

Acid-Base Balance This refers to regulation of the concentration of *hydrogen ions* (H+) in body fluids. An increased concentration of H+ makes this fluid more acid, while a decreased concentration of H+ makes the fluid more base. Acid-base balance has both metabolic and respiratory components, and a narrow range of H+ concentration is required for normal cellular function. To maintain this narrow range, the body has three systems of defense:

1. Buffer System (sodium bicarbonate/carbonic acid system)—The fastest-acting defense system (almost instantaneous). Carbonic acid (H_2CO_3) breaks down constantly into water (H_2O) and carbon dioxide (CO_2) *OR* into hydrogen ions (H+) and bicarbonate ions (HCO_3-):

$$H_2O + CO_2 \rightleftharpoons H_2CO_3 \rightleftharpoons H+ + HCO_3-$$

   The direction in which the reaction proceeds depends on the origin of excess.

2. Respiratory System—Backs up the buffer system and takes 1 to 3 minutes to be effective. If CO_2 *or* H+ increase, the rate and depth

of respirations are stimulated to increase, blowing off CO_2 and reducing carbonic acid until condition normalizes.

3. Renal System—Primarily for long-term maintenance of acid-base, this system (utilizing the kidneys) takes from several hours to several days to be effective. If the pH falls (H+ increase) beyond the capacity of respiratory system buffer, the kidneys excrete more hydrogen ions (and retain bicarbonate ions). If the pH rises (HCO_3− increase), the kidneys excrete more bicarbonate ions (and retain hydrogen ions).

torr torr is equal to mmHg (millimeters of mercury). It is used interchangeably with mmHg when reporting blood gases.

pH This is an expression of overall hydrogen ion (H+) concentration.

PaO_2 This is a measurement of arterial oxygen tension. Normal value is 80–100 mmHg (torr).

$PaCO_2$ This is a measurement of arterial carbon dioxide tension. Normal value is 35–45 mmHg (torr).

HCO_3 This stands for the bicarbonate level in arterial blood. Normal value is 22–26 mEq.

Neutral pH Neutral pH is usually considered to be 7.0.

Normal body pH Normal arterial pH is considered to be 7.35 to 7.45 (slightly alkaline).

Acidosis Refers to a pH measurement of less than 7.35 (increased H+ concentration).

Alkalosis Refers to a pH measurement of more than (decreased H+ concentration).

Respiratory Acidosis Inadequate ventilation (hypoventilation, trauma, pneumothorax, pulmonary edema, drug overdose) causes CO_2 retention, and thus an increase in the amount of carbonic acid (H_2CO_3) in the blood (pH DROPS).

Tx: Treat the cause and assist ventilations.

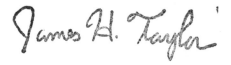

Respiratory Alkalosis Excessive ventilation (hyperventilation) causes CO_2 elimination, reducing the amount of carbonic acid (H_2CO_3) in the blood (pH RISES).

Tx: Treat the cause. With simple hyperventilation, rebreathe CO_2 (with the old "brown paper bag").

Metabolic Acidosis Excess amounts of acid produced by the body (diabetic ketoacidosis, ASA overdose) increase carbonic acid (H_2CO_3) in the blood while using up significant amounts of the bicarbonate (HCO_3-) buffer (pH DROPS).

Tx: Treat the cause and consider sodium bicarbonate IV.

Metabolic Alkalosis Excess amounts of base occur (overdose of antacid, overzealous administration of intravenous sodium bicarbonate), wiping out carbonic acid (H_2CO_3) in the blood and using up hydrogen ions ($H+$) (pH RISES).

Tx: Supportive care while waiting for the body's buffers to accomodate. (Kidneys will retain $H+$ to balance HCO_3-, lungs will retain CO_2 to a degree—watch ventilations carefully.)

Summary

Paramedics must thoroughly understand the pathophysiology of shock, and most importantly, the importance of *transport without delay* (not even for IVs) in those patients whose only chance of reversal lie in the operating room. Balancing the risk of further injury versus immediate extrication and transport is a determination that is difficult—even for those with many years in the field. One of our most important challenges lie in salvaging the many trauma patients that die before reaching an operating room. Understand shock, and you understand the hurry.

SELF-TEST

Chapter 11

1. Define shock.

   ANSWER: Simply put, inadequate tissue perfusion.

2. What are the four components needed to maintain normal tissue perfusion?

   ANSWER: a. adequate pump

   b. adequate fluid volume

   c. intact vascular system

   d. adequate ventilation

3. What is the difference between compensated and uncompensated shock?

   ANSWER: a. *Compensated shock is early shock,* when the heart rate and force of contractions are increased to compensate and maintain normal blood pressures and adequate tissue perfusion.

   b. *Uncompensated shock is late shock,* when the heart is unable to maintain normal blood pressure or adequate tissue perfusion by increases in the heart rate and strength of contractions.

4. What percentage of total body weight is ICF (intracellular fluid)?

   ANSWER: ICF is 40% of total body weight.

5. What percentage of total body weight is ECF (extracellular fluid)?

   ANSWER: ECF is 20% of total body weight.

6. The chief extracellular cation is Na+ (sodium). What is its function?

   ANSWER: Na+ (sodium) is responsible for water distribution throughout the body. Water tends to follow sodium.

7. The intracellular cation is K+ (potassium). What is its function?

   ANSWER: K+ (potassium) is the mediator of electrical impulses in nerves and muscles.

8. The process by which water moves from an area of low concentration to an area of high concentration (across a semipermeable membrane) in attempt to equalize the solute concentrations of each is called _____ .

   ANSWER: osmosis

9. What are the three systems used by the body to maintain acid-base balance?

   ANSWER: a. buffer system

   b. respiratory system

   c. renal system

10. Define acidosis.

ANSWER: An increase in H+ (hydrogen) ion concentration in the blood. A pH of less than 7.35 is considered acidosis.

11. A decrease in H+ (hydrogen) ion concentration in the blood is called

_____ .

ANSWER: alkalosis

12. What causes respiratory acidosis, and how is it treated?

ANSWER: Inadequate ventilation causes respiratory acidosis by allowing a build-up of carbon dioxide. Treatment is directed toward eliminating the cause—generally by increasing the rate and/or volume of assisted ventilations.

13. What causes respiratory alkalosis, and how is it treated?

ANSWER: Hyperventilation causes respiratory alkalosis by eliminating too much carbon dioxide. Treatment is directed toward decreasing the rate and/or volume of assisted ventilations, or to have the patient rebreathe CO_2.

14. Excess amounts of acid production in the body cause _____

_____ .

ANSWER: metabolic acidosis

15. Excess amounts of base cause _____ _____ , perhaps from antacid overdose or excessive administration of sodium bicarbonate.

ANSWER: metabolic alkalosis

16. Give two examples of relatively isotonic IV solutions used in pre-hospital care?

ANSWER: Normal saline and lactated ringers.

Pharmacology

Paramedics are entrusted (under the direction of a physician or his orders) with the administration of drugs. As we have come to know, this is a double-edged sword, with both beneficial and lethal potential. Those drugs we carry and administer must be thoroughly understood (it is not that unusual to receive orders in error) and often reviewed. Our patients have medicine cabinets crammed with a myriad of pharmacologic agents, and though we are not pharmacists or physicians, we must be familiar with the common medications of cardiac, respiratory, hypertensive, psychiatric, seizure, diabetic, and geriatric patients. This chapter provides a brief overview of pharmacologic standard and practices.

Overview

Our view of pharmacology is divided into five standard categories:

1. Drug information;
2. Action of drugs;
3. Weights and measures;
4. Administration of drugs; and
5. Techniques of administration.

Also included are pertinent definitions that relate to pharmacology. Chapter 16 (Cardiovascular) reviews the drugs paramedics often carry and encounter.

Drug Information (Category 1)

Drug Information

1. Effects.
2. Proper dosages.
3. Contraindications.
4. Side effects.
5. Route(s) of administration.

Drug Sources

1. Animal (pancreas).
2. Vegetable (flowers, roots, leaves).
3. Mineral (calcium, iron, magnesium).
4. Synthetic (man-made).

Drug Names

1. Official (name listed in the *United States Pharmacopeia*).
2. Chemical (description of chemical makeup).
3. Generic (name given by first manufacturer).
4. Trade name (registered name—first letter then capitalized).

Drug Standards and Legislation

1. Exist to regulate uniformity, strength, and purity.
2. *The Pure Food Act* (1906)—Requires labeling.
3. *The Federal Food, Drug and Cosmetic Act* (1938, 1952, 1962)—Spells out nature of label requirements, gives the FDA authority to test for safety before allowing distribution and requires prescriptions for "dangerous" drugs.

4. *The Harrison Narcotic Act* (1914)—Regulates the manufacture, sale, import and prescription of specified narcotics, requires record-keeping, registration of distributors, and punishments for specific violations.

5. *The Narcotic Control Act* (1956)—Increased penalties of violations and added marijuana to the controlled group.

6. Federal regulatory agencies:

   a. *Bureau of Narcotics and Dangerous Drugs* (BNDD) (Includes the *Drug Enforcement Agency* (DEA)).

   b. *Food and Drug Administration* (FDA).

   c. *Public Health Service* (PHS).

Drug Forms

1. Solids:

   a. *Extracts* (concentrated preparations of a drug made by putting the drug into solution and evaporating the excess solvent to a prescribed standard).

   b. *Powders* (drugs ground into a pulverized form).

   c. *Pills* (drugs shaped into forms for swallowing).

   d. *Capsules* (drugs packed within cylindrical gelatin containers).

   e. *Tablets* (drugs compressed into discs).

2. Liquids:

   a. *Fluidextracts* (standard concentrations of a drug (1 ml. = 1 gram), dissolved in the most appropriate fluid).

   b. *Tinctures* (extracts of a drug diluted in alcohol).

   c. *Spirits* (volatile substances dissolved in alcohol).

   d. *Syrups* (drugs suspended in sugar and water).

   e. Elixirs (syrups with alcohol and flavoring).

   f. *Milks* (aqueous suspensions of insoluble drugs).

   g. *Emulsions* (preparations of one liquid distributed in small globules in another).

   h. *Liniments* (preparation of drug in a soft base for external use).

   i. *Lotions* (preparation of drug for external application).

3. Not solids or liquids:

   a. *Ampules* (sealed glass containers for single-dose sterile drugs).

   b. *Vials* (glass containers for multiple-dose sterile drugs, sealed with rubber stopper).

   c. *Suppositories* (drugs mixed with meltable base, usually applied rectally).

   d. *Ointments* (drugs for external application, in semisolid base).

   e. *Lozenges* (drugs suspended in sugared solid base, dissolved orally).

Actions of Drugs (Category 2)

Action:

1. When to use.
2. What to look for after administration.

Sites of Action:

1. Local effects.
2. Systemic effects.

Factors Influencing Drug Actions:

1. Age and condition of the patient.
2. Dosage.
3. Rate of absorption: (from fastest to slowest)

   a. Intravenous (IV).

   b. Endotracheal (ET).

   c. Rectal (not predictable).

   d. Intramuscular (IM) (requires adequate blood flow).

   e. Subcutaneous (SQ or SC) (requires adequate blood flow).

   f. Oral (PO)—(sublingual [SL], intralingual, ingestion).

Drug Actions Defined:

Depression—Decrease of functional activity, often characterized by sadness, dejection, and/or lethargy.

Physiological—Action caused by a drug when given in the concentrations normally present in the body.

Therapeutic—Beneficial action of a drug.

Untoward Reaction—Side effect(s) regarded as harmful.

Irritation—Slight or temporary damage to tissues.

Antagonism—Opposition between the effects of multiple medications.

Cumulative Action—Increased intensity of effect experienced after several doses of a medication.

Tolerance—Progressive lessening of a drug's effect after repeated doses.

Synergism—Combined effect of multiple drugs such that their combined actions are greater than the sum of their individual action.

Potentiation—Enhancement of the effect of one drug by another.

Additive—Progressive increase in drug's effect after repeated doses.

Habituation—A situation in which the effects produced by a drug are necessary to maintain a person's feeling of well-being.

Idiosyncrasy—An abnormal sensitivity to a drug, peculiar to an individual.

Hypersensitivity—Reacting with characteristic symptoms to contact with specific substances (allergy).

Autonomic Nervous System Controls the involuntary (automatic) bodily functions (heartbeat, respirations, digestion) and consists of two separate parts—the *parasympathetic* and the *sympathetic* nervous systems.

Parasympathetic Nervous System (alias the cholinergic nervous system)

1. Responsible primarily for *vegetative functions.*
2. Mediates primarily through the *vagus nerve.*
3. Chief *chemical mediator acetylcholine* (ACh).
4. Chief *parasympathetic* blocker is *atropine*, which can oppose the actions of acetylcholine.

Sympathetic Nervous System (alias the *adrenergic nervous system*)

1. Responsible primarily for *stress response.*
2. Mediates primarily through nerves in the thoracic and lumbar ganglia, and through release of *epinephrine* from the adrenal glands.

3. Chief *chemical mediator* is *norepinephrine.*
4. Chief *sympathetic blocker* is *propranolol* (Inderal), which occupies drug receptor sites and prevents their activation.

Drugs that effect the sympathetic nervous system are classified according to the two receptor sites which with they interact—*alpha* and *beta.* Some drugs have pure alpha or pure beta effects, while some have a combination of both alpha and beta effects:

1. *Alpha* effects:
   a. Heart—none.
   b. Lungs—none (or mild bronchoconstriction).
   c. Arteries—vasoconstriction.
2. *Beta* effects:
   a. Heart—increased rate, force, and automaticity.
   b. Lungs—bronchodilation.
   c. Arteries—vasodilation.

Common Sympathetic Drugs:

1. Isoproterenol (Isuprel)—pure beta.
2. Epinephrine (Adrenalin)—mostly beta (some alpha at higher doses).
3. Norepinephrine (Levophed)—mostly alpha.
4. Dopamine (Intropin)—beta at low doses, alpha at high doses.
5. Metaraminol (Aramine)—mostly alpha.

When studying a drug, examine these characteristics:

1. *Dose* (usual, how to compute, and is dose dependent on patient history).
2. *Dilution* (amount and type of dilutant—strength of the drug).
3. *Action* (how a drug creates its effect).
4. *Indications* (when to properly consider use of the drug).
5. *Precautions* (factors to consider before and during administration).
6. *Contraindications* (under what conditions not to use).
7. *Incompatability* (whether the drug can be mixed without adverse effect).

8. *Side effects* (predictable effects which may occur in addition to expected therapeutic effects).
9. *Antidotes* (to counteract the drugs effects, if available).

Weights and Measures (Category 3)

Apothecary System This system is seldom used anymore by professionals or other countries.

1. *Solids* (grains, drams, ounces, pounds).
2. *Liquids* (minims, fluidrams, ounces, pints, gallons).

Metric System This is a universally accepted system because it is more logical in its construction and is based on decimals for easier computations.

1. *Solids* (weight only):
   a. Microgram (ug) or (mcg) = .001 milligram (1/1,000 mg).
   b. Milligram (mg) = 1,000 micrograms or .001 gram (1/1,000 gm).
   c. Gram (gm) = 1,000 milligrams or 1,000,000 micrograms.
   d. Kilogram (kg) = 1,000 grams.
2. *Liquids* (volume-capacity):
   a. Milliliter (ml) = .001 liter (1/1,000 L).
   b. Liter (L) = 1,000 milliliters.
   c. 1 cubic centimeter (cc = 1 milliliter (ml).

Note: 1 ml of H_2O *weighs* 1 gm and *occupies* 1 cc of volume, thus a cc and ml are considered *equivalent expressions.*

Conversions Often it is necessary to convert from one system to another.

Apothecary to Metric (approximations)

1 minim = .06 ml	1 grain = 60 mg
1 fluidram = 4 ml	1 dram = 4 gm
1 fluidounce = 30 ml	1 ounce = 30 gm
1 pint = 500 ml	1 pound = 500 gm
1 quart = 1 liter (1000 ml)	

Metric to Apothecary (approximations)

1 ml = 15 minims   1 gm = 15 grains

10 ml = 2.5 fluidrams   10 gm = 2.5 drams

100 ml = 3.5 fluidounces   100 gm = 3.3 ounces

1 L (1000 ml) = 1 quart   1 kg (1000 gm) = 2.2 pounds

Administration Sets

1. Macrodrip (regular) infusion set, 15 drops (gtt) = 1 cc (or ml). Check packaging, as some sets have 10 gtt/ml.
2. Microdrip (minidrip) infusion set, 60 drops (gtt) = 1 cc (or ml).

Computing Dosage

$$\frac{\text{Desired dose (in mg)}}{\text{Concentration on hand (mg/ml)}} = \text{ml to be administered}$$

Flow Rate

Drops per minute (gtt/min) = volume to be infused × gtt/ml of administration set.

Drug Administration (Category 4)

Safety Considerations

1. Concentrate on the task.
2. Be sure base physician understands the situation.
3. Be sure base physician's orders are clearly understood.
4. Repeat the orders for confirmation.
5. Read drug labels carefully.
6. Double-check all calculations.
7. Use correct, properly operating equipment.
8. Handle medications carefully (many are packaged in breakable glass).
9. Exercise asceptic procedures.
10. Always be alert for incompatibility problems.

11. Monitor for signs/symptoms of overdose.
12. Always record time of administration and agent(s) involved.

Administration Techniques (Category 5)

1. Syringes—Identify the syringe type and note the measurement scale.
2. Containers (vials, ampules, preloads)—
   a. *Ampules*—After tapping gently to remove any fluid from the necks, grasp both top and bottom firmly (protecting your fingers with a 4 × 4 or wipe) and break cleanly at scored neck. Withdraw contents via needle with syringe, without touching needle against sides of ampule. After withdrawing contents via needle and syringe, deposit in sharps container.
   b. *Vials*—Remove protective cap, wipe rubber stopper with ETOH wipe, insert needle with syringe through rubber stopper, inject amount of air equal to volume being withdrawn, draw up correct amount of fluid and withdraw needle. Dispose of needle/syringe after use.
   c. *Preloads*—Be familiar with the particular brand/type of preload and packaging that you are to use—some of them seem absolutely unworkable at first view. After "popping the tops", screwing halves together and unsheathing the needle, be sure to evacuate any extra air in the fluid before administering (besides, it looks great on the evening news. . .). Dispose of needle/syringe after use.
3. *Parenterel* (other than through digestive tract) administration:
   a. *IV injection:*
      (1) Directly into vein (using asceptic technique).
      (2) Injection to IV tubing (pinch tubing above injection site).
      (3) Adding medication to IV bag (or bottle) (mix and label).
   b. *Subcutaneous injection* (injecting medication into the subcutaneous tissue—use 45 degree angle).
   c. *Intramuscular injection* (injecting medication directly into a muscle—use 90 degree angle).
   d. *Transtracheal [endotracheal] administration* (introducing medication into the bloodstream via the trachea (epinephrine, lidocaine, atropine) spray forcefully down endotracheal tube, then bag vigorously).

FIGURE 12.1. Subcutaneous Injection

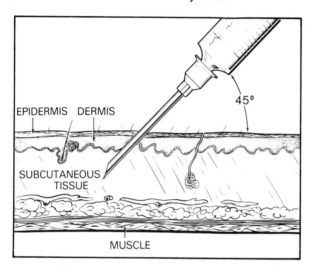

FIGURE 12.2. Intramuscular Injection

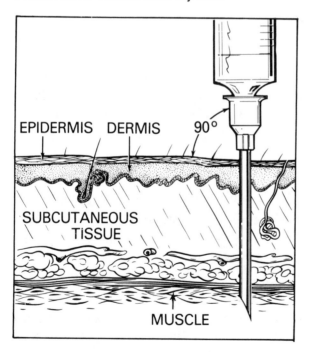

Summary

Paramedics must deal directly with their responsibility to handle and administer drugs. In this chapter we reviewed drug information, actions of drugs, weights and measures, administration of drugs and techniques of administration. Additionally, we presented some pertinent definitions related to pharmacology and the actions of drugs. In the last section of Chapter 16 (Cardiovascular) we offer a section reviewing some of the common drugs paramedics carry and encounter.

SELF-TEST

Chapter 12

1. What is the role of the autonomic nervous system and what are its two divisions?

   ANSWER: The autonomic nervous system controls involuntary body functions. It is divided into the parasympathetic and sympathetic nervous systems.

2. The parasympathetic nervous system is responsible primarily for vegetative functions, and is mediated through the vagus nerve. What is the chief chemical mediator of the parasympathetic nervous system?

   ANSWER: Acetylcholine.

3. The sympathetic nervous system is responsible primarily for stress response, often releasing epinephrine from the adrenal glands. What is the chief chemical mediator of the sympathetic nervous system?

   ANSWER: Norepinephrine.

4. State simply the difference between alpha and beta effects.

   ANSWER: Simply, alpha constricts and beta dilates.

5. What effect does beta stimulation have on the heart, lungs and arteries:

   ANSWER: a. Heart = increases rate, force and automaticity

                b. lungs = bronchodilation

                c. arteries = vasodilation

6. What effect does alpha stimulation have on the arteries?

   ANSWER: vasoconstriction

7. Name a medication that exhibits pure beta effects?

   ANSWER: Isuprel (isoproterenol)

8. Briefly explain the dosage-related effects of Dopamine.

   ANSWER: Dopamine exhibits beta effects at low doses and alpha effects at higher doses.

9. Define the term "tolerance" as it relates to drug actions.

   ANSWER: Tolerance is the progressive lessening of a drug's effect after repeated doses.

10. _____ refers to the enhancement of the effects of one drug by another drug.

    ANSWER: Potentiation

11. Define the term "idiosyncrasy" as it relates to drug actions.

    ANSWER: Idiosyncrasy is an abnormal sensitivity to a drug, peculiar to an individual.

12. There are _____ milligrams in one gram?

    ANSWER: 1,000 (1,000 mg = 1 gram)

13. How many micrograms are in one milligram?

    ANSWER: 1,000 micrograms = 1 milligram

14. A 220 pound (lb) patient weighs _____ kilograms (kg).

    ANSWER: 100 kg. Remember, 1 kg = 2.2 lb

15. How many drops equal 1 milliliter (ml) in standard macrodrip and microdrip infusion sets?

    ANSWER: a. macrodrip = 15 drops/ml (some sets have 10 drops/ml)

    b. microdrip = 60 drops/ml

CHAPTER 13

Trauma

The goal of emergency trauma care is to stabilize the ongoing pathologic process and reverse it as soon as possible. True reversal of significant trauma cannot be started in the field, as this requires oxygen-carrying IV fluids (blood) and (usually) operative correction of the injury. The field paramedic can begin the process by stabilizing the injury and providing rapid transportation to an appropriate facility (where the capabilities of reversal are immediately available). The steps necessary in treating the victims of trauma will include:

1. Assuring scene safety.
2. Providing adequate oxygenation/c-spine control (airway management—with initial in-line stabilization of the cervical spine).
3. Improving perfusion (control of severe bleeding and shock trousers at the scene—IV fluids enroute to the hospital).
4. Extrication from the site of injury.
5. Stabilization of possible fractures (c-collar, long spineboard, PASG if indicated—all other splinting done enroute with critical patients).
6. Immediate rapid transportation (critical patients) to a facility that has the equipment and personnel immediately available to intervene

in the pathological process—*Operating Room* (OR) via *Emergency Department* (ED/ER), then *Intensive Care Unit* (ICU).

Statistics

1. 150,000 trauma deaths per year in the United States (approx.).
2. Leading cause of death in ages 1–44.
3. Third leading cause of death overall.
4. Over 40,000 annual deaths due to motor vehicle accidents (MVAs).

Kinematics of Trauma

Kinematics refers to the examination of a traumatic event and prediction of the injuries that might possibly result from the forces and motion involved.

Newton's First Law of Motion "A body at rest will remain at rest and a body in motion will remain in motion until acted upon by some outside force."

Applicable Law of Physics "Energy can be neither created nor destroyed, but can only be changed in form." Some of the different forms that energy may take may include:

1. Thermal energy;
2. Electrical energy;
3. Chemical energy;
4. Radiant energy;
5. Mechanical energy.

Trauma Damage that results when *kinetic energy* (energy in motion) is transferred to body tissue. Trauma can be classified as either *blunt* or *penetrating.* For example, when an automobile comes to a sudden stop, the kinetic energy represented by the car (mass) in motion (velocity) is transferred to the vehicle and its occupants—and when that energy is absorbed there may be damage to both. There are actually three collisions involved:

FIGURE 13.1.

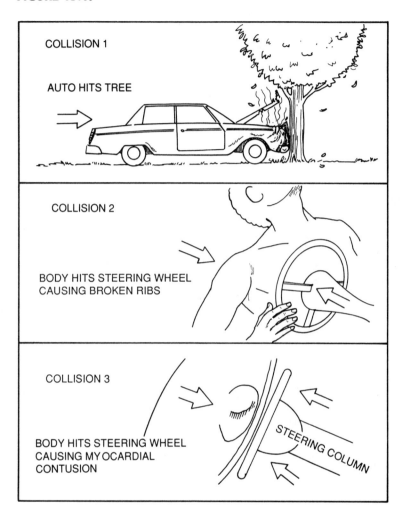

1. The automobile collides with an object;
2. The occupants collide with the inside of the stopped automobile;
3. The organs collide (within occupants).

Each of these collisions may result in damage, and must be considered independently when evaluating the mechanisms of injury for suspected injuries.

Kinetic Energy = One-half the mass times the velocity squared.

$$KE = \frac{M \times V^2}{2} \qquad KE = \frac{180 \times 40 \times 40}{2} \text{ or}$$

$$KE = \frac{288,000}{2} \quad KE = 144,000$$

If M (mass) = 180 lbs

If V (velocity) = 40 mph

Then KE (kinetic energy) = 144,000 units of energy

Blunt Trauma

Blunt trauma produces injuries by *deceleration* and *compression.*

Deceleration Injuries These are caused when the body decelerates and the organs continue forward. Some of the injuries that may occur include:

1. Head—Brain contusions/hematomas/contracoup injuries, brainstem or spinal cord injury at the point of attachment.
2. Thorax—Aorta torn by ligamentum arteriousum (80% mortality within first hour) and in other locations where organs attach.
3. Abdomen—Kidneys, small intestine, large intestine, spleen can all be torn at their points of attachment. The liver can be split in two by the ligamentum teres.

Compression Injuries These are caused when structures or organs are severely crushed or squeezed by compressing forces. Some of the injuries that may occur include:

1. Head—Skull fractures and brain contusions/bleeding/hematomas.
2. Thorax—Fractured ribs (even flail chest), myocardial contusion or rupture (as heart is compressed between sternum and spine), pulmonary contusions, pneumothorax (simple, open, tension), aortic rupture, and so forth.
3. Abdomen—Rupture of bladder, kidneys, pancreas, spleen, liver, and aorta (due to severe compression). Pelvic fractures (potential shock).

Motor Vehicle Accidents In the case of motor vehicle accidents (MVAs), injury patterns produced by these forces are relatively predictable. Because

MVAs comprise the majority of trauma cases seen by paramedics, a look at these injury patterns is in order:

1. Frontal Impact—Causes forward motion (car frame and body disrupted):
   a. Down-and-Under:
      1. Knees impact the dash—knee trauma, femur fractures, and hip dislocations.
      2. Upper body rotates forward into steering wheel or dash:
         a. Compression injuries—ribs, anterior flail chest, pulmonary contusions, ruptured liver or spleen.
         b. Deceleration injuries—torn aorta, lacerated liver.
      3. Head impacts steering wheel or dash:
         a. Hyperflexion/hyperextension—cervical spine injuries.
         b. Compression injuries—vertebral damage, facial bones, skull fractures, crushed larynx, further spinal cord damage.
   b. Up-and-Over:
      1. Chest/abdomen impact steering wheel (compression and deceleration injuries)—ribs, pneumothorax, flail chest, cardiac and pulmonary contusions, aortic tear, lacerated liver, ruptured spleen.
      2. Head impacts windshield—lacerations, skull fractures, cerebral contusions/hemorrhage, massive soft tissues damage. Hyperflexion/hyperextension/compression all cause cervical spine damage.
2. Rear Impact—Energy of impact is transferred as accelerated motion (the car shoots forward). If the headrest is improperly adjusted (or absent), hyperextension of the neck occurs with resultant cervical spine and/or connective tissue damage. If a frontal impact is also involved, look for two sets of injuries.
3. Side Impact (T-Bone)—Car moves out from under occupants (laterally):
   a. Chest impacts door—rib injuries, lateral flail chest, pulmonary contusion, ruptured liver or spleen (liver if right side impact, spleen if left side impact), shoulder injuries.
   b. Pelvis/femur impacts door—pelvis/femur fractures, knee injuries.
   c. Head/neck impacts door or frame—cervical spine fractures/sprains, cord damage, skull fractures, head/face lacerations, brain injuries.

4. Rotational Impact—One part of the vehicle impacts and stops, while the rest of the vehicle continues moving, pivoting around the point of impact. You may see a combination of possible injuries from both frontal and side impacts.

5. Rollover—In a vehicle rollover, multiple impacts may occur (often from several different angles). Obviously, predicting injury is very difficult, yet we know that statistically, rollover injuries are generally more serious. Victims ejected from the car are 300 times more likely to die and 1 out of 3 suffer cervical spine injury.

Seat Restraints These restraints have been proven to decisively minimize injury. Though injuries are sometimes due to seat restraints, they are certainly less severe than those that occur when victims are unrestrained. Seat restraints are most effective when combined with air bags.

Other Blunt Injuries A potpourri of other causes of blunt trauma would include:

1. Falls:
   a. Especially serious when from > 3 times the patient's height.
   b. Force is often transmitted from point of impact to other parts of the body (i.e., land on feet, fracturing both heels and lumbar spine).

FIGURE 13.2.

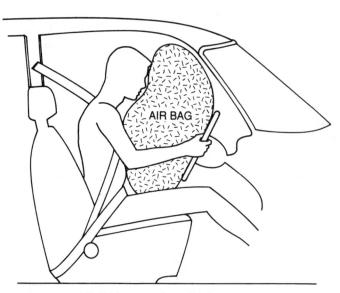

AIR BAG AND 3-POINT RESTRAINT

2. Pedestrian/Auto Accidents:

    a. Usually two impacts—first with car, then with ground or other object.

    b. High incidence of internal injuries and fractures.

    c. Low speed still dangerous because of large mass of automobile.

3. Motorcycle Accidents:

    a. 75% of all motorcycle deaths are due to head injury.

    b. Helmets are very important, but only partially effective.

    c. Victims often impact motorcycle (and/or other vehicle) before being ejected and impacting the ground (or other object).

    d. "Laying the bike down" in the face of impending impact may tend to minimize serious injuries.

4. Bicycle/Skateboard/Scooter Accidents:

    a. Head injuries, fractures and lacerations/abrasions most common.

    b. Helmets and knee/elbow pads provide important protection.

5. Sports Injuries:

    a. Mechanisms: falls, impact with other participants, impact with sports equipment, impact with boundaries of playing fields.

    b. Injuries: fractures, dislocations, sprains/strains, lacerations, contusions, abrasions.

6. Blast Injuries (injury due to three factors):

    a. Primary—caused by pressure wave of explosion. The air blast often injures air-containing organs (lungs, eardrums, stomach, GI tract).

    b. Secondary—caused by impact of debris propelled by blast force.

    c. Tertiary—caused when body is propelled into other objects or the ground (much like being ejected from an automobile or motorcycle).

7. Industrial Accidents:

    a. Mechanisms: Falls, twisting/shearing (caught in machinery), impacts, crushing, blast injuries.

Penetrating Trauma

The most common forms of significant penetrating trauma are knife and gunshot wounds. Other forms of penetrating trauma can be just as serious (such as an object thrown by a lawn mower, lawn darts, industrial fragments, and pneumatic nail guns). The principles of physics discussed earlier bear upon the seriousness of injury caused by penetrating objects. In this equation, velocity is the most important factor that affects kinetic energy.

$$KE = \frac{M \times V^2}{2}$$

KE = Impact (kinetic injury in foot-pounds)
M = Mass of object in pounds
V = Velocity in feet/second

Ballistical Terms

1. Caliber—The internal diameter of the barrel. This number is also usually given to the ammunition suited for the particular weapon. Example: A "38 Special" uses .38 caliber ammunition.
2. Rifling—Spiral grooves inside the barrel of some weapons that causes a bullet to spin, thus stabilizing its flight and increasing accuracy.
3. Cavitation—An area of damage that is produced by pressure waves that form when a bullet passes through body tissue at significant velocity. The tissues stretch and compress violently, causing a much larger cone of destruction than the mere track of the bullet would suggest. The higher the velocity, the larger the area of destruction.
4. Tumble—An end-over-end motion that occurs when a bullet impacts, as the center of gravity of the bullet seeks to become the leading edge. Obviously, more damage will occur if the side of the bullet is slicing through tissue.
5. Fragmentation—When a bullet breaks apart upon impact. Some bullets are designed to fragment, while others tend to fragment only when striking bone.
6. Profile Modification—Usually refers to the design of a bullet that will cause it to change shape upon impact. Example: Hollow-point bullets expand to a "mushroom" shape upon impact thereby increasing the area of contact (and damage) as they pass through tissue.

Classification by Energy Level Penetrating trauma can be classified as low, medium, or high energy depending upon the velocity of the penetrating object:

1. Low Energy—Low energy levels produce injury via sharp cutting edges, with very little secondary trauma. Example: A stab wound with a knife.

FIGURE 13.3.

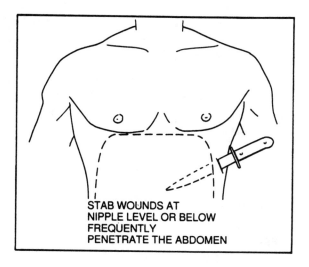

STAB WOUNDS AT
NIPPLE LEVEL OR BELOW
FREQUENTLY
PENETRATE THE ABDOMEN

FIGURE 13.4.

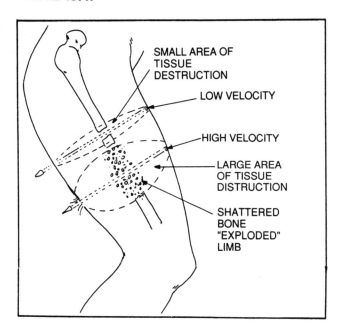

SMALL AREA OF
TISSUE
DESTRUCTION

LOW VELOCITY

HIGH VELOCITY

LARGE AREA
OF TISSUE
DISTRUCTION

SHATTERED
BONE
"EXPLODED"
LIMB

2. Medium Energy (muzzle velocity of < 1,500 feet per second)—Medium energy levels produce injury via cutting edges and cavitation (pressure waves that form around a missile and cause stretching and compression of tissues). The area of damage from cavitation may be 2-3 times the diameter of the penetrating medium velocity object. Example: A gunshot wound from a .38 Special.

3. High Energy (muzzle velocity > 1,500 feet per second)—High energy levels produce injury via the path of a penetrating object and cavitation, but the area of cavitation (and its injury) is much greater than with medium velocity projectiles. Example: A gunshot wound from a M-16 or AR-15.

Assessment and Management of Trauma Victims

Assessment and management of trauma victims is directed toward rapid recognition of life-threatening injuries, prioritized intervention, minimal "on-scene" times and rapid transport of critical patients to the emergency department/operating room.

Critical Injuries/Situations These situations require immediate rapid transport to the emergency department or operating room. These would include:

1. Severe respiratory difficulty:
   a. Airway obstruction (unrelieved by intervention);
   b. Sucking chest wound (open pneumothorax);
   c. Large flail chest;
   d. Tension pneumothorax;
   e. Major blunt chest injury.
2. Shock:
   a. Internal bleeding;
   b. Massive blood loss;
   c. Traumatic cardiopulmonary arrest (trauma code).
3. Decreased level of consciousness (LOC):
   a. Due to head injury (any of these):
      1. Unresponsive or responsive only to pain;

2. Unequal pupils;

3. Decreasing level of consciousness.

b. Due to shock or hypoxia.

Those who are not critical trauma patients (90-95%) may be more carefully evaluated and treated prior to transport to a medical facility. Assessing trauma patients should methodically include:

Scene Size-Up

Primary Survey

Vital Signs

Transport Decision:

  Critical = RAPID TRANSPORT

  Non-Critical = Continue Survey

Secondary Survey

Scene Size-Up

When you first arrive at the scene of a trauma event, there are three factors to be quickly evaluated:

1. Scene safety;

2. Mechanisms of injury; and

3. Number and severity of patients.

Primary Survey

When a patient has been safely accessed, the goal of a primary survey is to identify and treat life-threatening conditions. The A-B-C-D-E method provides a methodical approach:

A = Airway/C-Spine

B = Breathing

C = Circulation

D = Disability

E = Expose

1. Airway/C-Spine—Evaluate the airway. It is of primary importance that cervical spine immobility be maintained at all times in the trauma patient. If it is open and patent, move to the next step while protecting the cervical spine. If it is not open or patent, use one of the following methods to open and maintain the airway:

   a. Chin lift.

   b. Jaw lift.

   c. Jaw thrust.

   d. Mechanical airway (manual in-line c-spine immobilization must be maintained during insertion of *any* airway in trauma victims):

      1. Oropharyngeal airway.

      2. Nasopharyngeal airway.

      3. Needle cricothyroidotomy (in the presence of unrelieved complete airway obstruction).

2. Breathing—If the patient is breathing, note the following and move on to the next step:

   a. Labored?

   b. Fast or slow?

   c. Shallow or deep?

   d. Irregular?

   If the patient is not breathing, begin ventilations by one of the following methods:

   a. Mouth-to-Mouth—This method provides the benefit of immediate ventilation with high volume and a feel for lung compliance. It does not provide supplemental oxygen and can result in exposure to communicable diseases.

   b. Pocket Mask—The mask seals easily, ventilation is provided by the lungs of the rescuer—still with high potential volumes and a good feel for lung compliance. Most models have a one-way valve (to protect the rescuer) and oxygen port to allow relatively high concentrations of supplemental oxygen (60-80%).

   c. Bag-Valve-Mask—Allows moderate feel of lung compliance, low to moderate ventilation volumes, visualization of chest rise and high concentrations of supplemental oxygen (when properly equipped). This method is useless if a good mask seal is not maintained.

    d. Demand Valve/Mask—Allows high ventilation volumes of 100% oxygen when good mask seal is maintained, but must be utilized only by experienced rescuers. Lung compliance cannot be felt and lung damage from the pressures involved is a possibility. This method is contraindicated for pediatric and elderly patients.

3. Circulation—The neck can provide many vital clues to patient status within just a few seconds. Check:

    a. Carotid pulse. *If not present, begin cardiac compressions.* If present, note these qualities:

        1. Fast/slow.

        2. Strong/weak.

        3. Regular/irregular.

    b. Radial pulse (can be done while checking carotid). If present, it suggests that some tissue perfusion is still occurring, and that the systolic blood pressure is at least 80. If absent, suggests a lack of tissue perfusion (shock) and a systolic blood pressure less than 80.

    c. Capillary refill (CR). This can be easily noted when removing your fingers from checking the carotid pulse. Note the time it takes for the finger marks to return to normal color. This is an extremely important finding. If CR is:

    < 2 seconds = normal (TISSUE PERFUSION ADEQUATE)

    2-4 seconds = delayed (SHOCKY)

    > 4 seconds = absent, or profoundly delayed (PROFOUND SHOCK)

    d. Skin color/temperature/dryness. Can easily be done right at the neck, while checking pulse.

    e. Other pertinent findings:

        1. Swelling/lacerations/contusions/abrasions = TRAUMA.

        2. Subcutaneous emphysema = LARYNGEAL TRAUMA or PNEUMOTHORAX.

        3. Presence of JVD (jugular vein distension) = PERICARDIAL TAMPONADE or TENSION PNEUMOTHORAX (when combined with other signs/symptoms).

        4. Presence of tracheal shift = TENSION PNEUMOTHORAX.

Direct pressure should be applied to any active site of significant external bleeding with gloved hands until a pressure dressing can be applied. Some arterial bleeds will require direct hand pressure until arrival at the hospital. PASG (shock trousers) are useful in:

   a. Managing external bleeding below the umbilicus.

   b. Splinting the pelvis and lower extremities.

   c. Maintaining blood pressure in hypovolemic shock.

4. Disability—A simple check of the level of consciousness (LOC), using the A-V-P-U scale:

   A = ALERT

   V = responds to VERBAL stimuli

   P = responds to PAINFUL stimuli

   U = UNRESPONSIVE

5. Expose—It is essential to expose the chest of potentially critical trauma victims. Certain life-threatening conditions must be ruled out, and visualization/palpation/auscultation are necessary components of this procedure.
   LOOK for:

   a. Equal and adequate chest rise.

   b. Abrasions/punctures/lacerations/contusions.

   FEEL for:

   a. Symmetry.

   b. Fractures, unstable (flail) segments, tenderness.

   LISTEN bilaterally for:

   a. Air exchange.

   b. Rales (moist crackles), rhonchi, wheezing, hyperresonance.

   c. Absence of sounds on one or both sides.

Vital Signs

Should be taken immediately following the primary survey. A critical patient will be evident before this measurement, but the added information from quick measurement can be useful. This step may be justifiably delayed in some cases until rapid transport has begun.

Transport Decision

At this point in the assessment there should be enough information to categorize the trauma victim as *critical* or *non-critical*:

1. Critical Patient = IMMEDIATE RAPID TRANSPORT! pausing only for airway intervention, c-collar, quick extrication onto a long spine-board and application of PASG (shock trousers) if indicated. Other definitive care should be performed while enroute to the hospital. **Note:** ANY TRAUMA VICTIM who presents with a BP of < 90 systolic, pulse > 100, and a capillary refill time of > 2 seconds will require:
   a. O_2 supplement.
   b. PASG.
   c. Immediate rapid transport to the appropriate medical facility.
   d. 2 large bore IVs of lactated ringers (started enroute—NEVER DELAY TRANSPORT FOR THESE IVS).
2. Non-Critical Patient = Continue evaluation at the scene with the secondary survey.

Secondary Survey

The secondary survey is a head-to-toe examination designed to uncover other injuries. Non-critical patients will undergo this exam at the scene, while critical patients receive their secondary survey enroute to the hospital, if at all. Most clothing should be removed to perform this survey (ALL CLOTHING in serious patients). Common sense should dictate what may be left on while still in the public eye, but never sacrifice an adequate examination of the patient because of modesty. This has proved to be a fatal error for some patients and an inexcusable one for trained paramedics. The steps of the secondary survey include:

History

Mechanisms of Injury
A-M-P-L-E History

Head-to-Toe Exam

Head

Neck

Chest

Abdomen

Pelvis

Extremities

Back

Neurological Exam

Pupils .

Eye Opening

Verbal

Motor

Sensory

1. *History*—This can be obtained from the patient, bystanders, medic alert
   tags, witnesses, the family, police/fire/rescue personnel and observations of the paramedic. When working as a team, one EMT/EMT-P
   can elicit some points of history at the same time the other EMT/
   EMT-P is performing the secondary survey.
   a. *Mechanisms of Injury*—MVA (head-on, T-bone, rotational, rollover),
      fall, assault, gunshot, cutting, and so on.
   b. *A-M-P-L-E History:*
      A = Allergies (especially to medications)
      M = Medications (used by patient—include over the counter meds)
      P = Past medical history (significant illnesses, trauma, operations)
      L = Last oral intake (when, what and how much)
      E = Events preceding the injury
      Note: This data is subjective and can only be provided by the patient
         and/or significant others. With trauma patients, this informa-
         tion may not be readily available.
2. *Head-To-Toe Exam*—This assessment should be thorough but timely. The areas to be assessed are the:

a. *Head*—Check skull for depressions/deformities, scalp lacerations, impaled objects, hematomas, intact facial bones and mandible. Check pupils and re-check the airway. Note any blood or fluid from the ears and nose, "raccoons eyes" or Battles sign (bruising behind the ears). If there seems to be significant head injury in the presence of decreased level of consciousness—hyperventilate.

b. *Neck*—Check the carotid pulse, capillary refill, JVD, skin color/temperature/dryness. Note any tracheal deviation, JVD, subcutaneous emphysema, soft tissue injury or use of accessory muscles in respiration.

c. *Chest*—Check for equal chest rise, symmetry, flail segments, open wounds, paradoxical respirations, lacerations/punctures/abrasions/contusions, impaled objects (do not remove), presence and equality of bilateral breath sounds, tenderness and use of accessory muscles in respiration. Here are some of the traumatic chest problems you must be ready to identify:

(1) *Pneumothorax* (simple)—A defect in the pleura allows air into the pleural space, destroying the vacuum that normally causes the pleura to expand the lungs by following expansion of the ribs during inspiration. The lung collapses, presenting as pain and respiratory distress. Management is directed toward high-flow oxygen and supporting ventilations with positive pressure. This condition will sometimes progress to a tension pneumothorax.

(2) *Sucking Chest Wound* (open pneumothorax)—A defect in the external chest wall and the pleura, with air flowing directly in and out of the thorax. The normal mechanism for ventilation of the lungs (the creation of negative pressure in the thorax) is destroyed (directly proportional to the size of the hole). Management is directed toward covering the opening with an airtight seal (non-porous material). These injuries are life-threatening, and sometimes develop into a tension pneumothorax after successful initial treatment.

(3) *Tension Pneumothorax*—Air under compression on the injured side pushes against the good lung (inhibiting its function and decreasing ventilations) and the heart (inhibiting its pumping action and decreasing cardiac output). In the late stages, the trachea may deviate away from the injury and JVD (jugular vein distension) may be evident. If the patient has suffered

FIGURE 13.5. Open Pneumothorax

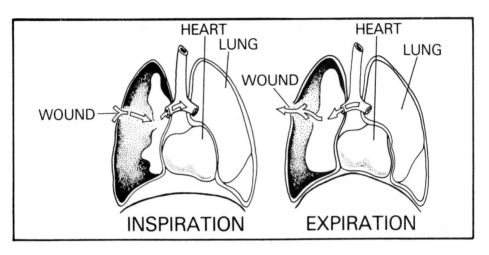

significant blood loss, there may be no JVD. Management is directed toward relieving thoracic pressure on the affected side by needle decompression in the second or third anterior intercostal space in the mid-clavicular line, supporting ventilations and high-flow oxygen. The needle decompression reduces the injury to a simple pneumothorax and vital signs should improve rapidly.

(4) *Hemothorax*—Blood loss into the pleural space, causing partial or total lung collapse. Essentially the same as a simple pneumothorax, except that blood (instead of air) enters the pleural space. Management is directed toward fluid volume replacement, supporting ventilations with positive pressure, and high-flow oxygen. More severe cases (with massive bleeding)

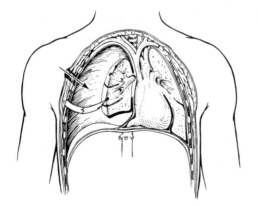

FIGURE 13.6. Tension Pneumothorax

may require chest decompression to remove blood under pressure.

(5) *Pulmonary Contusion*—Blood and swelling from bruised lung inhibits the exchange of gases in the alveoli at the affected location. Use high-flow oxygen.

(6) *Pericardial Tamponade*—Myocardial bleeding into pericardial sac causing a dcrease in cardiac refilling and a reduction in cardiac output. This presents with paradoxical pulses, narrowing pulse pressure, muffled heart sounds, distended neck veins (JVD) and hypotension. Management is directed toward high-flow oxygen, PASG (shock trousers) and fluid challenge enroute, but definitive treatment (subxiphoid pericardiocentesis) is usually reserved for the hospital.

(7) *Myocardial Contusion*—This injury, essentially a bruised heart, is very similar to an *acute myocardial infarction* (AMI). You may see cardiogenic shock, chest pain and dysrhythmias (such as multiple PVC's, atrial fibrillation, bundle branch blocks). Management is directed toward treating cardiac dysrhythmias (with drug therapy) and high-flow oxygen.

(8) *Flail Chest*—Three or more consecutive ribs, broken in at least two places, creating an unstable segment of the chest wall (and inhibiting normal ventilation). Presents with paradoxical respirations, pain, crepitus and severe respiratory difficulty.

FIGURE 13.7. Flail Chest

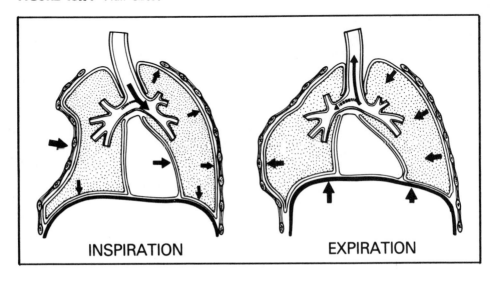

INSPIRATION   EXPIRATION

Management is directed toward stabilizing the flail segment, supporting ventilations with positive pressure and high-flow oxygen.

d. *Abdomen*—Palpate for tenderness, "guarding", rigidity, distension, and pulsating masses. Note any discoloration, impaled objects (do not remove) and lacerations/punctures/abrasions/contusions.

   Note: Shock vital signs—systolic BP < 90, poor capillary refill and pulse > 100—in the presence of abdominal tenderness and/or distension should be considered internal bleeding until proven otherwise. Internal bleeding can be life-threatening, so upgrade to rapid transport if it is strongly suspected.

e. *Pelvis*—Scan for soft tissue injuries. Palpate for stability ("grating", movement, deformity), pain and tenderness.

   Note: Pelvic fractures can be life-threatening, so upgrade to rapid transport if one is strongly suspected.

f. *Extremities*—Should be checked for fractures, dislocations, soft tissue injuries, strains/sprains, bleeding sites, peripheral pulses, sensation, movement, temperature, color and grip strength (hands).

   Note: Bilateral femur fractures can be life-threatening, so upgrade to rapid transport if present.

g. *Back*—If other injuries make it unwise to turn a patient, delay visualization of the back. Try to palpate the back as much as possible by sliding your hands along both sides. If log-rolling a patient for placement on long spineboard, use that opportunity to check the back for deformity, soft tissue injuries, bleeding, and so on.

3. *Neurological Exam*—This needs to be performed to determine the level of consciousness and possible neurological damage. TREAT ANY SUSPECTED SIGNIFICANT HEAD INJURY WITH HYPERVENTILATION AND HIGH-FLOW OXYGEN.

   Include the following checks:

   a. Re-check of the A-V-P-U level of consciousness status.

   b. *Pupils*—Check equality, size, shape, and response to light. Unequal pupils in an unconscious trauma patient are a very significant finding.

   c. *Eye Opening*—Note the level of stimulus required to cause the patient's eyes to open.

   d. *Verbal Response*—If the patient can talk, determine if his responses are appropriate or inappropriate. Note any slurring, expressive aphasia (difficulty speaking), snoring, etc.

e. *Sensory*—If awake, determine if the patient can feel your touch on fingers and toes. If unconscious, does the victim react to progressively more painful stimuli? If so, in what way (flexion, extension, withdrawal, localization)?

f. *Motor*—Determine if the patient can move any extremities (such as fingers and toes). If any patient movement can be elicited, note whether it is purposeful or non-purposeful?

g. *Glasgow Coma Scale* (optional)—Measures level of consciousness after assessing:

(1) Eye opening.

(2) Best motor response.

(3) Best verbal response.

h. *Champion Trauma Score* (optional)—Includes the value from the Glasgow Coma to figure its rating after assessing:

(1) Respiratory rate.

(2) Respiratory expansion.

(3) Systolic blood pressure.

(4) Capillary return.

It then predicts the survivability of trauma patients based upon similar statistical assessments.

Splinting

Critical Patients These patients should receive a cervical collar, be placed on a long spineboard (and immobilized), and be rapidly transported to the closest appropriate facility. When indicated, application of the PASG (shock trousers) provides additional stabilization AND MAY BE APPLIED QUICKLY AT THE SCENE OR ENROUTE. Any further splinting should be done in the ambulance enroute as time and management priorities permit.

Non-Critical Patients All fractures should be splinted before transport. Severely angulated fractures that *do not* involve joints should generally be straightened before splinting (unless significant resistance is encountered). Fractures/dislocations of and near joints should be splinted in the position found, unless there is an absence of distal pulse and ETA to hospital of over 30 minutes. In that case, careful straightening may be attempted, but if any resistance is encountered, straightening should be abandoned and the extremity splinted as found. Remember to:

1. Completely visualize the part of the body to be splinted.
2. Check distal pulse and sensation before and after splint is applied.
3. Immobilize one joint above and below the injury.
4. Pad the splint as necessary.

Transportation

Smooth RAPID TRANSPORT (lights and siren) is in order for critical patients as soon as they are loaded and strapped. Non-critical patients receive more treatment on the scene and merit average speeds within the legal limits. It is imperative that critical trauma patients be sent to facilities that have the immediate means to stabilize and reverse the pathological process of shock (blood replacement and surgical repair).

Communications

At the earliest opportunity, the receiving facility should be contacted with a clear summary of patient injuries and a recommendation to prepare for a critical trauma patient. In many areas, this is called *trauma team activation*. (The status of non-critical patients should also be communicated to the receiving hospital, but without any recommendation for a heightened response.)

Triage

Though most paramedics are not likely to confront *mass casualty incidents* (MCIs) with large numbers of victims (50 or more) in their careers, many will deal with smaller MCIs (10–20 victims, or even 2–10 victims) at some point. Most MCIs will be the result of trauma. Examples would include the following scenes:

1. Airplane crash.
2. Building/structure collapse.
3. Mass freeway trauma.
4. Explosion/fire.
5. Tornado, earthquake, or flood.
6. Automatic weapon fire into a crowd.
7. Bus crash.
8. Train derailment/crash.

When confronted with more than one victim per trained rescuer, how do EMT-Ps decide who is to be treated first? *Triage* is the process of sorting the victims into prioritized treatment categories with the aim of saving the greatest number of lives possible. Critical (but salvageable) victims are treated and transported first, severely injured (but non-critical) victims next, and victims with minor injuries (and the dead or mortally injured) last. Every agency has its own triage system, but the following is generic to many triage schemes:

1. IMMEDIATE—Critical patients requiring immediate intervention (within minutes) and transport for survival. These patients would exhibit:
   a. Airway problems (and severe respiratory distress).
   b. Significant chest injuries (especially with associated severe respiratory distress).
   c. Existing shock, signs of internal bleeding (such as tender distended abdomen) or severe external bleeding.
   d. Decreased and/or decreasing level of consciousness (due to head injury, shock, or hypoxia).
2. URGENT—Severely injured patients that will not die within 1-2 hours:
   a. Major or multiple fractures.
   b. Chest and abdominal injuries with stable vital signs (and no significant respiratory distress).
   c. Major burns.
   d. Significant obvious spinal injuries.
3. DELAYED—Patients whose injuries are relatively minor and who will survive without rapid intervention:

a. Minor fractures.

b. Lacerations and other soft tissue injuries.

c. Suspected spinal injuries.

d. Sprains, strains, and dislocations without circulation compromise.

e. Minor and moderate burns.

f. Other minor injuries and symptoms.

The DELAYED category also includes DOAs, full cardiac arrest (in the presence of other IMMEDIATE patients), and non-salvageable mortal injuries (such as through-and-through gunshot wound to the head with no neurological function). Time, personnel, and resources spent on these kinds of patients may well result in the death of salvageable patients.

Summary

Time is the enemy of the critical trauma victim. Effective prehospital assessment and treatment of trauma requires paramedics to differentiate between critical and non-critical trauma patients. Critical patients are quickly treated for shock and hypoxemia and immediately transported to an appropriate center for acute trauma care. Non-critical patients receive further systematic evaluation and treatment before transport and do not require the specialized care of a trauma center. Understanding the pathology and kinetics of trauma lead to a clearer awareness of the assessment and treatment priorities demanded by trauma victims.

SELF-TEST

Chapter 13

1. TRUE or FALSE. Less than half of all motor vehicle accident fatalities are alcohol-related.

   ANSWER: FALSE—*more* than half of all MVA fatalities are alcohol-related.

2. TRUE or FALSE. True reversal of significant trauma cannot be started in the field, as this requires oxygen-carrying IV fluids (blood) and (usually) operative correction of the injury.

   ANSWER: TRUE

3. Energy in motion is referred to as _____ energy.
   ANSWER: kinetic

4. Blunt trauma produces injuries by deceleration and _____ .
   ANSWER: compression

5. The study of a traumatic event to predict the injuries that may occur is called _____ .
   ANSWER: kinematics

6. TRUE or FALSE. Trauma is the leading cause of death in ages 1-44 in the United States.
   ANSWER: TRUE

7. Motor vehicle accidents produce a variety of injury patterns that are relatively predictable when the force and direction of impact can be determined. Name some of the directions of impact seen in MVAs.
   ANSWER: a. frontal impact   d. rotational impact
                    b. rear impact   e. rollover
                    c. side impact
                       (t-bone)

8. The most common forms of significant penetrating trauma are _____ and gunshot wounds.
   ANSWER: knife

9. _____ refers to an area of damage produced by pressure waves formed when a bullet passes through body tissue at significant velocity.
   a. Fragmentation
   b. Tumble
   c. Profile modification
   d. Cavitation

10. When determining kinetic energy, which is more significant; mass or velocity?
    ANSWER: Velocity

11. Critical trauma victims require immediate transport. Name three categories of trauma patients that might fit this description.
    ANSWER: a. severe respiratory distress
                     b. shock
                     c. decreased level of consciousness

12. What do the initials A-B-C-D-E in the trauma primary survey stand for?

    ANSWER: A = airway/c-spine

    B = breathing

    C = circulation

    D = disability (LOC)

    E = expose (the chest)

13. Name at least two ways to check perfusion without measuring the blood pressure.

    ANSWER: a. check a radial pulse

    b. check for capillary refill (CR)

    c. determine the level of consciousness

14. Name some of the things that must be checked once the chest of a trauma patient has been exposed.

    ANSWER: a. equal and adequate chest rise

    b. punctures/lacerations/abrasions/contusions

    c. bilateral lung sounds

    d. chest wall for fractures, flail segments, pain, tenderness

    e. use of accessory muscles

15. TRUE or FALSE. Critical trauma patients need 2 large-bore IV's in place before beginning transport.

    ANSWER: FALSE—transport of a critical trauma patient should *never* be delayed for placement of IVs.

16. Any trauma victim who presents with a BP of less than 90 systolic, pulse more than 100 and a capillary refill time of more than 2 seconds will require:

    a. supplemental oxygen

    b. PASG (shock trousers)

    c. immediate rapid transport

    d. 2 large-bore IVs enroute

    e c-collar and longboard (if needed)

    f. all of the above

    ANSWER: f. all of the above

17. Name at least three signs of a tension pneumothorax.

    ANSWER: a. severe dyspnea

    b. jugular vein distension (JVD)

     c. absent breath sounds on one side

     d. tracheal deviation (away from injured side)

     e. deteriorating vital signs

18. Blood loss into the pleural space is referred to as a _____ .

ANSWER: hemothorax

19. Blood and swelling from a bruised lung inhibits the exchange of gases in the alveoli at the affected location. This injury is technically called a _____ _____ .

ANSWER: pulmonary contusion

20. Myocardial bleeding into the pericardial sac can decrease filling of the ventricles and cardiac output. This is called _____ _____ .

ANSWER: pericardial tamponade

21. What traumatic injury to the heart mimics an acute myocardial infarction?

ANSWER: Myocardial contusion

22. Describe a "flail chest."

ANSWER: A flail chest means that three or more consecutive ribs are broken in two or more places, creating an unstable segment of chest wall interfering with the mechanics of ventilation.

23. List some signs of internal abdominal injury.

ANSWER: Tenderness, pain, "guarding", rigidity, distension, discoloration, abrasions/lacerations/contusions/punctures, or pulsating masses

24. How much splinting should a critical trauma patient receive?

ANSWER: Cervical collar, long spineboard, and PASG, if indicated.

25. Assuming that extensive extrication is not required, how long should be spent on the scene with a critical trauma patient?

ANSWER: Not more than 10 minutes—but as little time as possible.

26. Sorting multiple victims into prioritized treatment categories is called _____ . What is the goal of this process?

ANSWER: triage. The goal is to save the greatest number of lives possible

Burns

Burns account for a significant number of deaths and disability in this country. In this chapter we provide an overview of burn sources, evaluation of burn severity and extent, and priorities of prehospital treatment. The magnitude of burn injuries can be reduced by aggressively extinguishing the burn process, providing appropriate life support, treating the whole patient (not just the burns) and transportation to an appropriate medical facility.

Definitions

Epidermis—The outer layer of the skin, made of hardened non-living cells.

Dermis—The elastic inner layer of the skin—location of hair roots, glands, blood vessels and nerves.

Subcutaneous Tissue—Fatty layer beneath the dermis.

Fascia—Thin layer of tissue that covers the muscles.

Carbon Monoxide—Poisonous gas produced by burning materials. It is odorless and colorless, and binds rapidly to red blood cells, making them unable to carry oxygen.

A/C Current—Alternating current (may cause victim to prolong contact).

D/C Current—Direct current.

Insulator—Substance that prevents an electrical circuit from completing.

Conductor—Substance that allows current to flow through it.

Melanin—Pigment in the skin that protects against solar radiation.

Radioactivity—Spontaneous release of energy by atomic particles.

Alpha Radiation—Ionizing radiation of very low energy—can be stopped by paper, clothing, a few inches of air.

Beta Radiation—Ionizing radiation of relatively low energy—can be stopped by heavy clothing, glass, thin metal shielding.

Gamma Radiation—Similar to x-rays, gamma rays can easily penetrate the body and cause cellular damage. Lead shielding or thick concrete can effectively shield against gamma rays.

Roentgens—Units of measurement for determining gamma radiation levels.

Curies—Units of measurement for determining beta radiation levels.

Burn Sources

Thermal Thermal burns are the most common type of burns (12,000 die annually in fires). They are caused by radiation and conduction of heat via:

1. Hot liquid;
2. Hot solid;
3. Hot gas;
4. Direct flame.

Electrical Electrical burns are caused by electric current. The extent of an electrical injury is related to the intensity of current and the duration of exposure. Generally, damage to tissues is much more extensive than indicated by exterior burns.

1. *Contact*—Burns caused when tissue comes in contact with electrical current—usually an entrance and exit burn (current is more intense

at these locations), while damage can be extensive in structures between.

2. *Flash*—Burns caused when tissue is close to an electrical flash.
3. *Arcing*—Injuries received when electrical current jumps from surface to surface.
4. *Lightning*—Injuries received when the body is hit by lightning. Though superficial burns are often present, other systems (such as the nervous system and cardiac conduction systems) are often involved.

Chemical Chemical burns are caused when tissue contacts strong acids, alkalis, or other corrosives. The burn process continues as long as contact is maintained.

Radiation Radiation burns are caused by solar (sunburn) or nuclear (ionizing) radiation.

1. *Solar*—Ionizing radiation from atomic reactions on the sun that makes it past Earth's protective ozone layer and can burn skin tissue.
2. *Nuclear*—Ionizing radiation can cause significant internal (cellular) injury. Severity of contact depends upon type of radiation, strength of radiating source, distance from source, length of exposure and type of shielding available.

Burn Classifications

First Degree First degree burns involve a loss of epidermis, a redness of the skin, and pain. This type of burn should heal in 3-7 days.

Second Degree Second degree burns involve damage into the dermis with blistering of the skin and pain. The healing time is 6-14 days. *Deep* second degree burns can require skin grafts and usually heal in 14-21 days. These are usually painful, but sometimes nerve damage is deep enough to block pain impulses.

Third degree Third degree burns involve a total loss of the epidermis and dermis. They are painless due to the destruction of nerve endings. Skin grafting is required.

FIGURE 14.1.

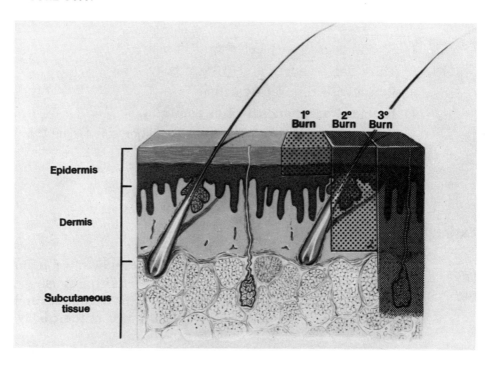

Burn Severity

Minor Burns
Minor burns include:

1. Second degree burns involving < 15% of body in adults and < 10% in children.
2. Third degree burns of < 2% of body.
3. First degree burns of < 20% of body excluding hands, feet, or face.

Moderate Burns
Moderate burns include:

1. Second degree burns of 15-30% of body, excluding hands, feet or face and 10-20% in children.
2. Third degree burns involving 2-10% of body.

Critical Burns

Critical burns include:

1. Second degree burns of > 30% of body.

2. Third degree burns of > 10% of body.

3. Burns with respiratory deficit.

4. Burns of face, hands, feet or genitalia.

5. Burns associated with fractures or major soft tissue trauma.

6. Electrical and deep acid burns.

7. Burns in the compromised patient.

Estimating The Extent of Burns

An easy way to estimate the extent of the body involved in burns is the *rule of nines,* which divides the body into sectors (most using a multiple of nine). The rule of nines is slightly different for infants and toddlers, who have a larger head in relation to the rest of their body.

Rule of Nines: (Adults)		Rule of Nines: (Kids)	
Head	9%	Head	18%
Arms (9% each)	18%	Arms (9% each)	18%
Chest and Abdomen	18%	Chest and Abdomen	18%
Back and Buttocks	18%	Back and Buttocks	18%
Legs (18% each)	36%	Legs (13.5% each)	27%
Genitalia	1%	Genitalia	1%
Total	100%	Total	100%

Management of Thermal Burns

To manage thermal burns:

1. Remove from the source of the burn.

   a. Cool the burn if < 10 minutes from contact and be sure clothing is entirely extinguished. Caution: It is easy to overcool the body and precipitate hypothermia.

   b. Remove any jewelry (and expect swelling).

2. Assure a patent airway, breathing, and circulation. Be prepared to utilize ET or EOA—edema develops swiftly and can fully occlude airway.

3. Assess level of consciousness.

4. Administer oxygen (assist ventilations if needed).

5. Secondary assessment.

6. Monitor ECG.

7. IV of LR or NS. There are several formulas available to compute the proper rate and volume of fluid administration. Be sure to place in an unburned site, if available.

8. Dress burns with dry sterile dressings.

9. Consider analgesics, but only if they can be given IV.

Management of Electrical Burns

To manage electrical burns:

1. Disengage the source—remove patient from the source of injury, if this can be done safely.

   a. Initiate cooling if seen within 30 minutes of event.

   b. Extinguish and remove clothing and jewelry.

   c. Do not overcool. Maintain core temperature.

2. Secure airway, breathing and circulation (use airway adjuncts as needed).

3. Assess level of consciousness.

4. Administer oxygen (assist ventilations if needed).

5. Secondary assessment.

6. Look for entrance and exit wound.

7. Carefully monitor ECG.

8. Iv of LR or NS. Utilize an unburned site if available—you may have to be creative. Fluid therapy and/or medication route is very important.

9. Dress burns with dry sterile dressings. (NO OINTMENTS OR GOOS)

10. Consider pain medication, such as morphine sulphate (2-10 mg IV), but watch for respiratory depression.

11. Treat for other injuries. Don't be mesmerized by the burn.

Management of Chemical Burns

1. Remove victim from the source of the burn, while avoiding contamination. The type of chemical must be identified as soon as possible.
2. Extinguish the burning process. Brush any excess agent from skin and clothing before flushing with water.
   b. Wet chemicals need to be flushed with large amounts of water and clothes removed.
   c. Some acids may contraindicate irrigation with water (i.e., sulfuric, hydrochloric, and muriatic acid).
   d. Special agents may require special techniques.
3. If chemicals involve the eye(s):
   a. Remove contact lens.
   b. Flush with H_2O for 10 minutes and cover both eyes with sterile dressing.
4. Secure airway, breathing, and circulation (if not already done).
5. Assess level of consciousness.
6. Administer oxygen (use airway adjuncts and assist ventilations if needed).
7. Monitor ECG.
8. If chemical has been ingested, determine the advisability of stimulating emesis before beginning the procedure.
9. IV of LR or NS.
10. Cover burn area with dry sterile dressings.
11. Consider pain medication such as morphine sulphate, but watch for respiratory depression.
12. Find and treat other injuries—don't be distracted by the burn.

Inhalation Injuries

Inhalation injuries often result from fires and flame in confined spaces, explosions, breathing toxic fumes, chemical vapors and super-heated steam. Upper airway edema can cause airway obstruction or compromise. There may be loss of surfactant (the chemical that helps keep the alveoli from collapsing) with resultant alveolar collapse and decrease in lung and tidal volumes.

Signs and Symptoms
The signs and symptoms of inhalation injuries include:

1. Visible signs:
   a. Singed nasal hairs;
   b. Facial burns;
   c. Blistering around lips and mouth;
   d. Soot on tongue, around mouth and nose, or in pharynx;
   e. Labored rapid breathing.
2. Symptoms:
   a. Restlessness, anxiety and confusion;
   b. Dyspnea.
3. Breath sounds:
   a. Rales (very significant);
   b. Clear initially—then abnormalities may develop;
   c. Stridor (may indicate a rapidly closing airway from swelling).

FIGURE 14.1.

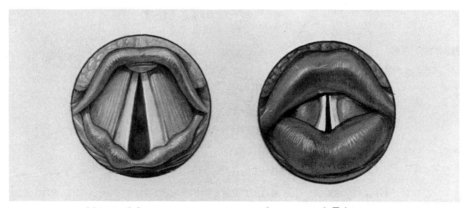

Normal Larynx   Laryngeal Edema

Prehospital Management:
Prehospital management for inhalation injuries should include the following steps:

1. Maintain open airway and administer high-flow hymidified oxygen;
2. Encourage coughing and deep-breathing;
3. Ventilatory assistance with adjuncts if indicated;
4. IV of LR or NS (bronchodilators may be needed);
5. Smooth transport, monitoring carefully for any changes and ready with intubation equipment. If intubation is unsuccessful in patients whose airways completely obstruct from edema, try forcing air past the obstruction with BVM or mouth-to-mouth forceful ventilations.

Summary

Though serious burns tend to be dramatic injuries, it is important for the paramedic to treat the whole patient, evaluating and supporting him in a systematic way. We reviewed thermal, chemical, electrical, radiation, and inhalation injuries, examined how to evaluate extent of burn involvement, classified burns as to severity and discussed priorities of prehospital management. A special note was made to avoid overcooling burn victims who are easy prey for hypothermia during (or as a result of) treatment.

SELF-TEST

Chapter 14

1. What are the four major types of burns?
   ANSWER: a. thermal
            b. electrical
            c. chemical
            d. radiation
2. Briefly note the difference between first, second, and third degree burns.
   ANSWER: a. first degree = redness, pain
            b. second degree = redness, blisters, pain
            c. third degree = charred, usually black, painless (nerve damage)

3. Give an example of a "minor" burn?

ANSWER: a. first degree = < 20% of body surface

b. second degree = < 15% of body surface

c. third degree = < 2% of body surface

4. What constitutes a "moderate" burn?

ANSWER: a. second degree = 15-30% of body surface

b. third degree = 2-10% of body surface

5. Give two examples of a "critical" burn?

ANSWER: a. second degree = > 30% of body surface

b. third degree = > 10% of body surface

c. burns with a respiratory deficit

d. burns of the face, hands, feet, or genitalia

e. burns associated with fractures or major soft tissue trauma

f. electrical and deep acid burns

g. burns in the compromised patient

6. Using the *rule of nines,* give the burn percentage estimate of a 5 year-old child with burns of the entire head and one entire leg.

ANSWER: 31.5% (18% for the head, 13.5% for the leg)

7. Using the *rule of nines,* give the burn percentage estimate for an adult with a burns of both entire arms and the front torso (chest and abdomen)

ANSWER: 36% (9% for each arm, 18% for the chest and abdomen)

8. When is it appropriate to pack a critical burn patient in ice?

ANSWER: Never! Ice application to a critical burn would probably cause hypothermia and tissue damage.

The Respiratory System

Definitions

Respiration—The exchange of gases between a living organism and its environment.

Pulmonary Ventilation—The process that moves air into and out of the lungs.

Lung Capacity—In the average adult male, the average lung capacity is about 6 liters.

Tidal Volume—The volume of gas inhaled or exhaled during a single respiratory cycle (500 cc).

Dead Air Space—Air remaining in the air passageways, unavailable for gas exchange (about 150 cc).

Alveolar Air—Air that actually reaches the alveoli for gas exchange (about 350 cc).

Minute Volume—The amount of gas moved in and out of the respiratory tract in one minute.

Vital Capacity—The amount of air that can forcefully be exhaled from the lungs.

Hypoxia—A state in which insufficient oxygen is available to meet the oxygen requirements of cells.

Hypoxemia—Reduced oxygen or a reduction in the partial pressure of oxygen in the arterial blood below normal limits.

Hypercarbia (hypercapnia)—Increased CO_2 or an increase in the partial pressure of CO_2 in the arterial blood above normal limits.

Respiratory Failure—This exists when the tension of respiratory gases in the blood is no longer within physiologic limits.

Cyanosis—Bluish discoloration of the skin due to an increase in carboxyhemoglobin in the blood.

Dyspnea—Difficult or labored breathing.

Tachypnea—Rapid respirations.

Hyperpnea—Deep inhalations.

Orthopnea—An increase in labored breathing while lying flat.

Apnea—Complete cessation of respiration.

Hypoventilation—A reduced rate and depth of breathing that can result in a rise in arterial carbon dioxide pressure.

Tracheal Tugging—This sign exists when tissue at the neck pulls inward due to significant respiratory distress.

Nasal Flaring—Excessive widening of the nostrils on inspiration due to severe respiratory distress.

FiO_2—An expression of the percentage of oxygen in inspired air.

Respiratory Assessment

History If you have a patient and the presenting history is of dyspnea, then you need to dig in and qualify the complaint:

1. Duration—how long has this been present?
2. Onset—was it gradual or sudden?
3. Does anything make it better or worse (laying down, sitting up)?
4. Is there a cough?
   a. Productive or non-productive?
   b. Sputum—character and color?
   c. Any blood coughed up?
5. What is the patient's past medical history?
6. Is the patient taking any medications (including oxygen)?
7. Does the patient have allergies?

Physical Examination

Observation Note the following as you initiate your exam:

1. Anxiety, restlessness, distress.
2. Shortness of breath—does it make speaking difficult?
3. Do symptoms continue while involving the patient in questioning?
4. Level of consciousness—is it compromised due to hypoxia?
5. What position does the patient favor to facilitate breathing.

Vital Signs Establish a baseline for:

1. Respirations:
    a. Rate, depth, character.
    b. Are there any abnormal breathing patterns?
2. Blood pressure.
3. Pulse—rate and character.

Inspection Look carefully for:

1. Skin:
    a. Color (cyanosis?), wet or dry, temperature.
    b. Is the capillary refill delayed (> 2 seconds is delayed)?
2. Nasal flaring or tracheal tugging?
3. Is there jugular vein distention (JVD)?
4. Are there retractions of intercostal, supraclavicular or suprasternal muscles?
5. Tracheal position (midline or deviated)?

Inspection of the Chest During your inspection of the chest look for:

1. Symmetrical movements.
2. Is the chest wall intact?
3. Are there any deformities, abrasions, lacerations, bruising, or subcutaneous emphysema?

Auscultation of the Chest

1. Are there any noises audible without the stethoscope?
2. Listen for at least one respiratory cycle in these locations:

    a. Posterior (between the eighth and ninth ribs is ideal).

    b. Anterior.

        1. Between the first and second ribs (mid-clavicular).

        2. Between the seventh and eighth ribs (mid-axillary).

3. Are the breath sounds equal bilaterally?

4. Does there seem to be adequate volume exchange?

5. Are there any *abnormal breath sounds*, such as:

    a. *Snoring*—A sound produced when the airway is partially obstructed by the tongue.

    b. *Stridor*—A harsh, high-pitched sound produced by upper airway obstruction.

    c. *Wheezing*—High-pitched whistling sounds produced by lower airway spasms or obstruction.

    d. *Rhonchi* (low wheezes)—Course rattling sounds produced by a buildup of secretions in the bronchial tubes.

    e. *Rales* (crackles)—Wet, fine crackling, popping or bubbling sounds produced by air moving through constricted, moist or fluid-filled small airways.

    f. *Friction rub* (pleural rub)—A creaking sort of sound produced by friction between the visceral and parietal pleura at some point in the respiratory cycle, probably due to inflammation, disease or injury.

Respiratory Disorders

Upper Airway Obstruction Some causes of upper airway obstruction may include:

1. The tongue (most common cause).

2. Foreign body (cafe coronary, especially with high ETOH levels).

3. Croup or epiglottitis in children.

4. Laryngeal edema (disease or trauma).

5. Facial trauma (broken teeth, bleeding in airway, tissue swelling).

Prehospital Management

1. Obstruction by tongue: Head tilt-chin lift, jaw thrust, jaw lift, nasopharyngeal airway, oropharyngeal airway.

2. Obstruction by foreign body: Heimlich maneuver (abdominal thrusts), visualization and removal (laryngoscope and Magill forceps).

3. Severe laryngeal edema:

   a. Maintain airway, administer O_2.

   b. IV (TKO).

   c. Administer epinephrine 0.3 mg of 1:1,000 solution sub-Q.

   d. Administer benadryl (diphenhydramine) 50 mg, slow IV push/deep IM.

   e. Consider vigorous BVM ventilation, tracheal intubation, or crico-thyroidotomy if the condition progresses to complete obstruction.

4. Facial trauma:

   a. Maintain airway (with neck immobolized) by positioning, allowing for drainage.

   b. Administer O_2 (cannula, mask or improvisation).

   c. Be prepared to perform tracheal intubation or cricothyrotomy.

Chronic Obstructive Pulmonary Disease (COPD) This disease is more common in men than women, more likely in urban environments and much more likely in long-term heavy cigarette smokers. In the normal healthy individual, *high levels of CO_2 are the primary stimulus for respiration*, with *low O_2 levels as a secondary or back-up stimulus to breathe*. Long-term COPD patients may not respond to high levels of CO_2 as their primary breathing stimulus, using instead low levels of O_2 as their stimulus to breathe. This is why we utilize supplemental oxygen cautiously in the long-term COPD patient. The high level of O_2 we usually provide might in some patients (rare) knock out their remaining breathing stimulus (low O_2 levels), tricking the body into apnea. However, *if COPD patients are in severe distress, they need oxygen badly. Do not withhold higher levels of O_2 in these distressed patients*! Simply be prepared to ventilate should apnea or bradypnea occur. Let's look at two types of COPD, emphysema and chronic bronchitis, keeping in mind that prehospital management is the same for each:

Emphysema/COPD This disease involves the gradual destruction of alveolar walls. Several changes occur in classic emphysema:

1. The destruction of alveolar walls results in:

   a. An increase in the ratio of air to lung tissue.

FIGURE 15.1.

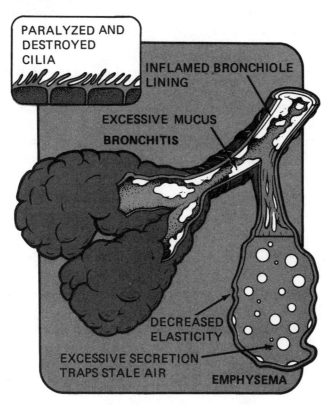

PARALYZED AND DESTROYED CILIA

INFLAMED BRONCHIOLE LINING

EXCESSIVE MUCUS

BRONCHITIS

DECREASED ELASTICITY

EXCESSIVE SECRETION TRAPS STALE AIR

EMPHYSEMA

b. A weakening of the walls in the small bronchioles.

c. Decreases in alveolar membrane area (less area available for gas exchange).

d. Decreases in the number of pulmonary capillaries (increasing the resistance to pulmonary blood flow).

2. Residual volume is increased (yet vital capacity remains about normal).

3. As the diseases progress, arterial PO_2 decreases and arterial PCO_2 increases (CO_2 retention).

4. Increased vascular resistance often leads to right heart failure.

5. Other complications are likely, including acute respiratory infections and cardiac dysrhythmias.

Hallmarks Markedly increased SOB upon exertion or excitement, barrel-chests and enlarged accessory respiratory muscles, "clubbed" fingers, pursed lips during prolonged expirations, chronic tachycardia and poor color, and decreased heart and lung sounds. A recent loss of appetite and subsequent weight loss often precedes a decompensation.

Chronic Bronchitis/COPD This disease is caused by increased numbers of mucous-secreting cells in the respiratory epithelium that produce excessive amounts of sputum. The alveolar walls are not seriously affected, but chronically large amounts of sputum tend to clog up the alveoli, causing hypoventilation, inhibiting gas exchange and stimulating CO_2 retention and arterial hypoxemia. Some other changes occur as well:

1. Increased PCO_2 levels cause constriction of pulmonary circulation, making right heart failure more likely.
2. Frequent acute respiratory infections cause scarring in the lungs.
3. Vital capacity is decreased, while residual volume is normal or somewhat decreased.
4. High PCO_2 levels may lead to irritability, decreased intellectual abilities, headaches, and personality changes.

Hallmarks Frequent respiratory tract infections, often a history of heavy cigarette smoking, productive cough between infections (at least 10 ccs of green or yellow sputum daily), SOB upon exertion or excitement, and victims often appear overweight and cyanotic.

Prehospital Management **(for both emphysema and chronic bronchitis)**

1. Maintain airway.
2. Administer oxygen, with the awareness that the respiratory drive may become diminished, requiring assisted ventilations. If distress is severe, use higher concentrations. If distress is low to moderate, begin at 2-3 liters/min. and increase as needed.
3. Start an IV of D5W (TKO).
4. Consider aminophylline administration by IV drip, 6 mg/kg added to 100 ccs D5W—give over 15-20 minutes or titrate to desired patient response.
5. NO sedatives or tranquilizers.
6. Monitor ECG carefully at scene and during transport.

Asthma Over 6 million Americans suffer from this disease, with 4-5 thousand deaths attributed each year. Half of asthma sufferers contract the condition before their 10th birthday, while another third of the victims suffer symptoms by age 30. Genetics seems to play a part in the likelihood of developing asthma. Asthma sufferers share an increased reactivity of the trachea, bronchi, and bronchioles to certain stimuli, which causes widespread (but fortunately reversible) narrowing of the airway passages (especially critical in the bronchioles). During an acute attack, the airway can become obstructed by bronchospasm, swelling of mucous membranes and thick mucous plugs in the bronchi. Predictably, there is a substantially reduced vital capacity, poor gas exchange, hypoventilation (and CO_2 retention) and progressive hyperinflation of the chest. Causes of an attack may include:

1. Allergic reaction to an inhaled irritant;
2. Excessive physical activity;
3. Emotional stress;
4. Respiratory infection.

Hallmarks Chronic nonproductive cough, dyspnea on expiration as the attack worsens and an asthma history.

Signs and Symptoms

1. Dyspnea, especially during exhalation;
2. Tightness in the chest;
3. Accessory muscles in use;
4. Patient often is sitting, leaning forward;
5. Usually coughs in attempt to gain relief—no sputum expelled;
6. Rapid breathing and pulse;
7. Wheezing (may *not* be present if attack is severe).

Note: All wheezing is not asthma. For example, pulmonary edema secondary to CHF/left heart failure produces wheezing.

Prehospital Management

1. Maintain airway.
2. Administer high-flow humidified oxygen (high concentration).

3. Start an IV of LR or NS (TKO or at rehydration rate ordered by physician).

4. Determine what medications, if any, have already been taken in response to the attack.

5. Administer 0.3–0.5 cc of 1:1,000 epinephrine (.3–.5 mg) subcutaneously,—repeat in 30 minutes if necessary (.01 mg/kg up to 0.3 ml).

6. Consider aminophylline, IV drip (6 mg/kg in 100 cc of D5W given over 15-20 minutes or titrated to desired patient response).

7. NO sedatives.

8. Monitor ECG carefully.

9. Smooth transport.

Static Asthmaticus This is a true emergency! Status asthmaticus is a severe prolonged asthma attack that cannot be broken with epinephrine. Exhaustion occurs quickly, as will acidosis and dehydration. Breath sounds and wheezes may disappear entirely as the chest becomes markedly hyperinflated.

Prehospital Management
Prehospital management for this condition is the same as for a severe asthma attack, but prompt aggressive treatment is even more critical. Rapid transport is indicated.

Pneumonia Pneumonia is a severe infection of the lower respiratory tract. Causes may include:

1. Bacteria;

2. Virus;

3. Fungus;

4. Inhalation of chemicals;

5. Parasite.

Signs and Symptoms

1. History of worsening respiratory distress, congestion, and coughing;

2. Fever;

3. Rales and/or ronchi (may be one-sided or bilateral);

4. Tachycardia;

5. Pleuritic chest pain;
6. Weakness upon exertion—may sweat easily;
7. Productive cough.

Prehospital Management

1. Maintain airway;
2. Administer oxygen (titrate flow and concentration to severity);
3. Consider IV for hydration and route for medication (elective);
4. Smooth transport.

Pulmonary Embolism This condition occurs when a clot (or shower of clots) or embolus occludes a pulmonary artery. Amazingly, there are 200,000 deaths per year due to this little-discussed disease process (many more deaths than from auto accidents). Women who smoke and take birth control pills are particularly susceptible. Causes of pulmonary emboli may include:

1. Prolonged immobilization;
2. Air, fat, or amniotic fluid emboli;
3. Congestive heart failure (CHF);
4. Recent significant surgical procedure;
5. Long-bone fractures;
6. Certain medications;
7. Thrombophlebitis.

When the blockage of pulmonary circulation occurs, the right heart pumps against increased vascular resistance, pulmonary capillary pressures increase and shunting of pulmonary blood away from occlusion occurs.

Hallmark Sudden onset of severe unexplained dyspnea, especially in a post-operative patient. Most of these occur in hospital setting. History is extremely important when considering this as a possibility.

Signs and Symptoms

1. Sudden onset of severe unexplained dyspnea (and/or chest pain);
2. If chest pain is present, it may be aggravated by deep breathing.

Prehospital Management

1. Maintain an airway;
2. Administer high-flow high-concentration oxygen and assist ventilations as needed;
3. Start an IV of D5W (TKO);
4. Monitor ECG;
5. Smooth rapid transport.

Pulmonary Edema This is a condition in which fluid in the lungs severely hampers respiration (see the chapter on the cardiovascular system (Chapter 16) for a complete discussion of this condition).

Inhalation Injuries

These injuries may be caused by super-heated air, toxic fumes, poisonous gases, and steam. Damage from chemical inhalation is covered in the chapter on burns.

Carbon Monoxide (CO) Carbon monoxide is an odorless, colorless gas produced during the incomplete combustion of organic fuels (such as gasoline, kerosene, and wood). CO occupies the same site on hemoglobin as oxygen, is 200 times more likely to grab that site and won't give it up easily once it is attached. If significant amounts of CO are inhaled, cellular hypoxia results as oxygen cannot be transported for cellular metabolism. CO poisoning is a common means of suicide and attempted suicide, is frequent in winter as a by-product of some home heating devices, and is a daily threat to firemen as they enter buildings full of smoke and toxic fumes due to combustion. Toxicity is directly related to the concentration of CO and the length of exposure.

Signs and Symptoms

1. Headache, irritability, agitation, and confusion;
2. Nausea and vomiting;
3. Errors in judgment;
4. Loss of coordination;
5. Chest pain;

6. Seizures;
7. Loss of consciousness.

Note: The famed "cherry-red" skin is rare and usually occurs after death.

Prehospital Management

1. Remove patient from the source of toxicity;
2. Maintain airway;
3. Administer high-flow, high-concentration oxygen;
4. Assist respirations;
5. Render supportive care while rapidly transporting to definitive care facility (preferably with hyperbaric chamber).

Hyperventilation

Hyperventilation occurs when rapid breathing blows off large amounts of carbon dioxide (CO_2), causing an electrolytic imbalance that leads to respiratory alkalosis. Usual causes would include:

1. Anxiety.
2. Central nervous system dysfunction:
   a. Head trauma;
   b. Stroke (CVA);
   c. Drug overdose (ASA, for example).
3. Pulmonary embolism.
4. Electrolyte imbalance.
5. Hypoxemia.

Hallmark Numbness, tingling, and shivering in patients having an anxiety reaction.

Note: Asthma has been known to be misdiagnosed as hyperventilation, with tragic results.

Signs and Symptoms

1. Rapid breathing;
2. Carpopedal spasms;

3. Numbness and tingling about the mouth, in the fingers and toes;
4. If prone to seizures, may exhibit seizure activity;
5. Anxiety.

Prehospital Management

1. Treat the underlying problem;
2. Rule out medical and traumatic causes;
3. Rebreathe CO_2 and/or talk patient into slowing down his or her respirations.

Summary

Shortness of breath (SOB) and respiratory distress account for a significant number of requests for emergency assistance. As 10-20 percent of the population are affected by respiratory disease/dysfunction, it is essential that paramedics thoroughly understand the diesase processes of these conditions and how they relate to signs and symptoms seen in the field. Prompt recognition, aggressive supportive care, and rapid administration of supplemental oxygen is the cornerstone of therapy for respiratory emergencies. Oxygen-hunger is a frightening condition and calm purposeful intervention is very reassuring to the victims of these disease processes.

SELF-TEST

Chapter 15

1. What is the lung capacity of an adult male?
   ANSWER: About 6 liters.
2. Normal tidal volume in the adult is about _____ cc.
   ANSWER: 500
3. Difficulty in breathing while laying flat is called _____ .
   ANSWER: orthopnea

4. The most common cause of an upper airway obstruction is
   _____ _____ .

   ANSWER: the tongue

5. Why must caution be used when administering oxygen to COPD
   patients?

   ANSWER: Some COPD patients may be using low oxygen levels to
   stimulate their respirations. If these patients receive high oxygen
   levels, they may quit breathing and require artificial ventilation.

6. What are the hallmark signs and symptoms of the patient with
   emphysema?

   ANSWER: a. shortness of breath upon exertion

                b. barrel chests (and perhaps clubbed fingers)

                c. prolonged expirations (often with wheezing)

                d. chronic tachycardia and poor color

                e. decreased heart and lung sounds

7. What are some signs and symptoms of an acute asthma attack?

   ANSWER: a. dyspnea, especially during exhalation

                b. tightness in the chest

                c. use of accessory muscles

                d. non-productive coughs (trying to clear airway)

                e. rapid respiratory and pulse rates

                f. wheezing (may disappear if attack is severe)

8. _____ _____ is a severe and prolonged asthma attack
   that cannot be broken with epinephrine. It is life-threatening.

   ANSWER: Status asthmaticus

9. What are the chief signs and symptoms of pulmonary embolism?

   ANSWER: Sudden onset of severe unexplained dyspnea (especially
   in post-operative patients). If chest pain is also present, it may be
   aggravated by deep breathing.

10. Why is exposure to carbon monoxide so dangerous?

   ANSWER: Carbon monoxide (CO) is 200 times more likely to bind
   to hemoglobin than is oxygen (O_2)—causing cellular asphyxia.

CHAPTER 16 _____

The Cardiovascular System

The initial impetus to train and equip paramedics was directly related to a high number of prehospital deaths from *coronary artery disease* (CAD) and the realization that specialized early intervention in acute events could greatly reduce mortality, myocardial damage, and recovery time. Appropriately, a significant portion of this text is devoted to an overview of the cardiovascular system. A brief review of ECG rhythm interpretation is included in this chapter for your reference.

Anatomy of The Heart

The heart is located near the center of the breastbone and is approximately the size of its owner's fist. The top of the heart is referred to as the *base,* the bottom is the *apex,* and it is surrounded by the *pericardium,* a double-walled sac composed of the:

1. *Visceral Pericardium*—The inner serous layer.
2. *Parietal Pericardium*—The outer fibrous layer.
3. *Parietal Fluid*—The lubricant between the pericardium and the epicardium.

Layers The heart muscle itself is composed of three layers:

1. *Epicardium*—The outer layer.
2. *Myocardium*—The thick middle layer. The myocardial muscle is extremely specialized, with muscle cells unique to the heart. It is striated like skeletal muscle, but shares the electrical properties of smooth muscle and is composed of contractile proteins arranged in parallel bands that slide together to cause cardiac contractions.
3. *Endocardium*—The smooth inner layer.

Chambers The heart is composed of four muscular chambers separated by connective tissue:

1. *Atria* (right and left)—Superior chambers that collect blood from the vascular system and feed it into the ventricles.
2. *Ventricles* (right and left)—Inferior chambers that receive blood from the atria and pump it forcefully back through the vascular system.
3. *Septum*—Connective tissue (and muscle) that separates the chambers.

Valves Special valves connect the chambers of the heart to each other and to the vascular system:

1. *Atrioventricular (AV) Valves*—Connect the atria and ventricles.
   a. *Tricuspid Valve*—Three-leaf valve that connects the right atrium and right ventricle.
   b. *Bicuspid (Mitral) Valve*—Two-leaf valve that connects the left atrium and left ventricle.
2. *Semilunar Valves*—Connect the ventricles to the vascular system.
   a. *Pulmonic (Pulmonary) Valve*—Connects the right ventricle and pulmonary artery.
   b. *Aortic Valve*—Connects the left ventricle and aorta.

Great Vessels The major blood vessels attached to the base of the heart:

1. *Vena Cava*—The superior and inferior vena cava meet in the right atrium, returning oxygen-poor blood from the body back to the heart.
2. *Pulmonary Artery*—Splits into left and right pulmonary artery and carries oxygen-poor blood from the right ventricle to the lungs for oxy-

genation. *Note:* This is the only artery in the body that carries oxygen-poor blood.

3. *Pulmonary Vein*—Collects oxygen-rich blood from the lungs (via four branches) and returns it to the left atrium. *Note:* This is the only vein in the body that carries oxygen-rich blood.

4. *Aorta*—Receives oxygen-rich blood pumped vigorously from the left ventricle and distributes it to the rest of the body.

Coronary Arteries The coronary arteries supply arterial (oxygen-rich) blood to the heart muscle and its electrical conduction system. Originating in the aorta immediately above the aortic valve, the coronary artery branches into the:

1. *Left Coronary Artery*—Supplies left ventricle, intraventricular septum, and part of the right ventricle. This artery further divides into the anterior descending and circumflex branches.

2. *Right Coronary Artery*—Supplies the right atrium, right ventricle, and part of the left ventricle.

Anatomy of the Peripheral Circulation

Blood Vessels Walls All blood vessel walls share similar characteristics. Some of these would include:

1. *Intima*—Smooth inner lining (single cell layer) of the vessel wall.

2. *Media*—Middle layer of the vessel wall containing elastic fibers and muscle that provides the ability to dilate (increase diameter) and constrict (decrease diameter).

3. *Adventitia*—The outer fibrous lining (provides strength for high pressure) of the vessel.

4. *Lumen*—The cavity within a blood vessel through which fluids pass which can vary greatly in size (due to a variety of factors).

Arteries Carry oxygenated blood from the left ventricle to the rest of the body. They are predominantly more muscular than veins and are under higher pressure. Arterioles are the smallest branches of the arteries, controlling blood flow to organs by their degree of resistance.

FIGURE 16.1.

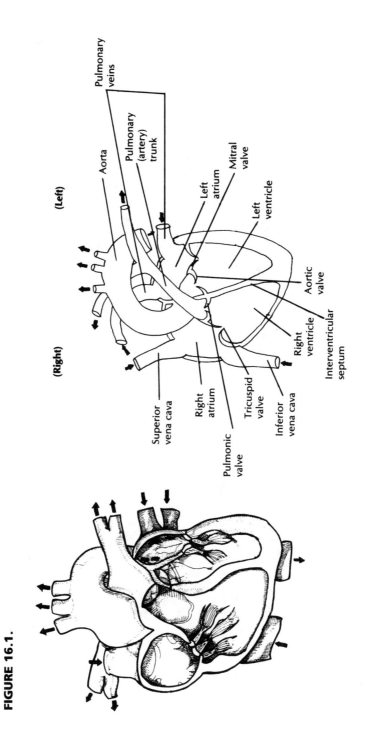

FIGURE 16.2.

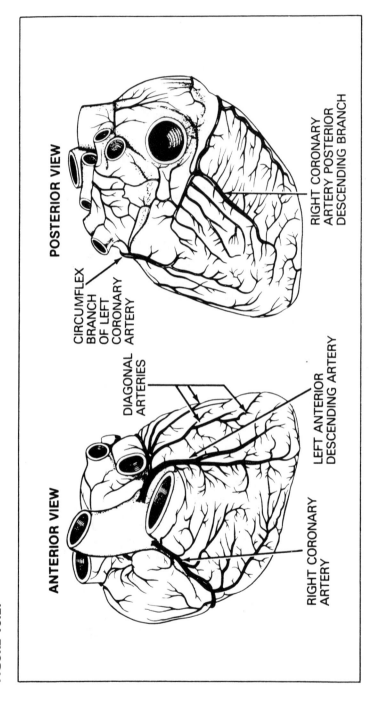

POSTERIOR VIEW

ANTERIOR VIEW

RIGHT CORONARY ARTERY POSTERIOR DESCENDING BRANCH

CIRCUMFLEX BRANCH OF LEFT CORONARY ARTERY

DIAGONAL ARTERIES

LEFT ANTERIOR DESCENDING ARTERY

RIGHT CORONARY ARTERY

Capillaries Connective vessels between the arterial and venous systems. In their walls (a mere single cell in thickness) all fluid, gas, and nutrient exchange occurs.

Veins Carry oxygen-poor blood back to the right atrium from the capillary level. They are less muscular than arteries and are under less pressure. Venules are the smallest branches of veins, bringing blood away from the capillaries.

FIGURE 16.3.

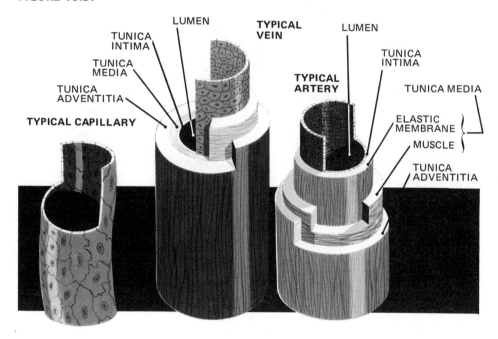

Physiology of the Heart

Blood Flow The SUPERIOR and INFERIOR VENA CAVA return blood from the venous system to the RIGHT ATRIUM, through the TRICUSPID VALVE and into the RIGHT VENTRICLE. From here it is pumped through the PULMONIC VALVE into the PULMONARY ARTERY, which carries the oxygen-poor blood to the LUNGS for reoxygenation (exchange of CO_2 for O_2) and returns via the PULMONARY VEIN to the LEFT ATRIUM, through the MITRAL (bicuspid) VALVE and into the

FIGURE 16.4.

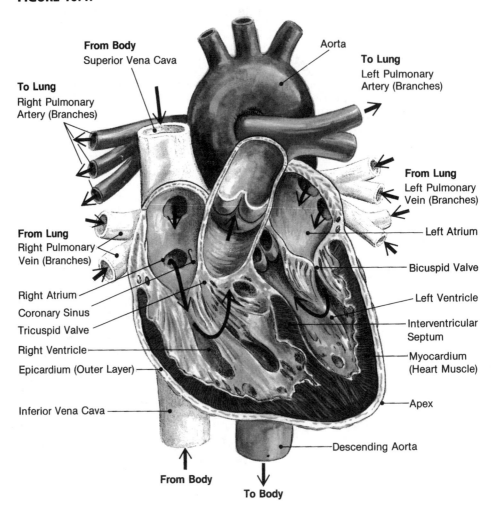

From Body
Superior Vena Cava

Aorta

To Lung
Right Pulmonary
Artery (Branches)

To Lung
Left Pulmonary
Artery (Branches)

From Lung
Left Pulmonary
Vein (Branches)

From Lung
Right Pulmonary
Vein (Branches)

Left Atrium

Bicuspid Valve

Right Atrium

Coronary Sinus

Tricuspid Valve

Left Ventricle

Interventricular
Septum

Right Ventricle

Epicardium (Outer Layer)

Myocardium
(Heart Muscle)

Inferior Vena Cava

Apex

Descending Aorta

From Body

To Body

LEFT VENTRICLE. This extremely muscular chamber pumps the now oxygen-rich blood through the AORTIC VALVE into the AORTA (where the coronary arteries are fed) for distribution to the rest of the body via the arterial system.

Systole Ventricular contraction (.28 seconds).

Diastole Ventricular relaxation (.52 seconds) and filling (atrial contraction). Seventy percent of the coronary artery filling occurs during this phase.

Right Heart The right atrium and ventricle pump against pulmonary resistance (low pressure).

Left Heart The left atrium and ventricle pump against systemic resistance (high pressure).

Heart Rate (HR) The number of ventricular contractions (heartbeats) per minute. The normal heart rate at rest is 60-100.

Starling's Law To a degree, the more that myocardial muscle is stretched (by filling of its chambers), the greater will be its force of contraction (and thus, its stroke volume).

Stroke Volume (SV) The amount of blood ejected from the ventricles during one contraction, normally about 60-100 ml. Stroke volume can be significantly increased in healthy hearts by:

1. Preload—The pressure under which the ventricle fills (influenced by venous return).
2. Afterload—The resistance against which the ventricle contracts (influenced by arterial resistance).
3. The ability of ventricular muscle to stretch (Starling's Law).

Cardiac Output (CO) Heart rate times stroke volume; the amount of blood pumped through the circulatory system in one minute. *Note:* Cardiac output in the healthy heart can be increased times *three* by an increase in rate alone.

Systemic Blood Pressure (BP) Cardiac output times peripheral resistance.

Nervous System Control Nerve fibers from the *autonomic nervous system* innervate the heart and exert a degree of control in several ways. The *parasympathetic nervous system* (mediated through the vagus nerve) and the *sympathetic nervous system* (mediated through nerves in the thoracic/lumbar ganglia) can have these effects:

1. *Parasympathetic Stimulation* (primarily affects atria):
   a. Chemical mediator—acetylcholine.
   b. Slows heart rate.
   c. Slows AV conduction.

2. *Sympathetic Stimulation* (affects both atria and ventricles):
   a. Chemical mediator—norepinephrine.
   b. *Alpha Effect:* Peripheral vasoconstriction.
   c. *Beta Effects:*
      1. Increase in rate, conduction and/or contractility.
      2. Bronchodilation.
      3. Peripheral vasodilation.

Function of Electrolytes Electrolyte imbalance can impair electrical and/or mechanical cardiac function. These electrolytes have major roles in the electromechanical process:

1. *Sodium* (Na+)— Needed for proper depolarization of myocardial cells.
2. *Calcium* (Ca++)—Needed for depolarization of pacemaker cells and myocardial contractility. (An increase in Ca++ [hypercalcemia] increases myocardial contractility, while a decrease in Ca++ [hypocalcemia] decreases contractility and increases electrical irritability)
3. *Potassium* (K+)—Needed during repolarization of myocardial cells. (An increase in K+ [hyperkalemia] decreases automaticity and conduction, while a decrease in K+ [hypokalemia] increases electrical irritability.)

Electrical Conduction

Automaticity The inherent ability to generate electrical impulses without outside stimulation (pacemaker cells).

Excitability The ability to respond to an electrical stimulus (all myocardial cells).

Conductivity The ability to transmit an electrical impulse from cell to cell.

Normal Conduction Pathways SA NODE—INTERNODAL PATHWAYS—AV NODE—BUNDLE OF HIS—BUNDLE BRANCHES—PURKINJE FIBERS.

FIGURE 16.5.

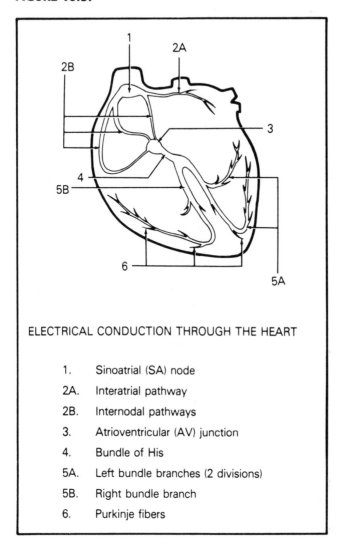

ELECTRICAL CONDUCTION THROUGH THE HEART

1. Sinoatrial (SA) node
2A. Interatrial pathway
2B. Internodal pathways
3. Atrioventricular (AV) junction
4. Bundle of His
5A. Left bundle branches (2 divisions)
5B. Right bundle branch
6. Purkinje fibers

SA (Sinoatrial) Node The heart's dominant pacemaker, located in the right atrium.

Internodal Pathways These pathways carry impulses from the SA Node to the AV node across both atria.

AV (Atrioventricular) Node The AV Node causes a slight conduction delay before stimulating the ventricles (the node itself has no pacemaking cells).

Bundle of His This is part of the AV Junction and provides the connection between atria and ventricles.

Bundle Branches These pathways carry electrical impulses very quickly to the purkinje fibers in each ventricle.

Purkinje Fibers These are the ends of the bundle branches and spread the electrical stimulus throughout the ventricular walls.

Depolarization The process by which muscle fibers are stimulated to contract. (caused by a change in cell's electrical charge due to electrolyte changes)

Cell Depolarization A resting (polarized) cell is negatively charged. Electrical stimulation of the cell wall alters its permeability to sodium ($Na+$); sodium rushes in, causing the cellular charge to become more positive (a slower influx of calcium ($Ca++$) also causes cell to become more positive); a muscle contraction occurs as a response to this depolarization (from negative to positive); and a depolarization wave is passed from cell to cell along conduction pathways.

Pacemaker Cell Depolarization Pacemaker cells capable of spontaneous self-depolarization (automaticity) are found all along the conduction system (except in the AV node)—some have their own intrinsic rate of discharge:

1. *SA Node*—60-100/minute (usually dominant because of faster rate).
2. *AV Junction*—40-60/minute.
3. *Ventricles*—20-40/minute.

Repolarization The return of the cell to a resting (polarized) state (and a return to an internal negative charge as electrolytes are redistributed by cell pumps).

ECG Electrical Physiology The electrocardiograph (EKG or ECG) represents electrical activity occurring in the heart (but not its effectiveness). It is interpreted by deviations from the *isoelectric line* (a flat line on the ECG that indicates an absence of electrical activity):

FIGURE 16.6.

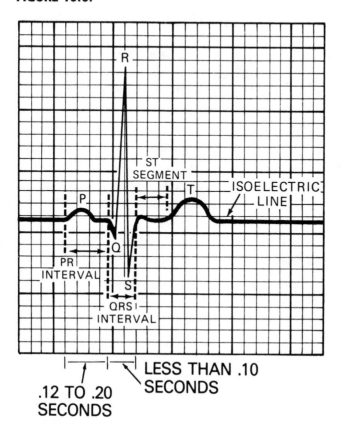

1. *P-Wave*—This represents depolarization of the atria. It is normally a small rounded upright (positive) wave that preceeds the QRS complex.

2. *QRS Complex*—This represents depolarization of the ventricles. It is normally composed of three distinct deflections:

   a. *Q-Wave*—The first downward (negative) deflection following the P-wave.

   b. *R-Wave*—The first upward (positive) deflection following the P-wave.

   c. *S-Wave*—The first downward (negative) deflection following the R-wave.

3. *T-Wave*—This represents ventricular repolarization. It is normally a rounded wave following the QRS complex (atrial repolarization is usually buried in the QRS complex and not detectable).

4. *P-R Interval*—This represents the duration of atrial depolarization (from pacemaker stimulus to beginning of ventricular depolarization). It is measured on the ECG from the beginning of the P-wave to the beginning of the QRS complex.

5. *S-T Segment*—The distance between the S-wave and the beginning of the T-wave. In some circumstances, an abnormality in this segment may indicate a degree of myocardial ischemia or injury.

6. *Refractory Period*—A time period between depolarization and repolarization when the myocardium is unable to respond to stimulation.

   a. *Absolute Refractory Period*—This is when a stimulus to the myocardium is unable to produce depolarization (contraction).

   b. *Relative Refractory Period*—A more vulnerable phase of the refractory period when a stimulus of sufficient strength *may* produce depolarization (at least in some of the cells).

ECG Rhythm Interpretation

Rapid interpretation of ECG rhythms is a skill that must be mastered by all paramedics. This section provides a brief review of the classic 5-step analysis of ECG strips, a review of normal and abnormal values, and examples of 24 cardiac rhythms (all 6-second strips in lead 2) recognized as essential for quick recognition by field paramedics.

ECG Graph Paper Each small box (horizontally) = 0.04 seconds. Each large box (5 small boxes) = 0.20 seconds. Five large boxes = 1 second. Standard strip for paramedic rapid interpretation = 6 seconds. Each small box (vertically) = 1 millivolt of amplitude. Ten small vertical boxes = 10 millivolts = standard calibration.

Systematic Analysis

1. Rate;
2. Rhythm;
3. P-waves;

4. P-R interval;
5. QRS complexes.

Rate This usually refers to the ventricular rate, but if atrial and ventricular rates are not the same, you must calculate both:

1. Normal = 60-100.
2. Bradycardia = less than 60.
3. Tachycardia = more than 100.

Rhythm Is it regular (normal)? Measure the R-R interval across the entire strip to determine. If *not* regular, is it:

1. Regularly irregular.
2. Occasionally irregular.
3. Totally irregular.

P-waves

1. Are they regular?
2. Is there one P-wave for each QRS?
3. Are they upright or inverted?
4. Are they related to the QRS?
5. Do they all look alike?

P-R Interval

1. Does it stay the same across the entire strip?
2. Is it prolonged or shortened?
3. Normal: .12-.20 seconds.

QRS Complex

1. Are they all alike in shape and duration?
2. Normal duration: less than .12 seconds.

Let's apply these criteria to the most common and benign of cardiac rhythms, the *normal sinus rhythm* (NSR):

Normal Sinus Rhythm (NSR)

FIGURE 16.7.

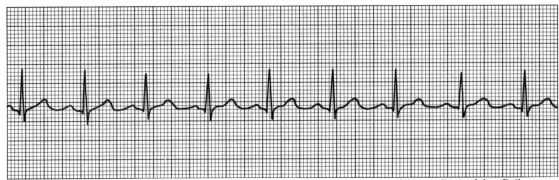

Reprinted with permission from *Basic Arrhythmias,* Second Edition, Revised by Gail Walraven, RN.

Rate: 60-100 per minute.

Rhythm: Regular (both P-P and R-R).

P-waves: Normal and upright, one P-wave before each QRS.

P-R interval: .12-.20 seconds and constant.

QRS: Less than .12 seconds.

Dysrhythmias Originating in the SA Node

Sinus Bradycardia

FIGURE 16.8.

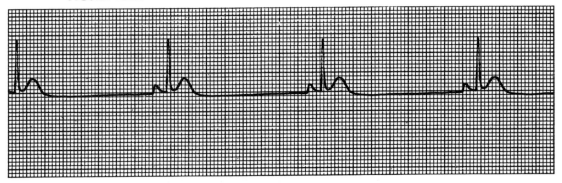

Rate: Less than 60 per minute.

Rhythm: Regular.

P-waves: Normal and upright, precede each QRS complex.

P-R interval: .12-.20 seconds and constant.

QRS complexes: Normal, each preceded by a P-wave.

Sinus Tachycardia

FIGURE 16.9.

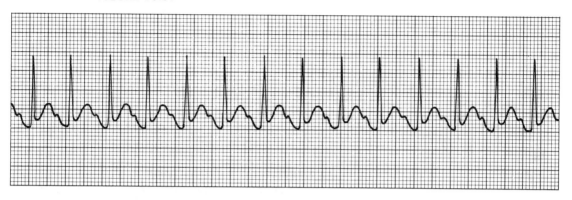

Rate: Greater than 100 per minute.

Rhythm: Regular.

P-waves: Normal and upright, one before each QRS (may be buried in preceding T-wave and be difficult to locate).

P-R interval: .12-.20 seconds.

QRS complexes: Normal, each preceded by a P-wave.

Sinus Arrhythmia

FIGURE 16.10.

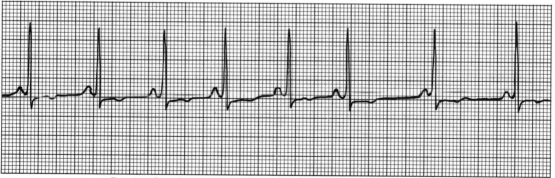

Reprinted with permission from *Basic Arrhythmias,* Second Edition, Revised by Gail Walraven, RN.

Rate: Usually 60-100 per minute (in respiratory form, rate *increases* with inspiration and *decreases* with expiration.

182

Rhythm: Irregular (if strip is long enough, you may see it as regularly or "cyclically" irregular). R-R will vary > 0.16 seconds.

P-waves: Normal and upright, one before each QRS.

P-R interval: .12-.20 seconds and constant.

QRS complexes: Normal, each preceded by a P-wave.

Sinus Arrest

FIGURE 16.11.

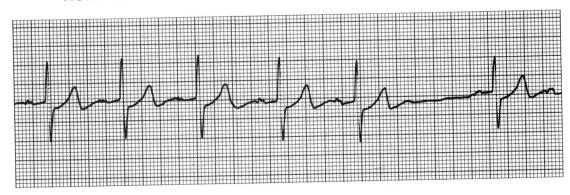

Rate: Normal or slow.

Rhythm: Irregular.

P-waves: Normal, where present, preceding each QRS. When the SA Node does *not* fire (or is blocked), the P-wave (& QRS-T complex) is absent.

P-R interval: .12-.20 seconds and constant.

QRS complexes: Normal (when present), each preceded by a P-wave.

Dysrhythmias Originating in the Atria

ECG features common to all atrial dysrhythmias include:

1. P-waves differ in appearance from sinus P-waves.
2. QRS complexes are of normal duration.

Wandering Pacemaker

FIGURE 16.12.

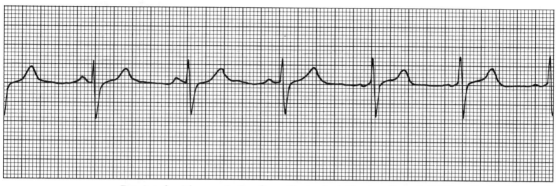

Reprinted with permission from *Basic Arrhythmias,* Second Edition, Revised by Gail Walraven, RN.

Rate: Usually 60-100.

Rhythm: Slightly irregular.

P-waves: May change in form from beat to beat or may disappear completely.

PR interval: May vary and may be less than .12 seconds.

QRS: Less than .12 seconds.

Premature Atrial Complex (PAC)

FIGURE 16.13.

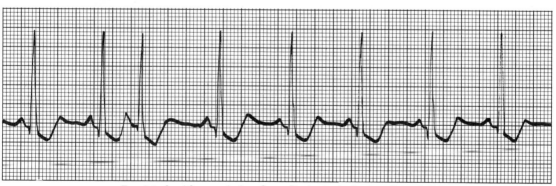

Reprinted with permission from *Basic Arrhythmias,* Second Edition, Revised by Gail Walraven, RN.

Rate: Depends on underlying rhythm.

Rhythm: Depends on underlying rhythm—usually regular except for PAC.

P-waves:

1. P-wave of PAC differs in shape from sinus P-wave.

2. Occurs earlier than next sinus P-wave would be expected.

3. May be hidden in preceding T-wave.

PR interval: Usually normal, but may be greater than .20 seconds.

QRS: Usually less than .12 seconds, but may be:

1. Greater than .12 seconds if PAC is abnormally conducted through partially refractory ventricles, or:

2. Absent, if PAC is nonconducted due to absolute refractoriness.

Paroxysmal Atrial Tachycardia (a form of PSVT)

FIGURE 16.14.

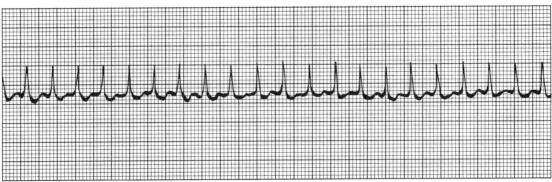

Reprinted with permission from *Basic Arrhythmias,* Second Edition, Revised by Gail Walraven, RN.

Rate: 150-250.

Rhythm: Characteristically regular, except at onset and termination.

P-waves:

1. Atrial P-wave looks different from a sinus P-wave.

2. They are frequently buried in the preceding T-waves.

PR interval: May be normal or prolonged.

QRS: Less than .12 seconds.

Atrial Flutter

Rate: Atrial 250-350, ventricular rate varies.

Rhythm: Atrial rhythm regular, ventricular rate usually regular but can be irregular if block varies.

FIGURE 16.15.

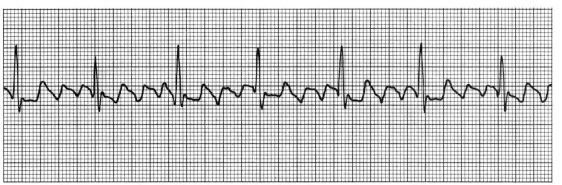

Reprinted with permission from *Basic Arrhythmias,* Second Edition, Revised by Gail Walraven, RN.

P-waves: Flutter (F) waves esemble "sawtooth" or "picket fence" pattern. (Suspect 2:1 flutter when the rhythm is regular and the ventricular rate is 150.)

PR interval: F-R interval is usually constant but may vary.

QRS: Less than .12 seconds.

Atrial Fibrillation

FIGURE 16.16.

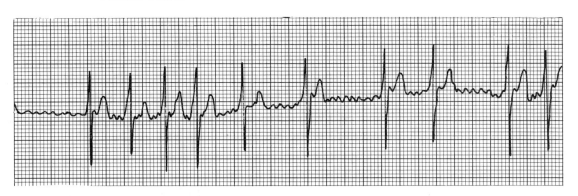

Rate: Atrial rate 350-700 (cannot be counted). Ventricular rate varies greatly.

Rhythm: Irregularly irregular.

P-waves: None discernible, chaotic atrial activity (or near flat line).

PR interval: None.

QRS: Less than .12 seconds.

Dysrhythmias Originating in the AV Junction

ECG features common to all junctional rhythms:

1. P-waves may be inverted in Lead II due to retrograde depolarization of the atria:

    a. The relationship of P-wave to QRS is dependent upon the timing of atrial depolarization to ventricular depolarization—P-wave may occur:

       1. Before QRS—atria depolarized first.

       2. After QRS—venticles depolarized first.

       3. During QRS—atria and ventricles depolarize together.

    Note that some low atrial impulses can also create inverted P-waves:

       1. QRS complexes are of normal duration.

       2. PR intervals will frequently be less than .12 seconds.

Premature Junctional Contractions (PJC)

FIGURE 16.17.

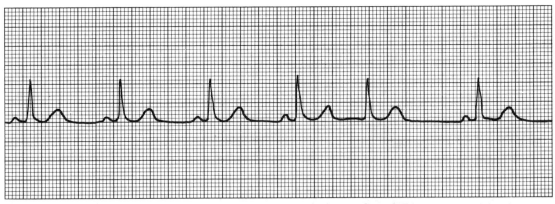

Reprinted with permission from *Basic Arrhythmias,* Second Edition, Revised by Gail Walraven, RN.

Rate: Depends on rate of underlying rhythm.

Rhythm: Depends on underlying rhythm—usually regular except for PJC.

P-waves: Inverted, before or after QRS—or absent.

PR interval: If P wave precedes QRS, it is usually less than .12 seconds.

QRS: Usually less than .12 seconds.

Junctional Escape Complexes and Rhythm

FIGURE 16.18.

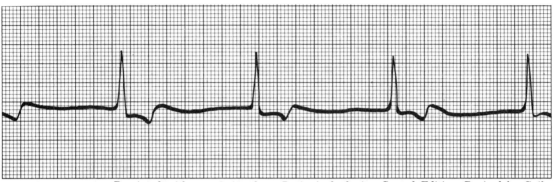

Reprinted with permission from *Basic Arrhythmias,* Second Edition, Revised by Gail Walraven, RN.

Rate: 40-60.

Rhythm:

1. Irregular if single junctional escape complex.

2. Regular if junctional escape rhythm.

P-waves: Inverted before or after QRS—or absent.

PR interval: If P wave precedes QRS, usually less than .12 seconds.

QRS: Usually less than .12 seconds.

Accelerated Junctional Rhythm

FIGURE 16.19.

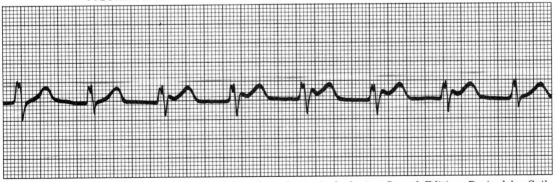

Reprinted with permission from *Basic Arrhythmias,* Second Edition, Revised by Gail Walraven, RN.

Rate: 60-100.

Rhythm:

1. Irregular if single junctional escape complex.
2. Regular if junctional escape rhythm.

P-waves: Inverted, before or after QRS—or absent.

PR interval: If P-wave precedes QRS, usually less than .12 seconds.

QRS: Usually less than .12 seconds.

Paroxysmal Junctional Tachycardia (a form of Paroxysmal Supraventricular Tachycardia—PSVT)

FIGURE 16.20.

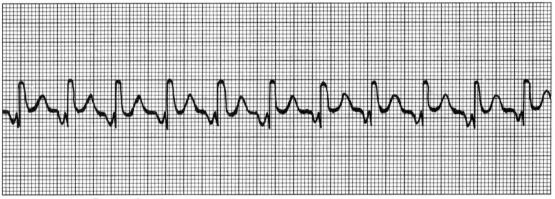

Reprinted with permission from *Basic Arrhythmias,* Second Edition, Revised by Gail Walraven, RN.

Rate: 100-180.

Rhythm: Regular.

P-waves: If visible, inverted—occur before or after QRS.

PR interval: If P-wave precedes QRS, usually less than .12 seconds.

QRS: Usually less than .12 seconds.

Dysrhythmias Originating in the Ventricles

ECG features common to all ventricular rhythms:

1. QRS complexes will be .12 seconds or greater in duration.
2. P-waves will be absent.

Ventricular Escape Complexes and Rhythm (Idioventricular Rhythm)

FIGURE 16.21.

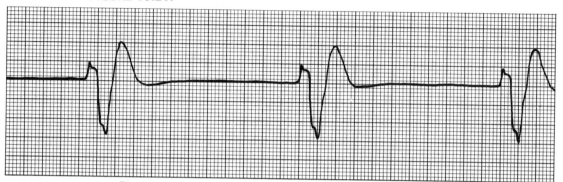

Reprinted with permission from *Basic Arrhythmias*, Second Edition, Revised by Gail Walraven, RN.

Rate: 20-40 (sometimes less).

Rhythm:

1. If a single escape beat—makes the rate's underlying rhythm irregular.

2. If an escape rhythm—usually regular, but a low pacemaker site can be unreliable.

P-waves: None.

PR interval: None.

QRS: .12 seconds or greater—looks bizarre.

Premature Ventricular Complex (PVC)

FIGURE 16.22.

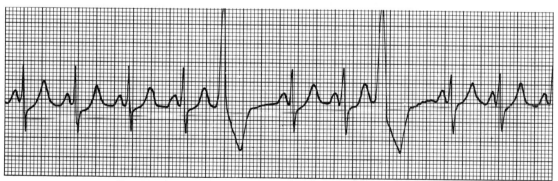

Reprinted with permission from *Basic Arrhythmias*, Second Edition, Revised by Gail Walraven, RN.

Rate: Depends on underlying rhythm and number of PVCs.

Rhythm: Interrupts regularity of underlying rhythm (occasionally irregular).

P-waves: None, although the normal sinus P-wave may be seen near PVC.

PR interval: None.

QRS: .12 seconds or greater—frequently looks bizarre.

Ventricular Tachycardia

FIGURE 16.23.

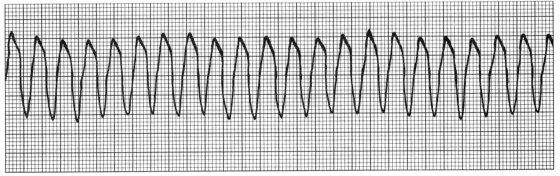

Reprinted with permission from *Basic Arrhythmias,* Second Edition, Revised by Gail Walraven, RN.

Rate: 100-250 (approximate).

Rhythm: Regular or slightly irregular.

P-waves: None associated with QRS complexes although some may be visible.

PR interval: None.

QRS: .12 seconds or greater—looks bizarre.

Ventricular Fibrillation

FIGURE 16.24.

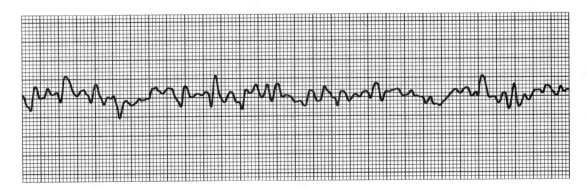

Rate: Cannot determine.

Rhythm: Totally chaotic undulations of varying amplitude and shape—no discernible waves or complexes.

P-waves: None.

PR interval: None.

QRS: None discernible.

Asystole

FIGURE 16.25.

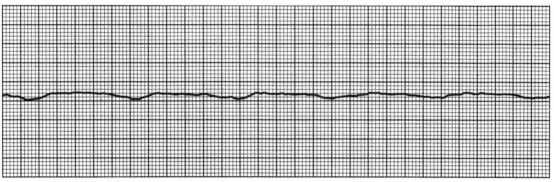

Reprinted with permission from *Basic Arrhythmias,* Second Edition, Revised by Gail Walraven, RN.

Rate: None.

Rhythm: No discernible waves or complexes—only an isoelectric line.

P-waves: None (straight line).

PR interval: None.

QRS: None.

Artificial Pacemaker Rhythm

Rate: Varies according to preset rate of pacemaker.

Rhythm: Regular if pacing constantly, possibly irregular if pacing only on demand.

P-waves:

1. None produced by ventricular pacemaker—sinus P-waves may be seen but are probably unrelated to QRS complexes.

2. Dual chambered pacemakers produce a P-wave following each atrial spike.

FIGURE 16.26.

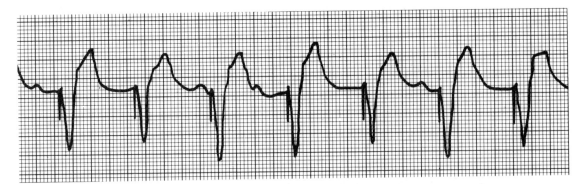

Pacemaker spike: A spike going upward or downward from the baseline which is an artifact created each time the pacemaker fires—this tells you only that the pacemaker is discharging.

QRS:

1. .12 seconds or greater and bizarre—appears identical to ventricular escape rhythm (idioventricular rhythm).

2. Each time ventricular pacemaker spike is seen, a QRS should follow— "capture."

3. With a demand pacemaker, some of patient's own QRSs may be seen (different contour)—no pacemaker spike should then be seen.

Dysrhythmias That are Disorders of Conduction

First-Degree AV Block

FIGURE 16.27.

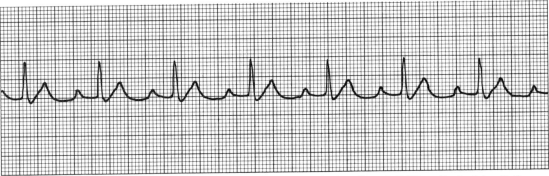

Reprinted with permission from *Basic Arrhythmias,* Second Edition, Revised by Gail Walraven, RN.

Rate: 60-100.

Rhythm: Regular.

P-waves: Precede each QRS.

PR interval: Greater than .20 seconds (prolonged)—usually constant.

QRS: Less than .12 seconds.

Second-Degree AV Block—Type I (Wenkebach)

FIGURE 16.28.

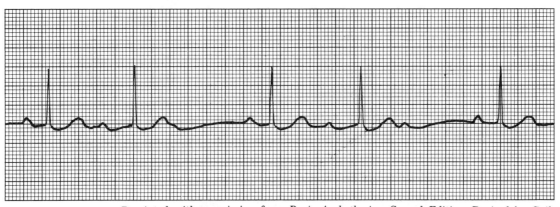

Reprinted with permission from *Basic Arrhythmias,* Second Edition, Revised by Gail Walraven, RN.

Rate: Atrial rate constant (usually 60-100), ventricular rate may be normal or slightly slow.

Rhythm: Atrial regular, ventricular irregular (look for group beating).

P-waves: Upright and uniform, some P-waves not followed by QRS complexes.

PR interval: Progressively lengthening prior to non-conducted P-wave.

QRS: Less than .12 seconds.

Second-Degree AV Block—Type II

Rate: Atrial rate constant (usually 60-100), ventricular rate usually bradycardia.

Rhythm: Regular or irregular depending on whether conduction ratio is constant or variable.

P-waves: Upright and uniform, more than one P-wave for each QRS.

FIGURE 16.29.

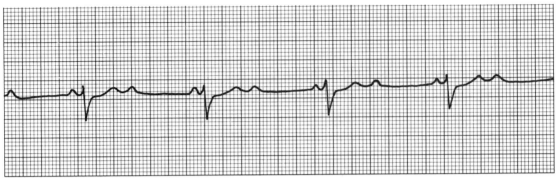

Reprinted with permission from *Basic Arrhythmias,* Second Edition, Revised by Gail Walraven, RN.

PR interval: Constant for conducted beats (may be prolonged).

QRS: May be normal, but often .12 seconds or greater due to abnormal ventricular depolarization sequence.

Third-Degree AV Block (Complete Heart Block)

FIGURE 16.30.

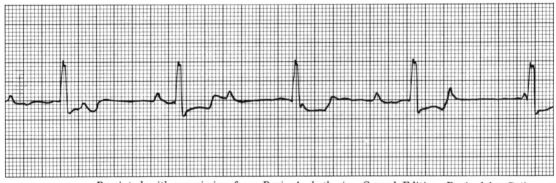

Reprinted with permission from *Basic Arrhythmias,* Second Edition, Revised by Gail Walraven, RN.

Rate: Atrial rate normal (60-100), ventricular rate 40-60 if escape focus is junctional—less than 40 if escape focus is ventricular.

Rhythm: Atrial and ventricular rates should both be regular.

P-waves: Upright and uniform, more P-waves than QRS complexes.

PR interval: No constant PR interval, P-waves may be superimposed on QRS complexes or T-waves (perhaps buried).

QRS: Less than .12 if escape focus is junctional—.12 seconds or greater if escape focus is ventricular.

Assessing the Cardiac Patient

Chief Complaints Any complaints should be quickly determined. Cardiac complaints may be few or multiple, but their importance is relative to overall patient condition and treatment.

Chest Pain This is the most common symptom associated with *myocardial infarction* (MI), yet 25% of patients suffering MIs do not complain of chest pain/discomfort. Try to determine:

1. Location of pain or discomfort (have them point).
2. Type or quality of pain (description):
   a. Sharp or dull (stabbing, cramping, ache)?
   b. Constant or intermittent (does it change)?
   c. Crushing, heavy or "just a feeling" (make them use *their* words)?
3. Duration (from first onset).
4. Is there any radiation (neck, arms, jaw, shoulder)?
5. Does anything make it better or worse (deep breathing, movement)?
6. Activity when pain began (at rest, asleep, exercising).
7. Associated symptoms (nausea/vomiting, sweating, weakness, pallor).
8. If any medication has been taken for the pain (Nitro, ASA/Tylenol, antacids, sedatives).
9. Any previous episodes (when, frequency, and how diagnosed).

Note: There are many causes of chest pain that are *not* cardiac.

Neck, Arm, Shoulder or Jaw Pain Some significant cardiac patients will present with this kind of pain instead of chest pain (history important).

Dyspnea/Shortness of Breath (SOB) The primary symptom in CHF (as blood backs up in the lungs due to a failing left ventricle), it is *very often* associated with myocardial infarction and is difficult to assess. Try to determine:

1. Onset (sudden or gradual) and activity at time of onset.
2. Duration.
3. If anything makes it better or worse (position, movement).
4. Any previous episodes (when, frequency, and how diagnosed).

Note: There are many causes of SOB that are *not* cardiac—use history to differentiate.

Syncope When present, it may be the only symptom of cardiac problems in the elderly patient. It is often caused by sudden changes in cardiac output due to transient arrhythmias, changes in heart rate and/or cerebral perfusion. Try to determine:

1. Activity and position at onset (at rest, standing quickly).
2. Duration (from first onset).
3. Associated symptoms (nausea/vomiting, SOB, sweating, skin color, weakness, dizziness, pain).
4. Any previous episodes (when, frequency, how diagnosed)?

Palpitations Feeling by patient that there are "skipped beats" or that "my heart is racing." This usually has no relation to any abnormal rhythm or irregularity, but should be evaluated in light of overall symptoms and history.

Other Complaints May include nausea, vomiting, weakness, dizziness, diaphoresis, change in pallor (pale, ashen, cyanotic), apprehension, and numbness.

Significant Medical History

This should be taken as soon as time allows, but must not cause any delay in management. Emergency treatment is necessarily based upon current signs and symptoms—not upon the past history. When taken, try to determine:

1. Current prescription medications (especially cardiac meds), dosages, frequency and routes of administration.
2. Current over-the-counter (OTC) medications.
3. Known allergies to medications.
4. Current medical problems.
5. Past significant medical problems (MIs, hypertension, diabetes, chronic lung diseases, heart failure).

Physical Examination

1. Primary survey:
   a. Airway (open, patent);
   b. Breathing (present, fast or slow);
   c. Circulation (palpable pulse and scan for serious bleeding).

2. Vital signs (and rough neurological status):
   a. Blood pressure;
   b. Respirations (rate, quality);
   c. Pulse (rate, regularity, quality);
   d. LOC (level of consciousness);
   e. ECG (dysrhythmias, abnormalities, ectopics).

3. Secondary survey: (Look, Listen and Feel)

LOOK for. . .
   a. Skin color (flushed, pale, normal, cyanotic, ashen);
   b. Capillary refill (0-2 normal, 2-4 delayed, > 4 absent);
   c. Jugular Vein Distension (JVD) (present or not—check at 45 degrees);
   d. Edema (peripheral/presacral—mild or pitting);
   e. Be alert for signs of cardiac treatment (nitro patch, pacemaker implantation, open heart surgery scars).

LISTEN to. . .
   a. Lungs (adequacy of volume, equality, use of accessory muscles, abnormal sounds—stridor, rales, rhonchi, wheezes);
   b. Heart (re-check ECG, identify pulse deficits or extra sounds, check for audibility and clearness of sound). DON'T WASTE MUCH TIME ON HEART SOUNDS—YOUR FINDINGS WILL NOT ALTER TREATMENT IN ANY WAY.

FEEL for. . .
   a. Skin condition (cool or hot, wet or dry);
   b. Edema (peripheral, presacral—mild or pitting);
   c. Pulses (fast or slow, regular or irregular, strong or weak);

Atherosclerosis

A progressive, degenerative disease of large and medium arteries, primarily affecting the:

1. Aorta (and its branches);
2. Cerebral arteries;
3. Coronary arteries:
    a. Especially prone to develop CAD (coronary artery disease) due to many bifurcations, constant torsion and movement (with heart beats) and right angles;
    b. May be obstructed by as much as 75% before decreased blood flow causes identifiable symptoms.

Development All males > 50 and females > 60 have atherosclerosis to some degree and evidence shows that many develop the condition early in adult life. Fats, lipids, and cholesterol in the bloodstream are deposited under the intima of blood vessels. As a result:

1. An injury response is stimulated in vessel walls, causing damage to the media.
2. Plaque formation begins (over time), as calcium deposits increase.
3. Small hemorrhages into the plaque may occur, followed by more scarring and fibrosis.
4. Collateral circulation develops to compensate for reduction of blood flow in partially obstructed arteries.

Major Risk Factors Several factors have been identified that increase the likelihood for early development of atherosclerosis, some of which are:

Modifiable

1. Hypertension;
2. Smoking;
3. Elevated blood lipids.

Non-Modifiable

1. Diabetes mellitus;
2. Male gender;
3. Advanced age;
4. Family history of early atherosclerosis development.

Results of atherosclerosis

1. Smooth intimal surface is disrupted, with a loss of vessel elasticity;
2. Reduction of blood flow;
3. Frequent bouts of thrombosis and total obstruction.

Coronary Artery Disease (CAD)

CAD is a condition in which atherosclerosis specifically attacks the coronary arteries, reducing potential blood flow. CAD eventually results in:

Angina Pectoris Chest pain that develops when oxygen demands of the heart (because of CAD) temporarily exceed the available blood supply and cause *ischemia*. Angina may also be caused by spasm of a coronary artery. Angina may be further classified as either stable or unstable.

Stable Angina

1. Usually the result of physical or emotional stress;
2. Short duration—usually 3-5 minutes, not more than 15;
3. May be relieved by rest, oxygen, and/or Nitro.

Unstable Angina (Preinfarction Angina)

1. Often occurs unpredictably, even at rest;
2. Does not respond as quickly to rest, oxygen, and/or Nitro;
3. May be the precursor of an MI.

Note: Angina pectoris mimics the pain of an MI. The difference is that anginal pain is temporary and indicates ischemia, while the pain of a

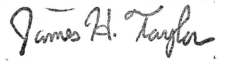

myocardial infarction lasts and results in damage and/or death of the heart muscle.

Prehospital Management

1. Keep patient at rest and try to lessen anxiety;
2. Administer high flow oxygen;
3. Monitor ECG;
4. Administer sub-L nitroglycerine (if *not* hypotensive);
5. If symptoms persist, treat as an MI and insist on hospital evaluation.

Myocardial Infarction (MI) Death of heart muscle (*necrosis*) due to absence of oxygenated arterial blood to a specific area or prolonged oxygen demand exceeding supply. Most MIs are associated with long-term *atherosclerotic heart disease* (ASHD), but may be caused by any of the following:

1. Coronary thrombosis (most common);
2. Coronary artery spasm;
3. Acute volume overload;
4. Persistent hypotension;
5. Acute hypoxia.

Signs and Symptoms

1. Substernal or epigastric pain/discomfort:
   a. Acts like anginal pain, but persists;
   b. Severe (crushing, aching, squeezing) or mild-to-moderate pain. May be improperly perceived as indigestion;
   c. Often radiates to arm, shoulder, neck, jaw, or back.
   d. Is not relieved by rest, oxygen, and/or nitroglycerine;
   e. Not affected by movement, deep breathing, change of position;
   f. Often occurs at rest, without physical exertion;
   g. May be "silent" (no pain at all).
2. Referred pain (may present as neck, shoulder, arm, or jaw pain *without* any chest pain).

3. Associated symptoms:
   a. Shortness of breath (dyspnea);
   b. Sweating (diaphoresis);
   c. Nausea;
   d. Pale skin color (pallor);
   e. Anxiety/apprehension;
   f. Extreme weakness/lethargy;
4. Vital signs:
   a. BP may be normal, elevated, or low (depends on underlying cause);
   b. Pulse may be normal, fast, slow, or irregular (depends upon underlying cause and possible arrhythmias);
   c. Respirations may be normal or increased.
5. Dysrhythmias offer the most common complications in the first few hours of a myocardial infarction. Watch especially for:
   a. Ventricular fibrillation;
   b. Ventricular tachycardia;
   c. Significant PVCs (premature ventricular contractions).

Note: All patients with chest pain and compatible history should be presumed to have an AMI (acute myocardial infarction) until proven otherwise. It can be a tragic mistake to assume that a younger patient is not suffering from an MI if signs/symptoms are present.

Prehospital Management

1. Place at rest, maintain good airway position;
2. Administer high-flow oxygen (exercise caution with COPD patients);
3. Monitor ECG (be prepared to treat dysrhythmias);
4. Vital signs and history (while conducting exam and treating);
5. Establish IV of D5W (TKO);
6. Sublingual nitroglycerine (if *not* hypotensive);
7. Consider morphine sulphate to achieve:
   a. Pain relief (which also reduces sympathetic discharge);
   b. Decrease in myocardial oxygen demand by decreasing venous return and systemic vascular resistance (SVR).
8. Calm transport to hospital. (if stable)

Left Ventricular Failure (Pulmonary Edema) Failure of the left ventricle to eject an adequate amount of blood forward with each contraction causes a back-up of blood into the pulmonary circulation. Eventually, fluid from the blood is forced from the capillaries into alveolar sacs, interfering with proper respiration (pulmonary edema) and resulting in significant hypoxia. Myocardial infarction is one common cause of left ventricular failure. Other causes include dysrhythmias, damage from previous MIs, chronic hypertension, disease/dysfunction of the heart valves, cardiac muscle disease, and trauma to the heart muscle. AN ACCURATE ASSESSMENT OF LUNG SOUNDS IS ESSENTIAL.

Signs and Symptoms

1. Severe respiratory distress, possibly including:
   a. Orthopnea (dyspnea when supine);
   b. Productive cough (white sputum = early stage, pink sputum = late);
   c. Paroxysmal nocturnal dyspnea (dyspnea at night, while sleeping).
2. Cyanosis (if severe).
3. Diaphoresis (sweating).
4. Abnormal lung sounds:
   a. Rales (fluid in alveoli, sounds like wet "popping" and doesn't clear with coughing;
   b. Rhonchi (fluid in the larger airways, harsher drier sound);
   c. Wheezes (airways spasm, high pitched whistling).
5. JVD (jugular vein distention) at 45 degrees of head elevation.
6. Vital signs:
   a. BP elevated;
   b. Pulse rapid (and possibly irregular);
   c. Respirations fast and labored.
7. LOC (level of consciousness) may or may not be diminished.

Prehospital Management

1. Sit up with feet dangling (to decrease venous return);
2. Administer high-flow oxygen (exercise caution with COPD patients);
3. Positive pressure ventilation (if patient can tolerate);

4. IV of D5W (TKO) (significant amounts of fluid must be withheld);
5. Monitor ECG;
6. Consider rotating tourniquets (rare—check local protocols);
7. Consider the following medications:
   a. Morphine sulfate (decreases venous return, reduces myocardial oxygen demands, reduces anxiety);
   b. Nitroglycerine—sublingually (for peripheral dilation);
   c. Furosemide (Lasix) (initial relaxant effect on venous system within 5 minutes, then diuretic effect to reduce intravascular volume);
   d. Aminophylline (bronchodilation).
8. Rapid transport (this is a true emergency).

Right Ventricular Failure This disorder is characterized by a failure of the right ventricle to eject an adequate amount of blood forward with each contraction, causing a back-up of blood into the venous system. Eventually, fluid from the blood is forced from the capillaries into the tissue, resulting in peripheral edema. The most common cause of right ventricular failure is left ventricular failure. Other causes include chronic hypertension, myocardial infarction, *chronic obstructive pulmonary disease* (COPD), pulmonary embolus, or trauma to the heart muscle.

Signs and Symptoms

1. Tachycardia (the body trying to compensate for reduced stroke volume);
2. JVD (jugular vein distention);
3. Peripheral edema (may be "pitting" if severe).

Prehospital Management

1. Place at rest with head elevated;
2. Administer high-flow oxygen (exercise caution with COPD patients);
3. Monitor ECG;
4. IV of D5W (TKO);
5. Watch for symptoms of left ventricular failure;
6. Smooth transport.

Cardiogenic Shock The most severe form of heart failure, cardiogenic shock occurs when the left ventricle fails to meet the metabolic needs of the body (even after correction of dysrhythmias, hypovolemia, and so on). All compensatory mechanisms have been exhausted. Usually this is the result of extensive myocardial infarction, but may be precipitated by accumulation of damage from previous MIs or trauma to the heart.

Signs and Symptoms

1. Signs and symptoms of acute myocardial infarction (AMI);
2. Hypotension (usually less than 80 systolic);
3. Rapid pulse (usual rhythm will be sinus tachycardia);
4. Rapid breathing (may have pronounced pulmonary edema);
5. Altered level of consciousness (LOC) (anywhere from apprehension to lethargy to unconsciousness);
6. Cyanosis or pronounced pallor;
7. Cool, clammy skin;
8. JVD (jugular vein distention).

Prehospital Management

1. Begin transport as soon as possible, place in supine position;
2. Administer high-flow oxygen;
3. IV of D5W (TKO);
4. Monitor ECG (be sure to document rhythm);
5. Watch for development of pulmonary edema;
6. Consider Dopamine (Intropin) to support blood pressure;
7. Consider PASG (pneumatic anti-shock garment) as fluid challenge—but only if pulmonary edema is *not* present). NOT universally accepted.
8. Rapid transportation. DO NOT DELAY IN THE FIELD—MORTALITY RATE OF CARDIOGENIC SHOCK IS 80-90%.

Other Cardiovascular Emergencies

Aneurysms A dilation of a blood vessel. We will discuss atherosclerotic, dissecting, and traumatic aneurysms.

Abdominal Aneurysm Atherosclerosis weakens the wall of the aorta (usually below the renal arteries) and causes a "ballooning" of the vessel. Men are much more likely to suffer this condition than women (10 times more likely).

Signs and Symptoms

1. Abdominal pain (possibility with accompanying back pain);
2. Hypotension (and related shock symptoms);
3. Palpable pulsatile mass (depending upon size and stage);
4. Decreased or absent femoral pulse;
5. May be masked as GI (gastrointestinal) bleed.

Prehospital Management

1. Begin transport as soon as possible, get definitive history;
2. Administer high-flow oxygen;
3. Apply PASG (pneumatic anti-shock garment);
4. Two large-bore IVs of LR (wide open)—after enroute;
5. Rapid transport.

Dissecting Aortic Aneurysm This disorder begins with a small tear in the inner wall (intima) of the aorta which allows blood to enter and travel under the intima—usually creating a hematoma. Two-thirds of these conditions involve the ascending aorta. Most are due to degenerative disease of connective tissue and are often accompanied by chronic hypertension. Once begun, these false passages may extend to the thoracic and abdominal aorta, coronary arteries, carotids, subclavian, and so on. They can rupture at any time.

Signs and Symptoms

1. Severe "tearing" substernal chest pain. It may radiate, perhaps to the back, "right between the shoulder blades."
2. Elevated blood pressure. This is a confusing sign, because the patient presents as "shocky" because of impaired perfusion.
3. Dissection into other arteries may precipitate some of the following:
   a. Syncope;
   b. CVA (cerebrovascular accident);

FIGURE 16.31.

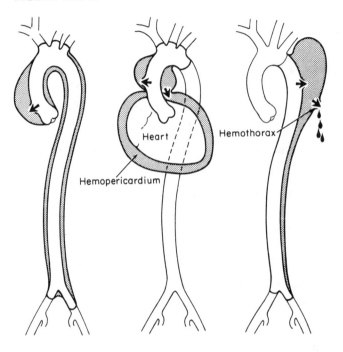

Heart

Hemothorax

Hemopericardium

c. Decreased or absent pulses;

d. Pericardial tamponade;

e. Heart failure;

f. AMI (acute myocardial infarction);

g. Different readings in arm blood pressure.

Prehospital Management

1. Limit movement, place immediately at rest;

2. Administer high-flow oxygen;

3. (PASG) pneumatic anti-shock garment in place—in case of rupture;

4. Two large-bore IVs of LR (after enroute);

5. Consider morphine sulfate if diagnoses seems solid;

6. Rapid, smooth transport.

Acute Arterial Occlusion This is a sudden occlusion of arterial blood flow due to trauma, thrombosis, or embolus.

Signs and Symptoms

1. Sudden excrutiating pain (in 80% of cases);
2. Pallor and cool skin (or cyanosis/mottling) below occlusion;
3. Shock present in some occlusions (such as mesenteric);
4. Decreased or absent pulses distal to the occlusion.

Prehospital Management

1. If mesenteric, treat shock with oxygen, IV fluids, morphine, and so on.
2. If extremity is involved, protect affected limb (do not allow weight-bearing). Flow must be re-established within 4-8 hours.
3. Rapid smooth transport.

Cardiac Arrest/Sudden Death Sudden death (death within one hour of onset of symptoms) has many causes other than cardiac disease, such as:

Drowning	Trauma
Electrocution	Acid-base imbalance
Electrolyte imbalance	Drug reactions
Hypothermia	Hypoxia

Cardiac arrest may be the first indication of cardiac disease in a significant number of patients, and risk factors for arrest are the same as for atherosclerotic heart disease (ASHD). Dysrhythmias associated with cardiac arrest include:

1. Ventricular fibrillation (V-fib)—60-70%;
2. Ventricular tachycardia;
3. Asystole;
4. Profound bradycardia/heart blocks;
5. Electromechanical dissociation (EMD).

Current ACLS (Advanced Cardiac Life Support) Algorithms as set forth by the American Heart Association are considered to be a reasonable blueprint of care for prehospital emergency cardiac care. These are contained in an appendix at the end of this text. Local medical control may choose to alter such protocols to the needs of their particular area.

Drug Review

Electrolyte Solutions

Sodium Bicarbonate (NaHCO₃)

Mechanism of Action: An alkalyzing agent used to treat metabolic acidosis.

Indications:

1. Cardiac arrest—in specific circumstances, after first line medications have been unsuccessful;
2. Other forms of metabolic acidosis;
3. Hyperkalemia.

Precautions:

1. May overcorrect acidosis (without blood gases);
2. Vigorous effective ventilation must occur concurrently;
3. Do not mix with catacholamines (will inactivate) or calcium (will precipitate);
4. Avoid use in the presence of hypokalemia.

Side Effects:

1. Metabolic alkalosis;
2. Acute hypokalemia;
3. Carbon dioxide retention (without vigorous ventilations);
4. Salt and water overload.

Dosage: 1 mEq/kg IV initially in *extended* cardiac arrest, followed by 1/2 mEq/kg in 10-15 minutes.

Pediatric Dosage: 1-2 mEq/kg in *extended* cardiac arrest.

How Supplied: Prefilled syringe—50 ml of 8.4% solution (1 mEq/ml).

Calcium Chloride (CaCl)—(NOT RECOMMENDED IN CARDIAC ARREST/ RESUSCITATION)

Mechanism of Action:

1. Increases myocardial contractility;
2. Neutralizes effects of calium channel-blockers.

Indications:

1. To reverse overdose of calium channel-blocker (or magnesium sulfate);
2. Acute hyperkalemia;
3. Hypocalcemia;
4. Calcium gluconate is sometimes used to relieve pain and muscle spasms caused by a black widow spider bite.

Precautions:

1. Use with caution in patients on digitalis (may precipitate digitalis toxicity);
2. Rapid administration while heart is beating may cause reflex slowing of heart rate;
3. Causes necrosis and tissue irritation if infiltrated at IV site;
4. Do not administer with Sodium Bicarbonate.

Side Effects:

1. May increase cardiac irritability in presence of digitalis;
2. May cause vasospasm in coronary and cerebral arteries;
3. See other precautions above.

Dosage: 2-4 mg/kg IV of 10% solution (100 mg/ml), IV. Repeat at 10 minute intervals if considered necessary.

How Supplied:

1. Prefilled syringe: 10 ml of a 10% solution;
2. Ampule: 10 ml of a 10% solution.

Antidysrhythmics

Atropine Sulphate

Mechanism of Action:

1. Parasympatholytic agent that reduces (blocks) vagal tone;
2. Increases sinus node discharge rate;
3. Improves AV conduction;

4. May reduce chances of ectopic ventricular activity (by increasing sinus rate);
5. May initiate a cardiac rhythm in asystole.

Indications:

1. Bradycardia (with marked hypotension or frequent ventricular ectopic beats);
2. Third degree AV block;
3. Ventricular asystole;
4. Antidote for organophosphate poisoning.

Precautions:

1. Increases myocardial oxygen demand (by > rate);
2. Not appropriate for bradycardia unless signs of poor perfusion or ventricular ectopics are present;
3. Be alert to history of glaucoma;
4. Do not give in doses < 0.5 mg—it may precipitate reflex bradycardia (or ventricular fibrillation).

Side Effects: Ventricular tachycardia/fibrillation have been reported after IV administration.
Dosage:

1. 0.5 mg IV repeated at 5-minute intervals until desired effect is achieved (up to 2.0 mg);
2. 1.0 mg as initial dose for asystole;
3. Higher doses may be ordered for organophosphate poisoning.

Note: May be given through endotracheal tube (1-2 mg diluted in 10 ml of normal saline or sterile water).
Pediatric Dosage: 0.01-0.03 mg/kg (0.1 mg minimum).
How Supplied: Usually in prefilled syringe with 1 mg in 10 ml (0.1 mg/ml).

Lidocaine Hydrochloride

Mechanism of Action:

1. Suppresses dysrhythmias of ventricular ectopic origin;
2. Elevates ventricular fibrillation threshold;
3. Depresses conduction and interrupts re-entry pathways in ischemic tissue.

Indications:

1. PVCs, if:
   a. Frequent (more than 5/minute);
   b. Multiformed;
   c. Close-coupled (R-on-T phenomenon);
   d. Salvos of V-Tach;
   e. PVCs of any frequency in the ischemic heart.
2. Ventricular tachycardia.
3. Recurrent ventricular fibrillation and ventricular fibrillation.
4. Prophylactically in the setting of acute MI (controversial).
5. Following successful defibrillation.

Precautions:

1. IV bolus must precede a drip (a drip by itself may take 20-30 minutes to obtain effect).
2. Lidocaine toxicity (adverse reactions usually related to CNS), may be indicated by:
   a. Seizures;
   b. Altered consciousness;
   c. Muscle twitching;
   d. Slurred speech;
   e. Hypotension;
   f. Decreased hearing;
   g. Numbness.
3. Allergy to lidocaine is not uncommon—check history.

Dosage:

1. 1 mg/kg IV bolus, followed by an immediate infusion of 2-4 mg/min IV drip. (put 1 gm lidocaine in 250 ml of D5W [4 mg/ml] and run at 30-60 gtt/min).
2. ACLS recommends an additional 0.5 mg/kg bolus be administered after 10 minutes. If ventricular ectopy persists, additional boluses of 50 mg can be given every 5 minutes up to a total dose of 225 mg.

Note: May be administered via ET tube.

Caution: Decrease dosage by 50% in the presence of reduced hepatic blood flow (AMI, CHF, shock), or if patient is > 70 years old.

Pediatric Dosage: 1 mg/kg IV bolus to a maximum of 50 mg.

How Supplied:

1. Bolus: usually in prefilled syringe containing 100 mg in 5 ml (2% solution);
2. For dilution: usually vial of 2 gm in 10 ml *or* 1 gm in 5 ml (both a 20% solution)—put in 250 ml or 500 ml of D5W with microdrip.

Bretylium Tosylate

Mechanism of Action:

1. Elevates ventricular fibrillation threshold;
2. May terminate re-entry pathways;
3. May initially increase rate and arterial pressure, then decreases same;
4. May convert ventricular fibrillation to a perfusing rhythm.
5. Does not appear to affect myocardial conductivity and contractility.

Indications:

1. Ventricular fibrillation that has not responded to defibrillation and lidocaine;
2. Recurrent ventricular fibrillation.
3. Refractory ventricular tachycardia, unresponsive to standard therapy.

Precautions:

1. Dosage should be reduced if using catacholamines;
2. Use with caution if digitalis toxicity is possible;
3. Watch for postural hypotension.

Side Effects:

1. Possible transient tachycardia and hypertension after injection;
2. Postural hypotension later;
3. Nausea and vomiting after rapid injection.

Dosage:

Ventricular fibrillation: 5 mg/kg IV (undiluted) if given rapidly. If V-fib persists (after defibrillation attempt), give 10 mg/kg IV and repeat at 15-30 minute intervals as needed to a maximum dose of 30 mg/kg (onset of action in about 2 minutes).

Recurrent ventricular tachycardia: 5-10 mg/kg (diluted to 50 ml) slow IV push over 8-10 minutes (especially in the conscious patient). This may be repeated in 1-2 hours with the same dose (onset of action 20 minutes or more).

How Supplied: Usually in ampule, 500 mg in 10 ml (50 mg/ml).

Verapamil **(Isoptin, Calan)**

Mechanism of Action:

1. Inhibits slow-channel calcium activity in cardiac and vascular smooth muscle;
2. Reduces both contractility and myocardial oxygen consumption;
3. Dilates peripheral and coronary blood vessels, reducing systemic vascular resistance;
4. Slows conduction and prolongs refractory period in AV node.

Indications:

1. Paroxysmal supraventricular tachycardia (that does not require cardioversion);

2. Atrial fibrillation/flutter (to control the rate of ventricular response);
3. May be of some benefit in treating arrhythmias due to ischemia (not proven).

Precautions:

1. May cause hypotension, so monitor BP closely;
2. Not to be used in conjunction with IV beta blockers;
3. Contraindicated in patients with AV block, sick sinus syndrome, or cardiac failure;
4. Contraindicated in patients with known WPW with atrial fibrillation/flutter.

Side Effects:

1. Transient hypotension;
2. AV block;
3. Bradycardia;
4. Heart failure.

Dosage:

1. 0.075-0.15 mg/kg IV (may be repeated in 30 minutes in 0.15 mg/kg dose), 10 mg is maximum single dose given over one minute;
2. Peak effect occurs within 3-5 minutes.

Pediatric Dosage: 0.1-0.2 mg/kg (total single dose: 0.75-2.0 mg).
How Supplied: Usually in ampule with 5.0 mg in 2 ml (2.5 mg/ml).

Procainamide
Mechanism of Action:

1. Suppresses ventricular ectopic activity (use after lidocaine has been ineffective);
2. May suppress re-entry pathways.

Indications:

1. PVCs and recurrent ventricular tachycardia (which cannot be controlled with lidocaine);
2. Persistent ventricular fibrillation.

Precautions:

1. Must monitor BP continuously, watching for hypotension caused by too rapid injection (warning signs include widening of the QRS and lengthening of the PR or QT interval);
2. May precipitate heart blocks or cardiac arrest.

Dosage: For PVCs and ventricular tachycardia, 100 mg every 5 minutes (20 mg/minute) until one of the following occurs:

1. The dysrhythmia is suppressed;
2. Hypotension ensues;
3. The QRS complex widens by 50%;
4. A total of 1 gram has been injected.

How Supplied: Usually in vials:

1. 1000 mg in 10 ml (100 mg/ml);
2. 1000 mg in 2 ml (500 mg/ml).

Sympathomimetic Agents

Epinephrine (Adrenalin)

Mechanism of Action: Endogenous catacholamine with both alpha and beta receptor stimulating actions:

1. Increases heart rate;
2. Increases myocardial contractility;
3. Increases systemic vascular resistance;
4. Increases arterial blood pressure;
5. Increases myocardial oxygen demand;

6. Increases automaticity of ectopic foci;
7. Bronchodilation;
8. May convert fine V-fib to coarse V-fib;
9. May help restore electrical activity in asystole.

Indications: First-line drug in cardiac arrest:

1. Ventricular fibrillation;
2. Asystole;
3. Electromechanical dissociation (EMD);
4. Severe bradycardias unresponsive to atropine;
5. Anaphylaxis.

Note: Epinephrine produces a desirable redistribution of blood flow during CPR and elevates coronary perfusion pressure.
Precautions:

1. Don't mix with sodium bicarbonate, as it may neutralize epinephrine;
2. Avoid intracardiac injection unless last resort—it can cause intractable V-fib (and other problems).

Side Effects: Ventricular dysrhythmias. BE AWARE of increased myocardial oxygen demand caused by the actions of epinephrine.
Dosage:

1. 0.5-1.0 mg of 1:10,000 solution IV, repeated at 5 minute intervals as needed;
2. As IV drip (to increase and sustain BP and heart rate), 1 mg. in 250 ml D5W—infuse at 1-4 mcg/min.

Note: May be given down ET tube—use 1 mg (10 ml of 1:10,000).
Pediatric Dosage: 0.01 mg/kg of 1:10,000 IV bolus; in anaphylaxis: 0.1 cc of 1:1,000 solution IM (or 0.01 mg/kg).
How Supplied:

Prefilled syringe—1.0 mg in 10 ml (0.1 mg/ml);
Ampule—1.0 mg in 1 ml [1:1,000 solution]—use in anaphylaxis.

Norepinephrine (Levophed)

Mechanism of Action: Has both alpha and beta effects, including:

1. Potent peripheral vasoconstriction;
2. Increased myocardial contractility (beta 1);
3. Renal and mesenteric constriction;
4. Increases BP very quickly.

Indications:

1. Hemodynamically significant hypotension (usually cardiogenic shock) that does not respond to other sympathomimetics;
2. Particularly effective when total peripheral resistance is low (as with neurogenic and anaphylactic shock).

Note: If used, norepinephrine should be strictly temporary, with treatment directed toward correction of the underlying problem.

Precautions:

1. Contraindicated in cases of hypovolemia;
2. Avoid use in hypotensive bradycardias—treat the bradycardia;
3. Increases myocardial oxygen demand significantly—potentially causing more damage in an AMI—thus it is used as a last resort in patients with ischemic heart disease;
4. Monitor BP closely—a decrease in cardiac output may occur in some cases (due to its primary action of increasing systemic vascular resistance);
5. Monitor ECG closely—norepinephrine may cause dysrhythmias;
6. Local tissue necrosis and sloughing occurs if IV infiltrates at injection site.

Side Effects:

1. Reflex bradycardia;
2. Severe hypertension;
3. Dysrhythmias.

Dosage: IV drip only: put 4 mg Levophed in 250 ml D5W (yields 16 mcg/ml). Begin at 2-3 ml/min, titrate to maintain BP at 90-100 systolic.

How Supplied: 4 ml ampule containing 4mg (1 mg/ml).

Isoproterenol (Isuprel)

Mechanism of Action: Isoproterenol is a pure beta stimulator which exhibits several dose-related effects:

1. Increased heart rate;
2. Increased contractility;
3. Increased myocardial oxygen demand;
4. Decreased peripheral vascular resistance;
5. Bronchodilation.

Indications: Hemodynamically significant bradycardia unresponsive to atropine (in the patient who still has a pulse).

Precautions:

1. Isoproterenol causes a significant increase in myocardial oxygen demand—do not use in patients with ischemic heart disease (AMI);
2. Monitor ECG—it can induce serious arrhythmias or worsen tachyarrhythmias.
3. Monitor blood pressure carefully when maintaining a drip—it can cause hypertension.

Side Effects:

1. Tachycardia;
2. Ventricular dysrhythmias (V-tach or V-fib)—IF SO, SLOW OR STOP INFUSION!;
3. Infarct extension.

Dosage: Put 1 or 2 mg Isuprel in 250 ml D5W (yields 4 mcg/ml or 8 mcg/ml), using microdrip. Drip 2-20 mcg/min, titrated to heart rate and BP response.

Pediatric Dosage: 0.1-1.0 mg/kg/min.—start drip at 0.1 mcg/kg/min.

How Supplied: Usually 1.0 mg in 5 ml ampule (0.2 mg/ml).

Dopamine (Intropin)
Mechanism of Action:

1. Stimulates alpha, beta and dopamine receptor sites—it's actions depend on dose level:
   a. 1-2 mcg/kg/min.—dilates renal and mesenteric vessels (with no appreciable effect on the heart rate or BP;
   b. 2-10 mcg/kg/min.—increases cardiac output (beta effect);
   c. 10-20 mcg/kg/min.—causes peripheral vasoconstriction (alpha effect) and an increase in BP—may begin to cause renal vasoconstriction;
   d. Above 20 mcg/kg/min.—alpha effect reverses dilation of renal and mesenteric vessels and decreases flow through these vessels.
2. Chemical precursor of epinephrine.
3. Increases myocardial oxygen demand (though less than Isoproterenol).

Indications:

1. Cardiogenic shock;
2. Shock syndrome (if not hypovolemic).

Precautions:

1. Do not mix with sodium bicarbonate (may be neutralized);
2. Contraindicated for hypovolemic shock and hypertensive crisis;
3. Monitor infusion rate carefully (this can easily get away from you in the field).
4. Infiltration at IV site can cause tissue necrosis and sloughing;
5. Potentiated by MAO inhibitors (Parnate, Marplan, Nardil)—so decrease dose if these drugs are in patient history.

Side Effects:

1. Tachydysrhythmias, ectopic beats;
2. Dyspnea, angina;
3. Nausea, vomiting;
4. Headache, excessive vasoconstriction.

Dosage: IV DRIP ONLY: Put 200 mg dopamine in 250 ml D5W (800 mcg/ml) with microdrip, begin infusion at 2-5 mcg/kg/min.—titrate upward to desired response (see mechanisms of action).

Pediatric Dosage: 2-10 mcg/kg/min.

How Supplied: 200 mg in 5 cc vial (40 mg/ml).

Drugs for Myocardial Ischemia and Pain

Oxygen

Mechanism of Action: An odorless, tasteless, and colorless gas necessary for proper cellular metabolism. By supplementing inspired air with oxygen, higher oxygen levels can be achieved in the blood and at the tissue level.

Indications:

1. Suspected hypoxemia or respiratory distress from any cause;
2. Acute chest pain in which AMI is suspected;
3. Shock from any cause;
4. Major trauma;
5. Carbon monoxide poisoning. Many other situations for appropriate oxygen use are conceivable.

Precautions: Use with caution in COPD patients, but do not withhold if needed. Instead, be ready to assist ventilations if necessary.

Note: Nasal cannulas are effective nose and mouth-breathing patients.

Side Effects:

1. Non-humidified oxygen may irritate mucous membranes;
2. No danger of "oxygen toxicity" exists in the prehospital setting.

Dosage/Administration:

1. Low flow = 1-2 L/min.;
2. Moderate flow = 4-6 L/min.;
3. High flow = 10-15 L/min.

May administer by all sizes of masks, cannulas, demand valve (mask or mouthpiece), and so forth.

How Supplied: Usually by various sizes of pressurized tanks (full = 2,000 lb pressure or greater). Regulators reduce the pressure and meter the flow.

Nitroglycerine
Mechanism of Action:

1. Relaxes vascular smooth muscle;
2. May increase coronary blood flow (by dilating coronary arteries and enhancing collateral circulation flow);
3. Relieves coronary artery spasm;
4. Reduces myocardial oxygen demand (and work) by dilation of peripheral vascular bed (and reduction of preload and afterload).

Indications:

1. Ischemic myocardial pain (angina, AMI);
2. Pulmonary edema, secondary to left ventricular failure;
3. Hypertensive crisis.

Precautions:

1. Do *not* use in hypotension/shock (may cause a sudden drop in BP);
2. Monitor BP closely before and after administration;
3. Rapidly deteriorates, especially with exposure to air, light or temperature extremes.

Side Effects:

COMMON: Headache, dizziness, flushing, burning under tongue;
SERIOUS: Hypotension and reflex tachycardia (may respond to leg elevation, lowering of head or anti-shock trousers).

Dosage: 0.3-0.4 mg (1/200-1/150 grains) sublingually every 3-5 minutes until discomfort is relieved (to a total of 3 tablets). Do not swallow.
How Supplied: 0.3 mg (1/200 grain), 0.4 mg (1/150 grain), 0.6 mg (1/100 grain) tablets, in bottles of 100. Preferred for field use: Nitrolingual Spray (provides metered spray of 0.4 mg and has long shelf life).

Nitrous Oxide (Nitronox)

Mechanism of Action: A 50:50 blending of nitrous oxide and oxygen.

1. Produces CNS depression and decreases sensitivity to many forms of pain;
2. Provides supplemental oxygen (50%) while relieving pain with a short-duration easily-reversible agent;
3. The beneficial effects of nitronox dissipate within 2-5 minutes after discontinuing use.

Indications: All types of pain, including:

1. Myocardial infarction;
2. Burns;
3. Fractures;
4. Internal tissue pain (kidney stones, appendicitis, and so on).

Precautions: Be sure ambulance is well-ventilated. Do not administer nitronox in the presence of these conditions:

1. Decreased level of consciousness;
2. Chest trauma;
3. ETOH intoxication;
4. Abdominal distension;
5. Respiratory problems (COPD, pulmonary edema, edema, pneumothorax, severe SOB);
6. Cyanosis with Nitronox administration;
7. Inability to comply with instructions;
8. Pregnancy;
9. Shock (when higher oxygen concentration levels are required).

Note: If using for myocardial pain, be sure to give O_2 by face mask during intervals of non-use and immediately after its use is terminated.

Side Effects: These symptoms are sometimes experienced while inhaling nitrous oxide:

1. Drowsiness (common);
2. Lightheadedness, numbness, tingling and/or slurred speech;
3. Nausea and vomiting;
4. Minor headache;
5. Amnesia, euphoria or confusion.

Dosage: Intermittently inhaled through a demand valve via mask or mouthpiece as needed for pain control (or until very drowsy). Should always be self-administered by patient and O_2 must be given during intervals that nitronox is not being used.

Note: Self-administration is a safety procedure—should the patient's level of consciousness drop, mask or mouthpiece falls away.

How Supplied: Usually as package of 2 tanks with pre-mix valve, demand valve and mask and/or mouthpiece.

Morphine Sulphate

Mechanism of Action:

1. Extremely potent narcotic analgesic;
2. Dilates peripheral vasculature (reducing preload and afterload and decreasing myocardial oxygen demand);
3. Reduces respiratory rate and tidal volume;
4. Reduces apprehension and anxiety.

Indications:

1. Acute myocardial infarction;
2. Acute pulmonary edema;
3. Pain control.

Precautions:

1. Must be administered slowly (2 mg/min IV);
2. Monitor BP closely;
3. Contraindicated in hypotension;
4. Use caution if respiratory depression already exists (or if patient has long-term COPD).

Side Effects:

1. Respiratory depression (be ready to assist ventilations);
2. Hypotension;
3. Nausea and vomiting;
4. Constricted pupils;
5. Decreased level of consciousness.

Note: Effects may be reversed with naloxone.

Dosage: 2-10 mg IV (given in 2-5 mg increments until pain relief or desired hemodynamic effects achieved). May be repeated in 5-30 minutes if needed.

How Supplied: Prefilled syringe: 20 mg in 10 ml (2 mg/ml). Tubex syringe: 10 mg in 1 ml. Vial: 8 mg in 1 ml. These ranges may vary.

Meperidine **(Demerol)**

Mechanism of Action: Narcotic analgesic used for pain control.

Indications: Moderate to severe pain.

Precautions: Contraindicated in the following:

1. MAO inhibitors;
2. Head injury;
3. CNS or respiratory depression. Use caution in undiagnosed abdominal pain and pregnant patients.

Side Effects:

1. Nausea and vomiting;
2. Respiratory depression.

Note: Effects may be reversed with naloxone.

Dosage: 50-100 mg IM or IV slowly—give in 5-10 mg increments and titrate to effect.

How Supplied: Prefilled syringe: 200 mg in 2 ml (100 mg/ml).

Other Important Drugs

Furosemide (Lasix)

Mechanism of Action: Potent diuretic that:

1. Inhibits sodium reabsorption in the kidneys;
2. Causes diuresis;
3. Decreases venous return (preload) through venous dilation. When given IV Lasix acts rapidly (5 minutes), with peak effect occurring in 30-60 minutes and a total duration of 2 hours.

Indications:

1. Acute pulmonary edema;
2. Cerebral edema following cardiac arrest;
3. CHF;
4. Acute hypertensive emergencies.

Precautions:

1. Can cause profound diuresis—so monitor BP closely;
2. Contraindicated for pregnant women;
3. Contraindicated in hypovolemic states;
4. Do not use in known hypokalemia.

Side Effects:

1. Nausea and vomiting.
2. Possible volume depletion and dehydration.
3. Potassium depletion (especially bad for digitalis patients).

Dosage: 0.5-2.0 mg/kg IV bolus, administered over 1-2 minutes. If there is no effect with the bolus, a drip of 0.25-0.75 mg/kg/hr may produce adequate diuresis, even in patients with renal problems.

Pediatric Dosage: 1 mg/kg IV bolus.

How Supplied: Ampules: 20 mg in 2 ml (10 mg/ml), 100 mg in 10 ml (10 mg/ml).

Naloxone (Narcan)

Mechanism of Action: A narcotic antagonist which aggressively binds to narcotic sites while exhibiting negligible effects of its own—effective duration is 1-4 hours.

Indications:

1. Reversal of narcotic effects (particularly respiratory depression) due to narcotic drugs (morphine, Demerol, heroin, Dilaudid, Percodan, codeine, Lomotil, Talwin, and so on);
2. Diagnostically in any coma of unknown origin (to rule out or reverse narcotic depression).

Precautions:

1. May precipitate frank withdrawal symptoms in patient physically dependent on narcotics;
2. Be prepared to restrain a violent patient (you may rouse him/her from an expensive "nod");
3. If the duration of the narcotic is longer than the duration of the Narcan, patient may slip back into coma—so monitor closely.

Side Effects: None significant.

Dosage: 0.4-2.0 mg slow IV push (may be repeated at 2-3 minute intervals for 2-3 doses). Some systems are using higher doses.

Note: Darvon overdose may require larger doses.

Pediatric Dosage: 0.01 mg/kg IV.

How Supplied:

Prefilled syringes: 0.4 mg in 1 ml, higher doses becoming available.
Ampules: 0.4 mg in 1 ml, 2.0 mg in 1 ml.

Diphenhydramine (Benadryl)

Mechanism of Action:

1. An antihistamine which blocks action of histamines released from cells during an allergic reaction;
2. Direct CNS effects, which may be stimulant or (more common) depressant, depending upon individual;

3. Anticholinergic, antiparkinsonism effect which is used to treat acute dystonic reactions to antipsychotic drugs;
4. May prevent or ease symptoms of motion sickness.

Indications:

1. Second-line drug in anaphylaxis/allergic reactions;
2. Counters some effects of antipsychotic drugs;
3. Parkinson's disease;
4. Sometimes used to sedate children.

Precautions:

1. Children may demonstrate excitability rather than drowsiness;
2. May depress respirations;
3. Additive effect may be seen with ETOH and other depressants;
4. Contraindicated in patients receiving MAO inhibitors, patients with COPD or asthma, pregnant patients and newborns;
5. Do not give subcutaneously (irritating).

Side Effects:

1. Drowsiness, sedation, confusion, headache;
2. Blurred vision, dizziness, headache, nausea, and vomiting;
3. Tremors, palpitations, convulsions;
4. Excitability in some (especially children);
5. May cause shortened diastole, atrial tachycardia and changes in T-waves.

Dosage: 50 mg slow IV push or deep IM.
Pediatric Dosage: Children up to 12: 1-2 mg/kg (should not exceed 50 mg).
How Supplied: Ampules: 50 mg in 2 ml (25 mg/ml), 50 mg in 1 ml (50 mg/ml). Prefilled syringes: 50 mg in 1 ml (50 mg/ml).

Aminophylline (Theophylline)

Mechanism of Action: This drug is a combination of theophylline and ethylene diamine that acts to:

1. Relax smooth muscle of the bronchial airways (bronchodilator);
2. Dilate peripheral blood vessels;
3. Stimulate cardiac, cerebral, and skeletal muscles;
4. Cause diuresis.

Indications:

1. Bronchospasm;
2. Respiratory distress due to:
   a. Cardiac PND and CHF;
   b. Asthma/status asthmaticus;
   c. Emphysema.

Precautions:

1. Monitor ECG during administration;
2. Decrease dose in patients with severe cardiac or hepatic disease;
3. Administer slowly (to avoid toxic and side effects);
4. If patient already takes oral theophylline preparations, document the regimen and last dose/time taken.

Side Effects:

1. Tachycardia and other dysrhythmias;
2. Hypotension;
3. Nausea and vomiting;
4. CNS—headache, nervousness, dizziness, agitation, and light-headedness.

Dosage: 250-500 mg (5-6 mg/kg) added to 50-100 ml of D5W (with microdrip) and administered IV over 20 minutes.

Note: Not a first-line cardiac drug.

Pediatric Dosage: 3-6 mg/kg.
How Supplied:

Ampules: 250 or 500 mg.

Diazepam (Valium)
Mechanism of Action:

1. Sedative effects;
2. Terminates seizure activity;
3. Relaxes skeletal muscle.

Indications:

1. Acute seizure disorders (such as status epilepticus);
2. Sedation for syncronized cardioversion;
3. Occasionally used in field for the control of extremely combative patients.
4. Reduction of anxiety.

Precautions:

1. Use with caution in hypotensive patients;
2. Monitor respiratory status—can cause respiratory depression;
3. Use with caution in COPD patients or patients with respiratory depression from any source;
4. Effects pronounced in patients who have taken depressant drugs (or ETOH);
5. Don't mix with other drugs;
6. Avoid use in pregnant patients.

Side Effects:

1. Respiratory depression;
2. Dizziness;
3. Transient hypotension.

Dosage: 2.0-10 mg slow IV bolus (5 mg/min.) until desired effect is achieved.

Pediatric Dosage: .05-.1 mg/kg IV slowly.

How Supplied: Prefilled syringe: 10 mg in 2 ml (5 mg/ml).

Propanolol Hydrochloride (Inderal)

Mechanism of Action: A beta-adrenergic receptor (beta 1 and 2) blocking agent that:

1. Decreases automaticity;
2. Decreases conductivity;
3. Decreases ventricular contractility (and thus stroke volume);
4. Causes bronchoconstriction;
5. Decreases cardiac work load and oxygen consumption.

Indications:

1. Recurrent ventricular tachycardia and fibrillation;
2. Rapid supraventricular dysrhythmias;
3. Prevention of angina pectoris (clinical).

Precautions:

1. Contraindicated in asthma and COPD;
2. Caution in patients with AMI (or post cardiac arrest).

Side Effects: May cause:

1. Acute heart failure (CHF);
2. Severe sinus bradycardia (correct with atropine and/or Isuprel);
3. AV block (all kinds).

Dosage: 1-3 mg IV slowly every 5 minutes (take the whole 5 minutes to give it), not to exceed a total dose of 0.1 mg/kg with careful monitoring of BP and ECG. Dose may be repeated to a total of 3-5 mg.

Note: Most areas do not use this drug in prehospital care—but you will find it frequently in patient homes as oral medication.

How Supplied: Ampules: 1 mg in 1 ml (dilute to 10 ml for better control).

Digitalis (Digoxin, Lanoxin)
Mechanism of Action:

1. Increases the force of ventricular contractions;
2. Slows impulse conduction through the AV node;
3. Slows cardiac rate;
4. Increases cardiac output in diseased hearts.

Indications:

1. CHF;
2. Rapid supraventricular dysrhythmias (atrial fib, atrial flutter, PAT).

Precautions: Digitalis toxicity is a common problem—most of the adverse effects reflect such toxicity.

Side Effects:

1. Loss of appetite, nausea and vomiting;
2. Yellow vision, blurred vision, spots, "shimmering";
3. Any cardiac dysrhythmia—may not respond to traditional antidys-rhythmic drugs;
4. Headache, weakness, insomnia and depression.

Dosage: 0.50-0.75 mg per 45 kg (100 lb) given in increments.

Note: Most areas do not use this drug in prehospital care—but you will find Digitalis frequently in patient homes as oral medication, usually 0.25 mg tablets.

How Supplied:

Tablets: 0.25 mg each.

50% Dextrose (D50W)
Mechanism of Action: The body's basic fuel, it is regulated by insulin, which stimulates storage of excess glucose from the bloodstream and glucagon, which mobilizes stored glucose into the bloodstream.

Indications:

1. Hypoglycemic states (usually associated with insulin shock in diabetes);

2. Coma or unconsciousness of unknown etiology;
3. Seizures of unknown origin;
4. CPR patients when cause of arrest unknown;
5. Chronic ETOH abusers;
6. Hypothermia.

Precautions:

1. Draw blood sample before administering;
2. If available quickly, test blood with reagent strip or glucometer before administration;
3. Use with caution in patients with suspected low potassium levels;
4. Contraindicated with intracranial (or intraspinal) bleeds;
5. Infiltration at injection site can cause necrosis (be aware while injecting);
6. With known alcoholic patients, administer 50 mg of IV Thiamine before giving dextrose.

Side Effects: Remarkably free of side effects—it should be utilized whenever a question exists. One bolus usually raises the blood sugar 50-100 mg%, and it is not uncommon for patients suffering from hypoglycemia to wake up almost immediately after injection.

Dosage: 50 cc of 50% Dextrose IV (after drawing blood, if possible) into a secure vein. Give orally if patient is awake and able to handle secretions.

How Supplied:

Prefilled syringes: 50 ml of 50% Dextrose (in water)—D50W.

Squeezable tubes: Tubes of glucose gel for oral administration (smearing on the mucosa).

Oxytocin (Pitocin)
Mechanism of Action:

1. Increases electrical and contractile activity in uterine smooth muscle;
2. Initiates (or enhances) rhythmic contractions at any time during pregnancy (uterus is more sensitive at term).

Pitocin exerts its effect within minutes, has a very short half-life and is rapidly inactivated and excreted.

Indications:

1. Control of severe postpartum uterine bleeding (especially if uterine massage is ineffective) by stimulating immediate contraction of the uterus;
2. Labor augmentation (in hospital only!).

Precautions:

1. Must consider the possibility of more than one fetus (can cause uterine rupture in these cases and death of second fetus);
2. Administration should follow delivery of placenta whenever possible;
3. Avoid use in patient with cardiovascular disease.

Side Effects:

1. In larger doses, Pitocin can cause a transient but marked vasodilating effect and reflex tachycardia;
2. May precipitate (or worsen) cardiac arrhythmias;
3. Uterine spasm, uterine tetanic contraction or uterine rupture.

Dosage:

1. Put 10 Units (20 mg) in 500 ml NS or LR (40 mcg/ml)—run at 20-30 gtts/min (microdrip), titrated to severity of hemorrhage and uterine response;
2. 10 Units (1 ml) IM (only if unable to start IV).

How Supplied:

Ampules: 10 Units in 1 ml (20 mg).
Prefilled syringes: 10 Units in 1 ml (20 mg).

Additional Medications

Syrup of Ipecac

Mechanisms of Action: Induces vomiting, partially emptying the stomach of ingested contents. Ipecac is considered most effective when given within 30 minutes of ingestion.

Indications:

1. Suspected (or confirmed) overdose of medication;
2. Accidental (or intentional) poisoning.

Contraindications:

1. Coma or decreased level of consciousness;
2. Seizures;
3. Pregnancy;
4. Possible AMI;
5. Child under 1 year;
6. Ingestion of petroleum products (but not motor oil), corrosives (strong acids or alkalis), mineral seal oil, signal oil or furniture polish oils.

Exceptions: DO USE IPECAC if ingestion was:

1. Pesticides;
2. Heavy metal halogenated hydrocarbons;
3. Camphor-based hydrocarbons;
4. Aromatic hydrocarbons.

Side Effects: None from occasional use. Aspiration is the biggest danger.

Adult Dosage: 30 cc by mouth, followed by 2-3 glasses of water.

Pediatric Dosage: 15 cc by mouth, followed by 2-3 glasses of water (must be at least 1 year old).

How Supplied: Usually in 15 cc and 30 cc bottles, available over the counter.

Physostigmine (Antilirium)

Mechanisms of Action: This parasympathetic (cholinergic) agent reverses toxic effects of anticholinergic drugs taken in overdose.

Indications: Treatment of anticholinergic poisoning from toxic doses of:

1. Atropine;
2. Tricyclic antidepressants;
3. Jimson seeds;
4. Certain nonprescription sleep aids.

Contraindications:

1. Asthma and/or COPD;
2. Bradycardia;
3. Coronary artery disease;
4. Obstruction of the GI or urinary tract.

Side Effects:

1. Bradycardia;
2. Diaphoresis;
3. Hypersalivation;
4. Seizures (if administered too fast).

Dosage: 2 mg diluted in 10 ml D5W and given IV over 2 minutes.
How Supplied: 2 ml ampules (1 mg/ml).

Mannitol

Mechanisms of Action: Mannitol is an osmotic diuretic, remaining in the vascular space to draw fluid from the cells for eventual excretion.
Indications:

1. Treatment of cerebral edema, following closed head injury or cardiac arrest;
2. Diuresis in some drug overdoses.

Contraindications:

1. CHF and pulmonary edema;
2. Serious renal impairment;

3. Intracranial hemorrhage;

4. Pregnancy;

5. Dehydration.

Side Effects:

1. Headache and nausea;

2. Fall in serum Na+;

3. Might precipitate CHF in borderline patients.

Dosage: 500 mg/kg IV.
How Supplied: 5% or 10% solution in 1000 ml, 15% or 20% solution in 500 ml.

Thiamine

Mechanisms of Action: The use of Thiamine before giving dextrose treats a possible B-vitamin deficiency that can result in irreversible neurological damage in some alcoholics (those with Wernicke's or Korsakoff's syndrome).

Indications:

1. Suspected alcoholics who are about to be treated with dextrose.

2. Suspected Wernicke's or Korsakoff's syndrome.

Contraindications: Known allergy to Thiamine.
Side Effects: None known within prescribed dosage limits.
Dosage: 100 mg IV push before administering dextrose. Thiamine can be given IM if intravenous route is not available.

Drug Categories Defined

Digitalis Preparations—Drugs used in treatment of congestive heart failure and certain atrial dysrhythmias.

Nitrates—Drugs used to relieve anginal pain.

Antiarrythmics—Drugs that control cardiac rhythm disturbances.

Diuretics—Drugs that stimulate fluid excretion.

Antihypertensives—Drugs intended to control high blood pressure.

Anticoagulants—Drugs that inhibit the blood clotting process.

Bronchodilators—Drugs that prevent and treat bronchospasm.

Antibiotics—Drugs that combat infection.

Anticonvulsants—Drugs that inhibit seizure activity.

Antacids—Medications taken to relieve gastric acidity.

Psychotropics—The category of drugs that alter mood and behavior.

Antidepressants—Drugs given to combat chronic depression.

Antipsychotics—Drugs that alter the behavior or mentally ill subjects.

Tranquilizers—Drugs that relieve anxiety.

Methadone—Oral narcotic used in management of heroin addiction.

Patient's Medicine Cabinet

Common Antiarrhythmic Drugs	*Common Antacids*
Digoxin	Alka-Seltzer
Dilantin	Gaviscon
Inderal	Gelusil
Lanoxin	Maalox
Pronestyl	Mylanta
Quinidex	Riopan
Quinidine	Rolaids
Common Diuretics	Silain-Gel
Aldactazide	Tums
Aldactone	*Common Antipsychotic Drugs*
Aquatensen	Haldol
Diuril	Lithane
Dyazide	Mellaril
Hydrochlorothiazide	Navane
Hydrodiuril	Prolixin
Lasix	Quide
Common Nitrates	Serentil
Iso-Bid	Sparine
Isordil	Stelazine
Nitranol	Taractan
Nitrobid	Thorazine
Nitroglycerin	Tindal
Nitrostat	Trilafon
Sorbitrate	Vesprin

Common Anticonvulsants	Inhalers
Dilantin	Asthma-meter
Mesantoin	Bronkosol
Mysoline	Isuprel
Nembutal	Medihaler
Tegretol	Allupent

Common Antihypertensive Drugs

	Common Oral Hypoglycemic Drugs
Aldomet	Diabinese
Apresoline	DBI
Catapres	Dymelor
Inderal	Orinase
Minipress	Tolinase
Serpasil	

Common Bronchodilators

Common Antidepressants

Tablets:

Actifed	Adapin
Bronchobid	Aventyl
Bronkodyl	Elavil
Bronkolixir	Imipramine
Bronkotabs	Norpramine
Elixophyllin	Parnate
Marax	Sinequan
Sudafed	Tofranil
TheoDur	Tegretol
	Triavil

Suppositories:

Common Tranquilizers

Aminophylline	Atarax
Somophyllin	Equanil
Theophylline	Librax
	Librium
	Miltown
	Valium
	Vistaril

Summary

We have reviewed the anatomy and physiology of the cardiovascular system, cardiovascular disease processes and their treatment, electrical activity in the heart, ECGs and their interpretation, and an abbreviated section of applicable medications. Further investigation is necessary for serious study, but the medications discussed in this chapter do cover most of what you will find on paramedic examinations. If you already have a basic grasp on the material, you should find this an adequate review.

SELF-TEST

Chapter 16

1. Which artery supplies blood to the left ventricle?

   ANSWER: The left coronary artery supplies the left ventricle.

2. 70% of coronary artery filling occurs during the _____ phase of cardiac contraction.

   ANSWER: diastolic

3. Trace blood flow through the heart, beginning with the return of blood via the superior and inferior vena cava to the right atrium.

   ANSWER: Right atrium, tricuspid valve, right ventricle, pulmonic valve, pulmonary artery, lungs, pulmonary vein, left atrium, mitral (bicuspid) valve, left ventricle, aortic valve, aorta.

4. The more that myocardial muscle is stretched, the greater is its force of contraction. This principle is known as _____ _____ .

   ANSWER: Starling's Law

5. Trace the normal electrical pathway through the heart that results in a normal cardiac contraction, beginning with the SA node.

   ANSWER: SA node, internodal pathways, AV node, bundle of HIS, bundle branches, Purkinje fibers.

6. Electrolyte imbalance can impair electrical and/or mechanical cardiac function. Name at least one of these electrolytes.

   ANSWER: Sodium (Na+), calcium (CA++), or potassium (K+).

7. What is the term that refers to the inherent ability of cells to generate electrical impulses without outside stimulation?

   ANSWER: Automaticity

8. The process by which muscle fibers are stimulated to contract is called _____ .

   ANSWER: depolarization

9. What are the inherent rates of discharge of the SA Node, the AV junction and the ventricles?

   ANSWER: SA Node = 60-100

   AV junction = 40-60

   ventricles = 20-40

10. What is the normal duration of the P-R interval?

    ANSWER: .12-.20 seconds

11. Which ECG rhythm has regular rates for both atrial and ventricular depolarization, which seem to be beating independent of each other?

    ANSWER: Third degree AV block.

12. Which ECG rhythm has a fast atrial rate that cannot be counted, no discernible P-waves and a ventricular rate that is usually irregular?

    ANSWER: Atrial fibrillation.

13. Which ECG rhythm demonstrates totally chaotic undulations of varying amplitude and shape—with no discernible waves or complexes?

    ANSWER: Ventricular fibrillation.

14. Which ECG rhythm presents with a P-R interval that progressively lengthens until a QRS complex is dropped?

    ANSWER: Second degree AV block, Type I (Wenkebach).

15. Which ECG rhythm presents as a "straight line?"

    ANSWER: asystole.

16. Which ECG rhythm presents with an abnormally long P-R interval?

    ANSWER: First degree AV block.

17. Excluding chest pain, list some other signs and symptoms of a possible myocardial infarction (MI).

    ANSWER: Pain in the neck, arm, shoulder or jaw. Shortness of breath, syncope, palpitations, nausea, vomiting, weakness, dizziness, diaphoresis, apprehension and numbness.

18. There are a number of myocardial infarction victims that present without chest pain. What percentage of MI patients does this represent?

    ANSWER: About 25% of MI patients present without chest pain.

19. Define "atherosclerosis", and list some of its identifiable risk factors.

    ANSWER: Atherosclerosis is a disease of the large arteries which causes narrowing and a predisposition to develop clots. Some of its risk factors would include hypertension, smoking, elevated blood lipids, diabetes, male gender and a family history of atherosclerosis.

20. Coronary artery disease (CAD) exists when atherosclerosis attacks the coronary arteries and reduces potential blood flow. This sets the

stage for a symptom that develops when the available blood supply is exceeded by a temporary demand. What is this symptom?

ANSWER: Chest pain (angina pectoris).

21. What is the difference between angina and myocardial infarction?

ANSWER: Anginal pain is temporary and indicates ischemia, while pain from an infarction persists and results in myocardial damage.

22. Define pulmonary edema, and describe its relationship to left ventricular failure.

ANSWER: Pulmonary edema is fluid in the alveoli that inhibits gas exchange. It may develop when the left ventricle fails to eject an adequate amount of blood forward with each contraction. This backs blood up into the pulmonary circulation, where some of the fluid is forced across capillary membranes into the alveoli.

23. Lung sounds that resemble "wet popping" or "crackles" are called _____ .

ANSWER: Rales (fluid in the alveoli).

24. What condition is the most severe form of heart failure?

ANSWER: Cardiogenic shock.

25. What are some of the drugs that can be used for managing myocardial ischemia and pain?

ANSWER: Oxygen, nitroglycerine, nitrous oxide, morphine sulphate, and Demerol.

26. Name a hallmark sign of right heart failure.

ANSWER: "Pitting" edema in the extremeties, jugular vein distension or tachycardia.

27. What is an aneurysm?

ANSWER: A dilation of a blood vessel (much like a defect in tire tube).

28. What is the most common dysrhythmia seen immediately after sudden cardiac arrest?

ANSWER: Ventricular fibrillation.

The Endocrine System

The endocrine system exerts specific effects on body organs and tissues by means of hormones secreted by its specialized glands. This chapter briefly reviews those glands and their purpose and specifically discusses diabetes mellitis.

Hormones Hormones are substances secreted by an endocrine gland that affect other glands or systems of the body. Hormone production is greatly affected by stress.

Pituitary Gland This is the master gland of the body. It is located at the base of the brain and is responsible for regulating the function of other endocrine glands. It secretes ADH and Oxytocin.

Thyroid Gland This gland secretes hormones that control the metabolic rate. It has two lobes and is located in the neck.

Parathyroid Glands The parathyroid glands control the metabolism of calcium and phosphorus. These four or five pea-sized glands are attached to the posterior surface of the thyroid glands.

Adrenal Glands These glands are located just above the kidneys. They include the:

Adrenal Cortex—This secretes steroids and sex hormones.

Adrenal Medulla—This secretes catecholamines (epinephrine and norepinephrine) to regulate organs controlled by the sympathetic nervous system.

Ovaries The ovaries play a major role in reproduction. There are two, located in the pelvic cavity. They release:

Estrogen—Estrogen helps the formation of the inner lining of the uterus and promotes breast development.

Progesterone—Progesterone is responsible for the retention of sodium and water. It is also called the hormone of pregnancy.

Testes The testes secrete testosterone and promote growth and development of secondary sex characteristics.

Pancreas The pancreas' Islets of Langerhans secrete hormones that regulate insulin and glucogen. It is located to the right of the spleen and behind the duodeum.

Islets of Langerhans This part of the pancreas secretes:

a. Insulin (beta) cells—lower glucose level. Insulin is produced in response to high blood sugar. It aids in the breakdown of glucose and its transport to the cells.

b. Glucagon (alpha) cells—increase glucose level.

Glucose Imbalance This may occur for a variety of reasons and is present when the blood glucose level is outside the normal physiologic range.

Hyperglycemia High blood sugar (usually a gradual onset).

Hypoglycemia Low blood sugar (may be a rapid onset).

Type I (insulin dependant) Diabetes—May appear anytime after birth.

Type II (noninsulin dependant) Diabetes—Occurs in adult life and often can be controlled with diet (because the pancreas usually produces some insulin).

Diabetes Mellitus

Body cells must utilize glucose (simple sugar) for energy production. The more complex sugars are converted into simpler sugar (glucose) for ab-

FIGURE 17.1.

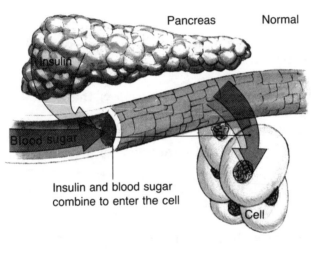

Pancreas   Normal

Insulin

Blood sugar

Insulin and blood sugar
combine to enter the cell

Cell

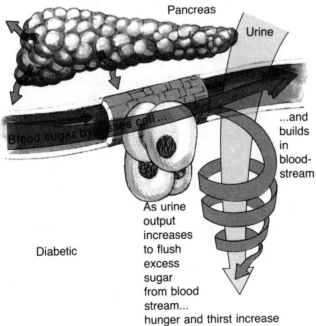

Pancreas

Urine

...and
builds
in
blood-
stream

Blood sugar bypasses cell ...

Diabetic

As urine
output
increases
to flush
excess
sugar
from blood
stream...
hunger and thirst increase

sorption and transport by the blood. Once circulating, glucose can be used by the cells of the body—BUT ONLY IF INSULIN IS PRESENT. Glucose cannot enter the cells without insulin, no matter how much glucose is present in the blood.

If there is a shortage of insulin, blood sugar levels climb, eventually triggering kidney action to excrete excess sugar through urination. Unable to utilize glucose, this person will experience hunger, despite high levels of sugar intake and will drink large amounts of fluids to try and offset the fluid loss being experienced because of excess urination. Over time, weight loss and weakness occur, while ketones and acids build up in the bloodstream as the body uses alternative energy sources for metabolism. Eventually, the blood can become so concentrated and toxic that coma will ensue (leading to death if untreated). No cure exists for diabetes, but it can usually be well controlled by diet and/or the addition of insulin (oral or injected) in an attempt to balance insulin and sugar levels in the blood. The two most serious potential hazards for the insulin-dependent diabetic are insulin shock and diabetic coma.

Insulin Shock (Severe Hypoglycemia) Insulin shock occurs when too much insulin is in the blood, which causes lots of sugar in the blood to enter the cells, leaving too little sugar in the bloodstream. This may be due to an overdose of insulin, failure to eat an adequate meal (to provide sugar levels) or excessive activity (that uses up sugar levels). The brain uses glucose in the bloodstream as its only fuel for metabolism, thus a severe lack of sugar in the blood may cause brain damage and death. PATIENT NEEDS SUGAR!

Signs and Symptoms

a. Rapid onset (can be within minutes).
b. Dizziness, headache, hunger, abnormal or bizarre behavior, speech slurring, uncoordinated movement.
c. Skin cool, pale and very diaphoretic.
d. Fainting, seizures, can become deeply comatose resulting in death or brain damage if not quickly treated.
e. Rapid pulse, BP normal or low, normal or "snoring" respirations if unconscious.
f. May mimic stroke or ETOH intoxication—BE CAREFUL.

Prehospital Management

a. Airway, oxygen (protect c-spine if possibility of injury exists).

b. IV of Normal Saline (D5W may be used if blood sample is taken before drip is established).

c. Draw a blood sample.

d. Use a Dextrostick or other glucose measuring device (if available).

e. If indicated, *or* if level of consciousness is decreased, administer 50 cc of D50W IV push.

   (1) If the patient is able to handle secretions, sublingual glucose may be appropriate (see your protocols).

   (2) If an IV cannot be established, sublingual glucose with patient on side in drainage/airway position may be appropriate.

f. If no result, administer Narcan 0.8-2.0 mg, IV push.

g. Monitor vital signs and transport smoothly.

Diabetic Coma (Severe Hyperglycemia) Diabetic coma occurs when too little insulin is in the blood causing a buildup of sugar in the bloodstream that cannot be utilized by body cells. Alternative fuel is used by the cells, producing acids and ketones as byproducts and concentrating the blood further until a coma is produced. This may be due to a failure to take insulin when needed, overeating, failure of the pancreas to produce enough insulin or an increase in metabolic rate (as in infection) that uses up insulin supplies faster. PATIENT NEEDS INSULIN!

Signs and Symptoms

a. Gradual onset (12-24 hours, even longer).

b. Nausea, vomiting, possibly abdominal pain, increasing restlessness, thirst, "dry mouth", excessive urination, "sweet breath" (like acetone or ETOH), uncoordinated movement, and speech slurring.

c. Dry red warm skin, confusion, stupor, bizarre behavior, and eventually coma and death (without intervention).

d. Weak rapid pulse, deep rapid respirations (Kussmaul), and normal/low BP.

e. May mimic stroke or ETOH intoxication—BE CAREFUL.

Prehospital Management

a. Airway, oxygen (protect c-spine if possibility of injury exists).

b. IV of Normal Saline (D5W may be used if blood sample is taken before drip is established).

c. Draw blood sample.

d. use a Dextrostick or other glucose measuring device (if available).

e. Though glucose is not technically indicated in this condition, IF THE LEVEL OF CONSCIOUSNESS IS DECREASED, administer 50 cc of D50W IV push (if an IV cannot be established, sublingual glucose with patient on side in drainage/airway position may be appropriate).

f. If no result, administer Narcan 0.8-2.0 mg. IV push.

g. Monitor vital signs and transport smoothly.

Note: It is often impossible to be make a differential diagnoses of these two diabetic emergencies. *When in doubt,* ALWAYS GIVE SUGAR! It won't hurt the patient in severe hyperglycemia, but may save the life of a patient suffering severe hypoglycemia.

Summary

The endocrine system and its glands control many body functions, one of which is the production of insulin. Insulin disorders are frequently seen by prehospital providers, and paramedics should be well-versed in its recognition and rapid treatment. Any patient exhibiting coma of unknown origin should receive prophylactic treatment of IV glucose to rule out blood sugar disorder. If the problem was low blood sugar, recovery after glucose administration is decisive and dramatic.

SELF-TEST

Chapter 17

1. Which gland is considered the master gland of the body?
   ANSWER: The pituitary gland.

2. What hormones are secreted by the pituitary gland?

   ANSWER: ADH and oxytocin.

3. Which gland secretes the catecholamines epinephrine and norepinephrine?

   ANSWER: The adrenal medulla.

4. Which hormone is called "the hormone of pregnancy?"

   ANSWER: Progesterone.

5. What part of the pancreas secretes hormones that regulate insulin and glucogen?

   ANSWER: The Islets of Langerhans.

6. A rapid onset of clammy skin, uncoordinated movements, speech slurring, irritability, bizarre behavior—perhaps even profound unconsciousness—might be an indication of what condition?

   ANSWER: Hypoglycemia (sometimes called insulin shock).

7. What is the most important need of the patient in insulin shock (hypoglycemia)?

   ANSWER: Sugar.

8. What is the most important need of the patient in a diabetic coma (hyperglycemia)?

   ANSWER: Insulin.

9. List some signs and symptoms of hyperglycemia.

   ANSWER: Slow onset (12-24 hours), nausea and vomiting, Kussmaul respirations (deep and rapid), fruity acetone breath, and eventual unconsciousness.

10. Any patient exhibiting coma of unknown origin should receive prophylactic administration of IV _____ . If there is no improvement, follow with IV _____ .

    ANSWER: a. glucose/dextrose (D50W for adult, D25W for child)

    　　　　　 b. Narcan

The Nervous System

This chapter provides an overview of the nervous system. Specifically, we concentrate on the *central nervous system* (CNS), the *peripheral nervous system,* and the two divisions of the *autonomic nervous system*—the sympathetic and parasympathetic. Included is basic assessment of CNS dysfunction and prehospital management of CNS emergencies.

Central Nervous System (CNS)

The central nervous system is composed of the brain, specialized nerve cells, and the spinal cord. It is responsible for interpreting, sending, and receiving messages that control all body functions.

Brain The brain is the center of consciousness and is the controlling (as well as the largest) organ of the body. It is covered by three protective layers, or *meninges*:

1. *Dura Mater* (outer)—Extremely strong fibrous tissue ("tough mother");
2. *Arachnoid* (middle)—Delicate membrane which contains circulating cerebrospinal fluid (CSF);
3. *Pia Mater* (inner)—Inner layer covering the brain and spinal cord.

FIGURE 18.1.

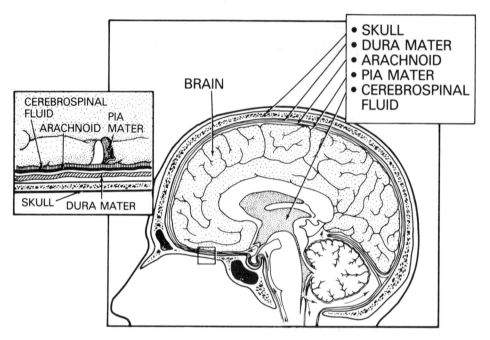

BRAIN

- SKULL
- DURA MATER
- ARACHNOID
- PIA MATER
- CEREBROSPINAL FLUID

CEREBROSPINAL FLUID
PIA
ARACHNOID MATER
SKULL DURA MATER

The brain is divided into three major regions:

1. *Cerebrum;*
2. *Cerebellum;*
3. *Brain Stem* (and medulla).

The brain floats within the protection of the bony skull, well-cushioned from most traumatic injuries. However, the very protection of that confined hard space can be a detriment when injury does occur. Like most body tissues, the brain swells when injured. In the tight confines of the skull, there is no room for significant swelling or bleeding—and when it occurs, *intracranial pressure* pushes the brain against sharp ridges in the cranium and squeezes brain tissue toward the only exit from the skull (the foramen magnum), thus compromising the brain stem as well as brain tissue in general. Early suspicion of brain injury and intracranial pressure is essential for proper management of CNS injuries.

Cerebrum The largest of the three lobes of the brain, the cerebrum is responsible for the higher functions (such as reasoning) and is composed of several lobes:

1. *Frontal*—Personality and motor functions;
2. *Parietal*—Sensory;
3. *Temporal*—Speech;
4. *Occipital*—Vision.

Cerebellum Located underneath the cerebrum, this lobe of the brain is mostly concerned with maintaining posture and equilibrium and coordination of skilled movements.

Medulla Located in the brainstem, this lobe contains control centers for regulating respiration and heart rate.

Spinal Cord A continuation of the brain, the spinal cord exits the skull through the foramen magnum and is encased within the bony spinal column and contains nerve tracts (31) that connect the brain with the other organs of the body. The spinal cord is also covered by meninges, like the brain, and serves as a *reflex center* and a *pathway for conduction* of impulses. It extends to the level of the second lumbar vertebrae.

Spinal Column The spinal column protects the spinal cord and provides support for the skeletal system. It is made up of 33 vertebrae, connective tissue and has five well-defined divisions:

1. *Cervical*—(seven vertebrae);
2. *Thoracic*—(twelve vertebrae);
3. *Lumbar*—(five vertebrae);
4. *Sacral*—(five vertebrae); and
5. *Coccygeal*—(four vertebrae).

Vertebrae These are bony coverings, connected by joints and ligaments, that comprise the spinal column and protect the spinal cord. Through the vertebrae, nerves innervate the spinal cord. Injury to the vertebrae often means underlying spinal cord injury.

Nerve Cells Nerve cells are classified into three types:

1. *Sensory* (afferent)—Sends messages toward the brain;
2. *Motor* (efferent)—Sends messages away from the brain; and
3. *Connector Neurons*—Unite sensory and motor input.

FIGURE 18.2.

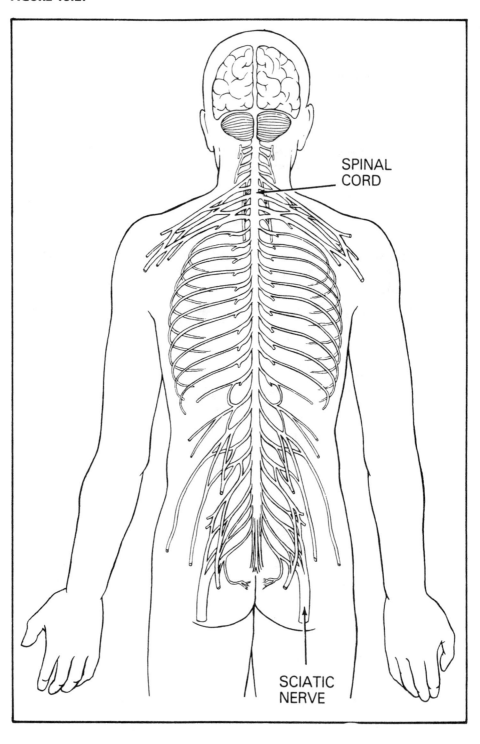

SPINAL
CORD

SCIATIC
NERVE

FIGURE 18.3.

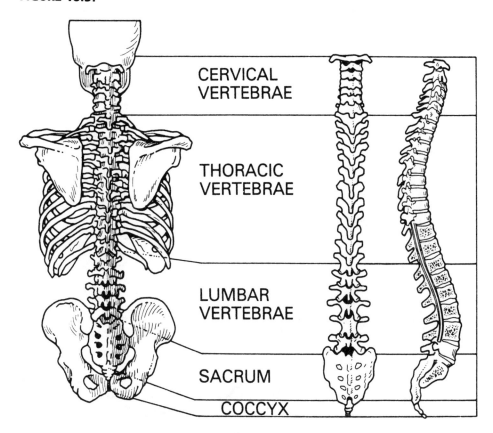

CERVICAL
VERTEBRAE

THORACIC
VERTEBRAE

LUMBAR
VERTEBRAE

SACRUM

COCCYX

Nerve Impulses These impulses are transmitted in two ways:

1. *Electrically* (through synapses); and
2. *Chemically* (through neurotransmitters).

Peripheral Nervous System

The peripheral nervous system is composed of peripheral nerves:

1. *Cranial Nerves*—Twelve pairs of nerves which exit the brain through holes in the skull and provide for specific functions in the head and face.

FIGURE 18.4.

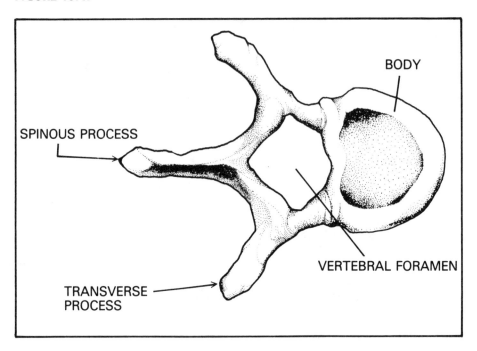

SPINOUS PROCESS

BODY

VERTEBRAL FORAMEN

TRANSVERSE
PROCESS

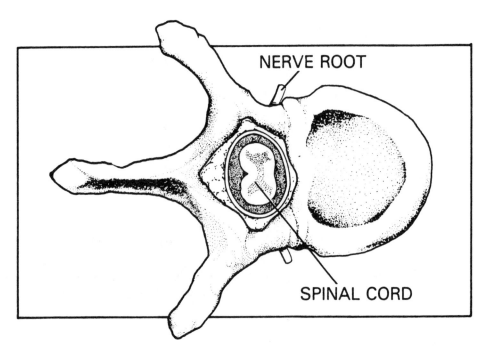

NERVE ROOT

SPINAL CORD

2. *Spinal Nerves*—Thirty-one pairs of nerves which exit through the spinal column between each vertebrae, providing pathways for sensory and motor impulses and connecting the two when appropriate (to bypass the brain).

The peripheral nerves can be categorized as:

1. *Sensory* (afferent)—Specialized nerves that provide information to the brain from other parts of the body. The impulses travel first to the spinal cord, are processed, and then travel to the brain.
2. *Motor* (efferent)—Specialized nerves that stimulate muscle contraction. Motor impulses are received from the brain by cell bodies in the spinal cord that then generate a motor command to a specific peripheral muscle.
3. *Connecting*—Provide a "bridge" between sensory and motor nerves in the brain and spinal cord. In the spinal cord, they connect these nerves directly, allowing for bypass of the brain when certain reflex arcs are stimulated (such as pulling away from an intense heat source).

Autonomic Nervous System (ANS)

The autonomic nervous system functions independently of conscious control. It is divided into the sympathetic and parasympathetic nervous systems, which tend to counterbalance each other.

Sympathetic Nervous System This system prepares the body to respond to threatening situations ("fight or flight"). When stimulated, it causes these effects:

1. Increases heart rate;
2. Increases strength of contractions;
3. Peripheral vasoconstriction;
4. Dilates bronchials;
5. Dilates pupils; and
6. Increases production of epinephrine.

Parasympathetic Nervous System This system acts in opposition to the sympathetic nervous system. When stimulated, it causes these effects:

1. Slows heart rate;
2. Causes bronchial constriction;
3. Constricts pupils; and
4. Relaxes muscle sphincters.

Nervous System Activity This can be divided into three categories:

1. *Voluntary*—Willed acts, signalled by voluntary activation of skeletal muscles.
2. *Involuntary*—Actions initiated independent of conscious thought, such as baseline respirations, baseline heart rate and force, and digestion.
3. *Reflex activity*—Reflex arcs function when a sensory impulse is transmitted by an afferent nerve pathway to a cell body in the spinal cord—where the impulse is bridged across directly to a motor nerve (WITHOUT FIRST BEING TRANSMITTED TO THE BRAIN), which generates a motor impulse that travels down an efferent nerve pathway to stimulate a peripheral muscle response.

Assessment of CNS Problems

Rapid accurate assessment of CNS problems is critical for paramedics.

History Though often difficult to obtain, an accurate history is vital—especially mechanisms of injury and any changes in LOC. Use bystanders, family members, and witnesses—and when possible, take an AMPLE history:

A = Allergies to medications.
M = Medications used or prescribed.
P = Past medical history.
L = Last oral intake.
E = Events preceding the illness or injury.

Physical Examination

1. *Assure and maintain airway* while *protecting cervical spine* (if patient is unconscious use chin lift, modified jaw thrust, and nasal or oral airways).
2. *Assess breathing:*
   a. If breathless, utilize in-line stabilization while ventilating and/or while inserting an endotracheal tube (or EOA/EGTA/PTL airway if unable to use ET) for ventilation).
   b. If breathing, watch closely for any change in respiratory patterns that might indicate CNS problems such as:
      1. Cheyne–Stokes respirations;
      2. Central neurogenic hyperventilation;
      3. Diaphramatic breathing;
      4. Periods of apnea or any other breathing irregularity.
3. *Assess circulatory status.* Watch for changes in pulse or blood pressure that might indicate developing *intracranial pressure. Early* signs of increasing intracranial pressure are:
      1. Rise in blood pressure;
      2. Bradycardia; and
      3. Elevated temperature.
   Late stage signs of intracranial pressure are:
      1. Tachycardia;
      2. Drop in blood pressure; and
      3. Elevated temperature.

Neuro Physical Exam

1. *Assess level of consciousness* (LOC)—Level of consciousness (LOC) is most important sign when evaluating injury to or dysfunction of the central nervous system. It is extremely important to note not only the baseline LOC, but any changes that occur (increase or decrease) during your care. Also assess:
   a. Orientation to person, time and place;
   b. Speech patterns;

c. Responses to questions;

d. Movement—purposeful or nonpurposeful;

e. Take a Glasgow Coma Scale.

FIGURE 18.5.

Glasgow Coma Scale	(Score the best response from each category and add the three scores)
A. Eye Opening	
Spontaneous 4	
To Voice 3	
To Pain 2	_____ Score for A
None 1	
B. Verbal Response	
Oriented 5	
Confused 4	
Inappropriate Words 3	_____ Score for B
Incomprehensible Words . 2	
None 1	
C. Motor Response	
Obeys Command 6	
Localizes Pain 5	
Withdraw (pain) 4	+ _____ Score for C
Flexion (pain) 3	
Extension (pain) 2	= _____ *Total Points* for
None 1	Glasgow Coma Scale (three scores combined)

This may be combined with other assessment factors to determine the Trauma Score—a method to predict survivability in trauma cases.

FIGURE 18.6.

TRAUMA SCORE

Respiratory Rate	10-24/min	4	
	24-35/min	3	
	36/min or greater	2	
	1-9/min	1	
	None	0	
Respiratory Expansion	Normal	1	
	Retractive	0	
Systolic Blood Pressure	90 mmHg or greater	4	
	70-89 mmHg	3	
	50-69 mmHg	2	
	0-49 mmHg	1	
	No Pulse	0	
Capillary Refill	Normal	2	
	Delayed	1	
	None	0	
Cardiopulmonary Assessment			

Total Trauma Score = Cardiopulmonary + Neurologic ⟶

GLASGOW COMA SCALE

Eye Opening	Spontaneous	4	
	To Voice	3	
	To Pain	2	
	None	1	
Verbal Response	Oriented	5	
	Confused	4	
	Inappropriate Words	3	
	Incomprehensible Words	2	
	None	1	
Motor Response	Obeys Command	6	
	Localizes Pain	5	
	Withdraw (pain)	4	
	Flexion (pain)	3	
	Extension (pain)	2	
	None	1	
Glasgow Coma Score Total			

TOTAL GLASGOW COMA SCALE POINTS

14 – 15 = 5	
11 – 13 = 4	**CONVERSION =**
8 – 10 = 3	**APPROXIMATELY**
5 – 7 = 2	**ONE-THIRD**
3 – 4 = 1	**TOTAL VALUE**

Neurologic Assessment

2. *Complete Secondary Survey* (head-to-toe)—While performing the secondary survey, don't forget these special components that have a bearing on CNS dysfunction:

   a. *Pupil size* (watch for contact lenses):
     1. Equality, roundness;
     2. Abnormal dilation/constriction;
     3. Reaction to light (together).

   b. *Extraocular movements:*
     1. Dysconjugate gaze;
     2. Uncoordinated movements.

   c. *Abnormal head and skull exam:*
     1. Depressions or irregularities in skull;
     2. Blood or fluid from the ears and nose;
     3. Battles sign (bruising behind the ears) or "raccoon eyes;"

   d. *Any deficits in peripheral sensory or motor function.*

Disorders Involving The CNS

Coma Coma is a deep state of unconsciousness from which the patient cannot be aroused by external stimuli.
*Mneumonic for common causes of coma:

A—Acidosis, Alcohol
E—Epilepsy
I—Infection
O—Overdose
U—Uremia
T—Trauma
I—Insulin
P—Psychosis
S—Stroke

Prehospital Management

1. Open and maintain airway and support ventilation as needed.
2. Protect cervical spine (if any possibility of injury).
3. IV of NS (TKO).
4. Draw a blood sample.
5. Use a Dextrostick or other glucose measuring device, if available.
6. Administer 50cc of D50, IV push.
7. If no result, administer Narcan 0.8-2.0 mg, IV push.

Seizures Massive disorganized electrical discharging of neurons in the brain. Causes can include:

1. Idopathic epilepsy (most common cause of seizures in adults);
2. CVA (stroke);
3. Trauma;
4. Alcohol or drug withdrawal;
5. Hypoxia;
6. Hypoglycemia;
7. Infections (severe);
8. Brain Tumors.
9. Eclampsia.

Types of Seizures

1. *Grand Mal*—Presents with a loss of consciousness, tonic-clonic movements, incontinence and confusion followed by coma or drowsiness.
2. *Petit Mal*—Occur mostly in children and are manifested by a brief loss of motor tone.

Prehospital Treatment

1. Maintain airway—use padded tongue blade or bite block—do not force between teeth (or use fingers).

2. Administer O_2.

3. Protect the patient from environmental objects, but do not rigidly restrain.

4. Place on side and suction as needed after tonic-clonic phase is over.

Status Epilecticus This is two or more seizures without a period of consciousness between them (the most common cause of status epilepticus in adults is failure to take prescribed medications).

Prehospital Management

1. Maintain airway, administer O_2 and assist ventilations as needed;

2. Establish IV D5W (TKO);

3. Administer 50cc of D50W, IV push;

4. Administer Valium 2-10 mg, IV push.

Cerebrovascular Accident (CVA/Stroke) This is an illness (acute) due to interruption of cerebral blood flow. It is the third leading cause of adult death in the United States.

Causes of CVA

1. Thrombus—Stationary blood clot;

2. Embolus—Clot or foreign body in motion;

3. Hemorrhage—Bleeding.

Transient Ischemic Attack (TIA) This is a brief episode of cerebral dysfunction that mimics a CVA, but lasts from a few minutes to a few hours (always < 24 hours).

Prehospital Management

1. Maintain airway, assist ventilations as needed;

2. Administer high-flow O_2;

3. Keep patient supine with head elevated 15 degrees;

4. IV NS (TKO);

5. Draw a blood sample and measure glucose (if equipment is available);

6. Monitor for cardiac dysrhythmias;

7. Consider 50 cc of D50W if known diabetic (or if dextrostick indicates hypoglycemia).

Summary

The various components of the nervous system totally control the functions of the body and an understanding of this system is essential to proper patient assessment and management. Most important to the paramedic is the central nervous system—and the most significant sign of CNS function is level of consciousness. Careful assessment, cervical spine immobilization, oxygenation and hyperventilation of head-injury patients, minimal on-scene time, early activation of hospital trauma teams, rapid transportation to the hospital/operating room—all these things combine to maximize appropriate treatment for patients with damage or dysfunction of the nervous system.

SELF-TEST

Chapter 19

1. What are the main components of the central nervous system?
   ANSWER: The brain, specialized nerve cells, and the spinal cord.
2. Name the three layers (meninges) covering the brain and spinal cord).
   ANSWER: Dura mater (outer), arachnoid (middle), and pia mater (inner).
3. The brain is divided into three major lobes—the cerebrum, the cerebullum and the brain stem (which includes the medulla). Which one of these is the largest?
   ANSWER: The cerebrum.
4. The control centers for regulation of heart rate and respirations is located in the _____ .
   ANSWER: medulla (or brain stem)
5. What is the function of the spinal cord?
   ANSWER: The spinal cord serves as a reflex center and a pathway for conduction of nerve impulses.

6. What are the five divisions of the spinal column?

   ANSWER: Cervical, thoracic, lumbar, sacral, and coccygeal.

7. How are nerve impulses transmitted?

   ANSWER: Electrically (through synapses) and chemically (through neurotransmitters).

8. What kind of nerve cells send messages to the brain (sensory input)?

   ANSWER: Afferent nerve cells.

9. What kind of nerve cells send messages away from the brain to stimulate muscle contractions (motor input)?

   ANSWER: Efferent nerve cells.

10. List some of the effects of sympathetic nervous system stimulation.

    ANSWER: a. increased heart rate and force of contractions

    b. peripheral vasoconstriction

    c. bronchial dilation

    d. pupil dilation

    e. increased production of epinephrine

11. List some of the effects of parasympathetic nervous system stimulation.

    ANSWER: a. decreased heart rate

    b. bronchial constriction

    c. pupil constriction

    d. relaxation of muscle sphincters

12. Name some respiratory patterns and changes that might indicate central nervous system (CNS) injury or dysfunction.

    ANSWER: a. Cheyne-Stokes respirations

    b. central neurogenic hyperventilation

    c. diaphramatic breathing

    d. periods of apnea

    e. other irregular respiratory patterns

13. Name some early signs of increasing intracranial pressure.

    ANSWER: a. hypertension

    b. bradycardia

    c. elevated temperature

14. A deep state of unconsciousness (from which the patient cannot be aroused by external stimuli) is called a _____ .

ANSWER: coma

15. Massive disorganized electrical discharging of neurons in the brain is called a _____ .

ANSWER: seizure

16. Two or more consecutive seizures (without a period of consciousness in between) is considered _____ _____ .

ANSWER: status epilepticus

17. What is the primary difference between a stroke (CVA) and a transient ischemic attack (TIA)?

ANSWER: A TIA is temporary, lasting from a few minutes to a few hours (less than 24 hours).

The Acute Abdomen

There are many conditions that present some degree of abdominal pain, and that pain (along with a good patient history) is often the most significant symptom in identifying the underlying problem. There is little use, however, for the field paramedic to spend much time trying to hammer down a close diagnoses—generally it will have no effect on the treatment rendered. It is important to have a general understanding of the abdomen and the kind of injuries and disease processes that cause abdominal pain. Most importantly, it is vital to know which of these conditions are (or may become) life-threatening, and how they present. We will briefly review the structures and organs in the abdomen, and then concentrate on assessing and treating the life-threatening.

Gastrointestinal Structures

Esophagus Portion of the digestive tract that connects the pharynx and the stomach.

Intestines

Small—The portion of the digestive tube between stomach and cecum, composed of the duodenum, jejunum, and ileum.

Large—The portion of digestive tube from ileocecal valve to anus, composed of cecum, colon, and rectum.

Rectum Distal portion of the large intestine.

Peritoneum Lining of the abdominal cavity.

Salivary Glands Produce and secrete saliva (connected to mouth by ducts).

Veriform Appendix A hollow appendage attached to the large intestine.

Contents of Abdominal Cavity

The boundaries of the abdominal cavity are the diaphragm on top, the pelvis on the bottom, the spine in the back and the muscular abdominal wall in the front.

Major Blood Vessels

1. *Aorta*—Largest artery in the body, carries oxygenated blood from the left ventricle and distributes it through the body—travels downward through the abdomen. (SITE OF LIFE-THREATENING AORTIC ANEURYSMS.)
2. *Inferior Vena Cava*—Large vein that returns blood from the lower extremities to the right atrium.

Solid Organs

1. *Liver*—Large and extremely vascular solid organ, often injured in blunt trauma. It secretes bile, produces essential proteins, stores glycogen and detoxifies the blood.
2. *Spleen*—Smaller, extremely vascular solid organ, often injured in blunt trauma.
3. *Pancreas*—Intra-abdominal gland that secretes insulin and digestive enzymes.
4. *Kidneys*—Filter blood and produce urine. Two, located in the retroperitoneum.

Hollow Organs

1. *Stomach*—Hollow digestive organ that receives food from the esophagus.
2. *Intestines*—Hollow digestives tubes that receive food from the stomach and move it (through the small and large intestine) to the rectum.
3. *Gallbladder*—Located beneath the liver, it stores and concentrates bile.
4. *Urinary Bladder*—Stores urine produced by the kidneys. It lies within the pelvic cavity behind the pubic bone.
5. *Uterus* (female)—Muscular organ that adapts to house a developing fetus. It normally lies within the pelvic cavity.

FIGURE 19.1.

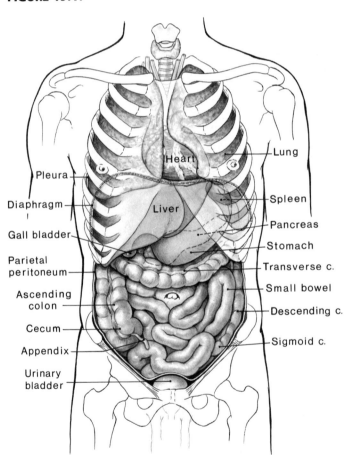

Location of Organs

Right Upper Quadrant

1. Liver;
2. Gallbladder;
3. Duodenum.

Left Upper Quadrant (LUQ)

1. Stomach;
2. Liver (part of);
3. Pancreas;
4. Spleen.

Right Lower Quadrant (RLQ)

1. Ascending colon;
2. Transverse colon (part);
3. Veriform appendix;
4. Ovary (female).

Left Lower Quadrant (LLQ)

1. Transverse colon (part);
2. Descending colon;
3. Ovary (female).

Urinary System

Kidneys These filter the blood and produce urine. There are two, located in the retroperitoneum.

Ureter The tube that connects the kidneys with the bladder.

Bladder Storage site for urine produced by the kidneys. It lies within the pelvic cavity, behind the pubic bone.

Urethra The tube leading from the bladder to outside of the body.

Reproductive System

Male

1. *Testes*—Secrete testosterone. There are two, located outside the body cavity in a sac called the scrotum (hangs below the penis).
2. *Prostate*—Gland situated at the base of the bladder. It sometimes becomes enlarged, restricting urine flow.
3. *Penile Urethra*—The tube in the penis that leads to the outside of the body.
4. *Epididymis*—Small organ located behind the testes (and in the scrotum). It serves as a reservoir for sperm cells.
5. *Vas Deferens*—Small muscular tube that conducts sperm from the epididymis to the urethra.

Female

1. *Ovaries*—Secrete estrogen. Two, located on each side of the uterus.
2. *Fallopian Tubes*—Tubes that extend from each ovary to the uterus through which eggs travel for possible fertilization.
3. *Uterus*—Muscular organ that protects a fetus while it grows and matures inside the body. It normally lies within the pelvic girdle, but grows upward and outward as fetus develops.
4. *Vagina*—Extends from the uterus to the birth canal (vulva).
5. *Vulva*—External genitalia.

Abdominal Pain

Nonhemorrhagic Causes

1. Local inflammation;
2. Peritoneal inflammation;
3. General inflammation.

Nonhemorraghic Disease Processes (Examples)

1. Peptic ulcer;
2. Appendicitis;

FIGURE 19.2.

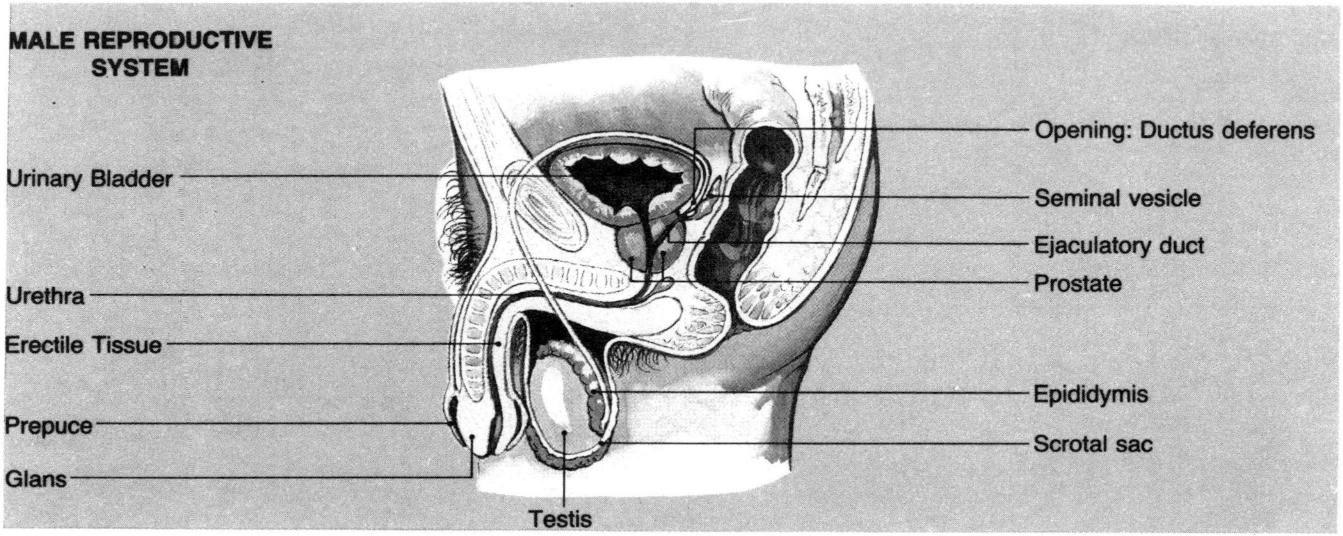

MALE REPRODUCTIVE
SYSTEM

Opening: Ductus deferens

Seminal vesicle

Ejaculatory duct

Prostate

Epididymis

Scrotal sac

Urinary Bladder

Urethra

Erectile Tissue

Prepuce

Glans

Testis

271

FIGURE 19.3.

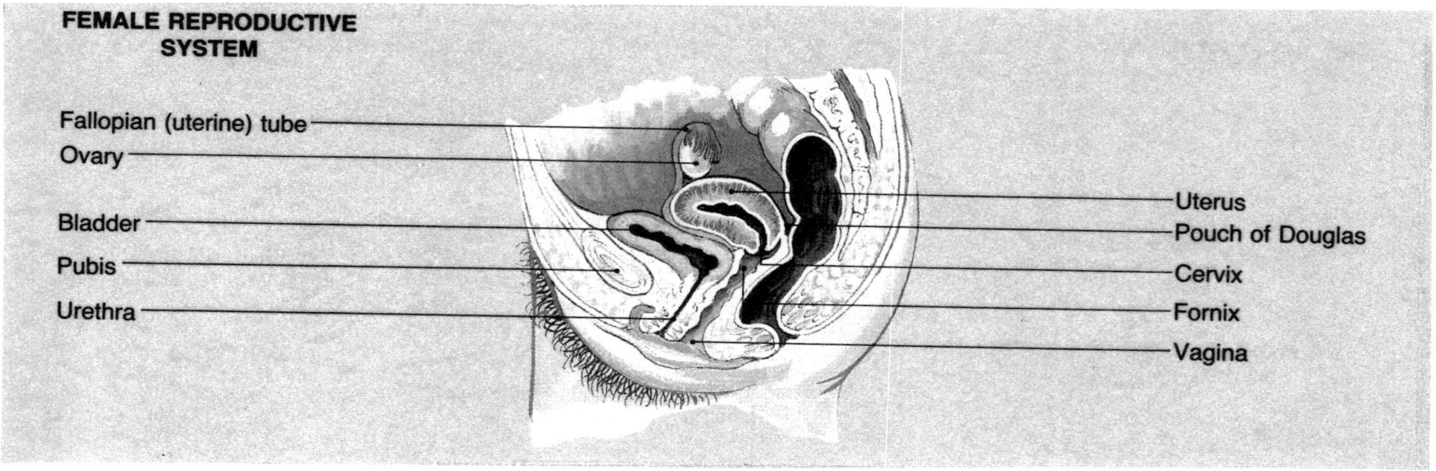

FEMALE REPRODUCTIVE SYSTEM

Fallopian (uterine) tube

Ovary

Bladder

Pubis

Urethra

Uterus

Pouch of Douglas

Cervix

Fornix

Vagina

3. Diverticulitis;
4. Kidney stone;
5. Pelvic inflammatory disease (PID);
6. Gallbladder disease;
7. Ovarian cyst.

Hemorrhagic Causes (Examples)

1. Esophageal varices;
2. Bleeding ulcer;
3. Diverticulitis;
4. Cancer of the colon;
5. Ectopic pregnancy;
6. Aortic aneurysm;
7. Trauma to organs or structures.

Assessment of Acute Abdomen

History Take an AMPLE history and concentrate in learning about the abdominal pain:

1. *Location*—Is it localized or general in nature? Have them point.
2. *Radiation*—Does it radiate through to the back (pancreatitis, aortic aneurysm), around the right side to shoulder (gallbladder), from the right lower quadrant across the lower abdomen (appendix) or to the left shoulder (spleen)?
3. *Quality*—Constant or intermittent, sharp, dull, "tearing" or ache? Cramping, intermittent pain often concerns obstruction of a hollow organ, while constant pain often suggests inflammation or malfunction of an organ.
4. *Duration*—Sudden onset? Associated with trauma or fall? Gradually occurring over several hours?
5. *Intensity*—Have the patient "rate" the pain, then you "rate" the pain subjectively, based upon your experience.
6. *Vomiting*—If present, what color (ask about coffee grounds, blood, or dark vomitus), how often, how forceful—save a sample, if possible.
7. *Bowels*—Any diarrhea? Blood, dark clots, dark or tarry stools?

Physical Examination The physical exam should include a primary survey, vital signs check, and a secondary survey. When palapating the abdomen in the secondary survey, be gentle but thorough. IF THE PATIENT IS IN SHOCK (FROM ABDOMINAL PROBLEM), TRANSPORT WILL BEGIN BEFORE THE SECONDARY SURVEY! Don't forget to look for pulsatile masses in patients at risk for aortic aneurysms.

Signs/Symptoms of Abdominal Pain

1. *Pain* (could be local, referred or generalized throughout abdomen).
2. *Vomiting* (may vomit blood—if so, get description or sample—is it bright red, fresh coffee grounds, old dark clots, and so on).
3. *Diarrhea* (again, look for blood in stool).
4. *"Guarding"* (protective reaction to palpation).
5. *"Rigidity"* (when palpation of an abdominal region reveals a hard rigid character).
6. *Vital signs:*
   a. Increased heart rate;
   b. Decreased blood pressure (may have orthostatic changes);
   c. Respirations (can be normal or increased).

General Prehospital Management

1. Airway and oxygen therapy.
2. IV of LR or NS (large bore).
3. Continued monitoring of vital signs and ECG.
4. Shock position—if tolerated (many of these patients will insist on a fetal position, or lying on their side).
5. Shock trousers, if indicated (MAST, PASG, PAST, PCPD—they all mean the same thing).
6. Immediate transport.

Note: IF PATIENT IS IN PROFOUND SHOCK, DO NOT DELAY TRANSPORT TO START IV(S)—GET THE SHOCK TROUSERS ON AND BEGIN TRANSPORT IMMEDIATELY!

Specific Abdominal Emergencies

Abdominal Aortic Aneurysm This is a large dilation (ballooning) of the aorta as it passes through the abdominal region, generally caused by atherosclerosis. Men are more likely to suffer this than women, especially as they get older (60–70). If the aneurysm ruptures badly before repair in the operating room, mortality can be high—but condition can often be surgically repaired.

Signs and Symptoms of Rupture

1. Abdominal pain;
2. Back (flank) pain;
3. Hypotension—possibly severe;
4. May have urge to defecate (caused by blood irritating peritoneum);
5. Pulsatile mass in abdomen (often can be palpated or seen);
6. Decreased femoral pulse;
7. May mimic GI bleed depending upon area of bleeding.

Prehospital Management

1. High index of suspicion is EXTREMELY important;
2. Airway and high-flow oxygen therapy;
3. Shock trousers;
4. Begin rapid transport to hospital/operating room;
5. Large-bore IVs of LR, wide open (two, if there is time);
6. Monitor vitals and ECG carefully enroute.

Ectopic Pregnancy This is a pregnancy that ensues when a fertilized egg implants anywhere other than the uterus (1 out of 200). Usually, that place will be in a fallopian tube (because that's where the egg is fertilized), after an egg does not make it down the tube to be implanted in the uterine wall. As the egg grows, the tube stretches and eventually ruptures, bleeding profusely. If the fallopian tube ruptures within its own intima, the blood will follow the tube to the uterus and present itself as severe vaginal bleeding. If the tube ruptures externally, dumping blood into the abdominal cavity, it presents as abdominal pain (perhaps with fever and spotting). In either case, the problem quickly becomes one of hypovolemic shock and can be fatal.

Signs and Symptoms of Rupture (or near-rupture)

1. Lower abdominal pain (may have rebound tenderness);
2. Significant history (symptoms of early pregnancy, skipped period, previous ectopic pregnancy, previous pelvic infection, intermittent spotting);
3. Possible severe vaginal bleeding (but may only be spotting);
4. Signs of hypovolemic shock (pale cold clammy skin, rapid thready pulse, and eventually hypotension and decreased LOC).

Prehospital Management

1. High index of suspicion;
2. Airway and high-flow oxygen therapy;
3. Shock trousers;
4. Begin rapid transport to hospital/operating room;
5. Large-bore IVs of LR, wide open (two, if there is time);
6. Monitor vital signs and ECG carefully enroute.

Note: Other OB/Gynecological emergencies can be just as life-threatening, such as abruptio placenta, third-trimester severe bleeding, and abdominal trauma in pregnancy, but ectopic pregnancy is mired in the "acute abdominal pain" category because the pregnancy is usually undiagnosed.

Summary

The acute abdomen presents a difficult problem for paramedics, due to the wide variety of problems that can exist, ranging from minor to life-threatening. Most of them present with abdominal pain of some kind, making it easy for some conditions to go undiagnosed (in both the prehospital and hospital phase). The field paramedic must have an understanding of the structures and systems involved, a constant suspicion of the abdominal conditions that are or can become life-threatening—and an ability to shift into high gear when signs or symptoms of severe abdominal bleeding are present.

SELF-TEST

Chapter 19

1. Which portion of the digestive system is comprised of the duodenum, jejunem and ileum?

    ANSWER: the small intestines

2. Which portion of the digestive system is comprised of the cecum, colon and rectum?

    ANSWER: the large intestines

3. The _____ secretes bile, stores glycogen and detoxifies the blood.

    ANSWER: liver

4. Bile is stored in the _____ _____ .

    ANSWER: gall bladder

5. What might you suspect if a pulsatile mass in the abdomen can be seen or palpated?

    ANSWER: an abdominal aortic aneurysm

6. The _____ is an organ that secretes insulin and digestive enzymes?

    ANSWER: pancreas

7. The _____ are located in the retroperitoneum, where they filter blood and produce urine?

    ANSWER: kidneys

8. The lining of the abdominal cavity is called the _____ .

    ANSWER: peritoneum

9. Which quadrant of the abdomen contains the spleen?

    ANSWER: the left upper quadrant (LUQ)

10. The fallopian tubes connect each _____ with the _____ .

    ANSWER: ovary, uterus

11. Briefly describe the appropriate prehospital management of a ruptured abdominal aortic aneurysm.

    ANSWER: airway, high-flow O_2, shock trousers, rapid transportation, large-bore IVs enroute and monitoring of vital signs and ECG

12. In *most* ectopic pregnancies, a fertilized egg implants in one of the _____ _____ .

ANSWER: fallopian tubes

13. Briefly describe proper prehospital management of an ectopic pregnancy.

ANSWER: airway, high-flow O_2, shock trousers, rapid transportation, large-bore IVs enroute and monitoring of vital signs and ECG

Anaphylaxis

Anaphylaxis is the most severe form of an allergic reaction and is truly an emergency. Death can occur within minutes of exposure. Most of what we see in the field (and what commonly gets lumped with anaphylaxis) can be classified as milder allergic reactions and will vary greatly in severity. It is important that paramedics understand the processes involved in an anaphylactic reaction and the nature and treatment of anaphylactic shock.

Definitions

Antigen An antigen is a foreign protein that, when introduced into the body, stimulates the production of specific protective proteins called antibodies.

Antibody An antibody is a protein produced in the body in response to a specific antigen (foreign protein) that attempts to destroy or inactivate the antigen.

Anaphylaxis Anaphylaxis is a massive allergic reaction that develops within seconds or minutes after introduction of an antigen to which the body is hypersensitive. Anaphylactic shock and death can occur within minutes (without intervention).

Antihistamine This is a drug that counteracts the effects of histamines and helps relieve the symptoms of an allergic reaction.

Histamine A histamine is a substance that, when released by the body, causes vasodilation, constriction of bronchial muscles and leakage of fluid from capillaries into tissues (edema).

Urticaria Also known as hives, these are bumps on the skin that indicate an allergic reaction.

Pathophysiology

Antigens that may cause allergic reactions can be introduced into the system in four ways:

1. Injection (through skin or via bloodstream—drugs, stings, bites).
2. Ingestion (by mouth—foods, drugs).
3. Inhalation (through the lungs—gases, pollens, airborne antigenics).
4. Absorption (through the skin—drugs, irritants, chemicals).

When an antigen is introduced into the body, it stimulates the production of specific antibodies, which attach to the antigen and try to neutralize it. During sensitization, antibodies specific to the sensitizing antigen attach to MAST cells (basophils). When a second exposure occurs, these antigens cause a release of histamines and heparin from the MAST cells into the circulation. The histamines attack vessel walls and cause pronounced vasodilation, as well as severe constriction of bronchial muscles in the lungs (causing bronchospasm and narrowing of the air passages) and significant leakage of fluid from capillaries into body tissues (edema).

Assessment

History is extremely important, but must be taken rapidly. In the severe case, intervention must be done while or before a history is gained. A significant portion of these patients (or their families/friends) will know what caused the allergic reaction. The trick is recognizing anaphylaxis in the non-suspecting victim.

Signs and Symptoms (Multi-system)

Respiratory System—Dyspnea, wheezing, sneezing, and coughing—respiratory distress may progress to complete airway obstruction.

Cardiovascular System—Vasodilation, increased heart rate and profoundly decreased blood pressure.

Gastrointestinal System—Cramping, nausea/vomiting and diarrhea.

Nervous System—Headache and convulsions.

Skin—Itching and hives (urticaria), swelling (facial, airway and site of introduction—if injected or absorbed), flushed face (with urticaria) and cyanosis.

Prehospital Management

1. Maintain airway and administer high-flow oxygen via bag-valve mask. It may become necessary to ventilate these patients, so ANTICIPATE.
2. Consider endotracheal intubation (as swelling may soon occlude airway) or transtracheal ventilation (if necessary and indicated).
3. Mild constricting band if exposure was on an extremity.
4. Shock trousers if indicated.
5. Begin rapid transport, unless local protocols suggest on-scene medication before transport.
6. Large-bore IV of LR or NS. (may need to expand volume)
7. Administer Epinephrine:
    a. Mild case: .3-.5 mg of Epinephrine (1:1000), Sub-Q (.3-.5 ml of solution);
    b. Severe case: .3-.5 mg of Epinephrine (1:10,000), IV push (3-5 ml of solution).
8. Consider additional medications:
    a. Benadryl, IV push (usually 50 mg);
    b. Aminophylline drip (if symptoms persist).
9. Monitor ECG and vital signs frequently enroute.

Summary

Anaphylaxis is a true emergency and one in which appropriate rapid intervention by paramedics can save a life. Recognizing the signs of anaphylactic shock in patients that do not suspect an allergic reaction and airway management by anticipation is crucial to successful management. Local protocols should address the special situation of anaphylaxis, with an eye toward early administration of epinephrine.

SELF-TEST

Chapter 20

1. An _____ is a foreign protein that, when introduced into the body, stimulates the production of specific protective proteins called antibodies.

   ANSWER: antigen

2. What factor must precede any anaphylactic reaction?

   ANSWER: The body must develop a hypersensitivity to a particular antigen.

3. What is "urticaria?"

   ANSWER: Hives—bumps on the skin that are one indication of an allergic reaction.

4. During an anaphylactic reaction the body releases histamines. What are some of the effects of histamines?

   ANSWER: Histamines cause vasodilation, bronchial constriction and leakage of fluid from the capillaries into tissues (edema).

5. Name four ways that antigens may be introduced to the body.

   ANSWER: injection, ingestion, inhalation, and absorption

6. List some possible signs and symptoms of anaphylaxis.

   ANSWER: a. dyspnea, wheezing, sneezing, coughing—sometimes swelling of the airway may progress to complete airway obstruction

   b. cramping, nausea, vomiting, diarrhea, itching, hives

   c. profound shock

       d. headache, convulsions

       e. flushed swollen face, cyanosis, edema at site of introduction

7. Briefly describe appropriate prehospital management of anaphylaxis.

ANSWER: Airway, high-flow O_2, ventilate if needed (consider ET tube), shock trousers, begin rapid transport (unless protocols suggest on-scene IV's and meds), large-bore IV (LR or NS), epinephrine (sub-Q if mild, IV if severe), consider benadryl, consider an aminophylline drip if symptoms persist, monitor vital signs and ECG.

Toxicology and Substance Abuse

This chapter addresses the assessment and treatment of toxicological emergencies. The number and diversity of potential toxins in our environment is staggering, but by identifying routes of entry into the body and determining appropriate general treatment priorities, a systematic approach to management can begin. In the case of drugs and other substances that are commonly abused, paramedics must be able to identify which patients are seriously affected, treat the treatable, and transport the rest to a facility that can provide treatment/evaluation.

Overview

Poisonings Over a million poisonings are reported each year in the United States, with approximately 70% of the victims under the age of five. Accidental poisonings account for about 10% of all emergency department visits and involve a variety of agents, including:

1. Household products (especially cleaning agents).
2. Food (bacteria).
3. Medications (over-the-counter and prescription).

4. Alcohol (especially in combination with medications).
5. Toxic plants.
6. Bites and stings.

Overdose An overdose can be classified as:

1. *Accidental*—Usually occurs when taking combinations of medications, giving or taking the wrong dosage, taking medication too often or combining medication with alcohol.
2. *Intentional*—Usually occurs when abusing therapeutic drugs for a desired effect or when attempting to commit suicide. Seventy to 90% of all suicides involve the ingestion or injection of drugs.

Drug Abuse Drug abuse usually leads to a wide range of behavioral, physical, and psychological effects. Often drug abuse begins with the overuse of pain or mood-altering medications, but the increased presence and usage of "recreational" drugs—many of which are in some way addictive and extremely dangerous—has severely compounded the problem for the individual abuser and society as a whole.

Alcoholism Considered by some as a form of drug abuse, alcoholism is currently being scrutinized and debated as either a "disease", "willful misbehavior", "psychological defect", "character weakness", or some combination thereof. The excessive use of alcohol while operating motor vehicles is a serious problem, as evidenced by the fact that more than half of all fatal accidents are alcohol-related.

Assessment

Effective assessment of poisonings will include the following:

1. *Primary Survey;*
2. *Vital Signs;*
3. *Transport Decision:* Critical (transport immediately); Non-Critical (continue assessment);
4. *History;*
5. *Secondary Survey.*

Primary Survey This survey is performed to uncover and treat any life-threatening condition (*A-B-C-D-E*):

1. *Airway/C-Spine*—If unconscious—or if any trauma is suspected, use precautionary measures to open and maintain the airway. (chin lift, jaw lift, jaw thrust)
2. *Breathing*—If breathing is present, note the rate, effort, and quality of respirations. Also be alert for breath odor and burns of the lips.
3. *Circulation:*
   a. Check carotid pulse—if present, note the rate and quality.
   b. Check a radial pulse—its presence indicates a probable systolic blood pressure of at least 80, while its absence indicates a probable systolic pressure of less than 80 (shock).
   c. Check capillary refill (CR)—if over 2 seconds, it is delayed, indicating poor tissue perfusion.
   d. Check skin color and temperature—an additional indication of respiratory function and tissue perfusion.
4. *Disability*—Check level of consciousness (LOC), using the A-V-P-U method:

   A = Alert;
   V = responds to Verbal stimuli;
   P = responds to Painful stimuli;
   U = Unresponsive.

5. *Expose*—Expose the chest to evaluate:
   a. Adequacy of ventilation;
   b. Integrity of the chest wall;
   c. Auscultate bilateral lung sounds.

Vital Signs Vital signs, including the cuff pressure, pulse, and respiratory rates and the presence or absence of fever (optional) should quickly be determined.

Transport Decision If at this time the patient is judged to be:

1. *Critical*—The patient should immediately be transported to the hospital, with all other assessment and treatment performed enroute. **Note:** Critical conditions would include:
    a. Severe respiratory distress/injury;
    b. Shock;
    c. Decreased level of consciousness.
2. *Non-Critical*—The patient examination should be continued.

History

1. *Identification of Poison:*
    a. Scene evaluation (medicine containers, paraphernalia, ETOH bottles, odors, method of entrance to the body);
    b. Patient or family information;
    c. Law enforcement or other rescue personnel;
    d. Bystanders/witnesses;
    e. Obtain containers and sample of substance(s) and vomitus.
2. *Current Event:*
    a. When was substance taken? *OR* When did exposure occur?
    b. How much of the substance(s) was taken? *OR* Duration of exposure?
    c. Has patient vomited (or has ipecac been given)?
    d. Has activated charcoal been given?
    e. Has any care been given?
    f. Is there a pertinent history of mental illness or recent stress?
3. *AMPLE History:*
    A = Allergies;
    M = Medications;
    P = Past medical history;
    L = Last oral intake;
    E = Events leading up to the emergency.

Secondary Survey Conduct a head-to-toe examination to rule out other injuries and assess the impact of the poison on the rest of the body. Check clothing for evidence of contamination.

Management

The principals of poisoning management include:

1. *Airway Control.*
2. *Identification of Poison.*
3. *Prevention of Absorption:*
   a. Ingested Poisons:
      (1) Emesis;
      (2) Activated charcoal;
      (3) Gastric lavage;
      (4) Dilution.
   b. Inhaled Poisons:
      (1) Removal from source;
      (2) Removal of contaminated clothing;
      (3) Protective respiratory apparatus;
      (4) Flushing lungs with oxygen;
      (5) Intubation (when indicated to protect airway).
   c. Injected Poisons:
      (1) Removal from further danger of injection;
      (2) Constricting band;
      (3) Immobilization;
      (4) Cold application;
      (5) Restrict movement.
   d. Absorbed Poisons:
      (1) Remove from exposure;
      (2) Brush off excess solids;
      (3) Flush with large amounts of water (when appropriate);
      (4) Remove contaminated clothing;
      (5) Re-flush with water.
4. *Antidote or Antivenom* (if available).
5. *Intravenous Access* (fluids and medications as needed).

Airway Control Maintain open patent airway and provide oxygen as appropriate. Patients with decreased level of consciousness may require intubation for protection of the airway. Always be ready to ventilate or suction the poisoning patient as needed.

Identification of Poison Use all available information, bring samples of poison, any containers and emesis to the hospital. Determine the route of entry into the body (ingestion, injection, inhalation, tissue contact).

Prevention of Absorption Using all the information at hand (which will usually include the advice of medical or poison control) a decision must be made on the most appropriate method of preventing absorption of the poison.

1. *Ingested Poisons*—There are four basic techniques employed to reduce absorption:

   a. Induced Emesis—Ingestion of ipecac is the method of choice for inducing emesis and is most effective when utilized within 30 minutes of ingestion (but may be of use for up to six hours). Obviously, inducing emesis is not appropriate in all cases. Guidance should always be obtained from local protocols, but these are general considerations:

   Induce emesis when:

   (1) Poison control or medical control has indicated that inducing emesis would be beneficial.

   (2) Substance has been in the body for less than 3-6 hours.

   (3) Large amounts of specific products have been ingested that will be extremely harmful if allowed to stay in the system.

   (4) Patient has ingested most pesticides, heavy metals, halogenated hydrocarbons and aromatic hydrocarbons.

   (5) Substance(s) ingested are unknown, but potentially significant.

   Do not induce emesis when:

   (1) Patient has a decreased level of consciousness. (or is unable to handle secretions)

   (2) Patient is convulsing.

   (3) Patient is pregnant.

(4) Patient may have an AMI (acute myocardial infarction).

(5) Patient has ingested corrosive substances.

(6) Patient has ingested small amounts of hydrocarbons.

(7) Patient has ingested tar, asphalt, motor or transmission oil, fuel or diesel oil, mineral oil, or baby and suntan oil.

(8) Patient has ingested mineral seal oil, signal oil or furniture polish oils (high risk of harmful vapor aspiration)

b. Gastric Lavage—As an alternative to (or following) inducement of emesis, gastric lavage removes some of the stomach contents via nasogastric tube, thus eliminating many of the contraindications for inducement of emesis. Gastric lavage varies greatly in effectiveness.

c. Activated Charcoal—Absorbs and binds toxins so they cannot be absorbed by the gastrointestinal tract. It should not be given before or with ipecac, as it inactivates the emetic. Activated charcoal is often given after emesis or gastric lavage as a way of neutralizing the remaining toxic agent(s). Though rarely used in prehospital care, recent studies suggest that activated charcoal is the most effective way to retard absorption of poisons by the body. It's use in the prehospital phase of emergency care will probably increase greatly in the near future. Dosage is as follows:

(1) Adults = 30-100 grams in a water slurry (can be obtained as a pre-mix).

(2) Children = 1-2 grams/kg in a water slurry.

d. Dilution—Some ingested poisons are better managed by dilution with water, milk, mineral oil or other appropriate fluids until the concentrations in the body are rendered less toxic. Selection of the dilute fluid must be done on a case by case basis.

2. *Inhaled Poisons*—The following techniques should be utilized as necessary to inhibit absorption of inhaled poisons:

a. Removal from source—The victim must be removed from contact before assessment or definitive treatment begins—BUT ONLY IF RESCUER IS PROTECTED AND CAN ACCOMPLISH THIS SAFELY.

b. Removal of contaminated clothing.

c. High-flow oxygen (and positive pressure ventilation if needed).

d. Intubation (if unconscious).

3. *Injected Poisons*—These techniques may be utilized to inhibit the absorption of injected poisons:
   a. Removal from danger of further injection—IF IT CAN BE DONE SAFELY.
   b. Constricting band above wound site (in certain cases).
   c. Immobilization of affected part.
   d. Cold application (selectively).
4. *Absorbed Poisons:*
   a. Remove from exposure—IF IT CAN BE DONE WHILE ENSURING THE SAFETY OF THE RESCUER.
   b. Brush off excess solid contaminants before flushing with water.
   c. Flush with large amounts of water (if appropriate).
   d. Remove contaminated clothing.
   e. Flush again with large amounts of water.

Poisonings

A poison can be defined as a substance that produces harmful physiological or psychological effects. Poison can enter the body by being ingested, injected, inhaled, or absorbed.

Ingested Poisons Poisons make their way into the body by being swallowed. Toxic effects on the body can be:

1. *Delayed*—Because of varied absorption rates from the gastrointestinal (GI) tract, many substances will exhibit delayed effects. While little is absorbed by the stomach wall (where a substance may remain for several hours), the walls of the small intestine absorb agents quickly.
2. *Immediate*—Corrosive substances (such as strong acids and alkalis) cause immediate damage to the lips, tongue, throat, esophagus, and upper GI tract—primarily through burns.

Ingested poisons are not all treated the same way. The following categories of substances require special handling:

1. Strong Acids and Alkalis—Acids (toilet bowl cleaner, and so on) and alkalis (ammonia, drain cleaner, bleach) may cause significant burns

on the lips and tongue and in the mouth, throat, esophagus, stomach, GI tract, and respiratory tract. *Do not induce vomiting,* as the amount of tissue damage can be increased. Dilution with milk or water is recommended, but in carefully controlled amounts to minimize the likelihood of vomiting. *Do not attempt to neutralize.* The chemical reaction that must occur creates heat and may cause internal burns.

2. Hydrocarbons—These account for a significant number of pediatric poison ingestions. The usual small amounts accidentally ingested by adults (as in syphoning gasoline) are seldom a problem.

   Signs and Symptoms: There are a wide variety such as coughing, labored breathing, tachypnea, cyanosis, nausea/vomiting, stomach pain, seizures, lethargy, coma, or fever.

   Management: Confirm the ABCs. Whether or not to induce vomiting after the ingestion of petroleum-based products will depend upon local protocols and the type and amount of product ingested. Following are some general guidelines.

   Induce vomiting in the case of:

   a. Large amounts (more than 1 ml/kg) of gasoline, kerosene, turpentine, lighter fluid, mineral spirits, and the like.
   b. Large amounts of halogenated hydrocarbons (carbon tetrachloride, trichloroethane, trichlorethylene, methylene chloride).
   c. Large amounts of aromatic hydrocarbons (benzene, toluene, zylene).
   d. Any hydrocarbon with heavy metals, insecticides, nitrobenzene, or aniline.

3. Methyl Alcohol (methanol, wood alcohol)—An alcohol contained in products such as varnishes, paints, paint removers, sterno and antifreeze. Alcoholics have been known to drink methanol when ethanol is unavailable—often with tragic results.

   Signs and Symptoms: Rapid breathing, hypotension (perhaps shock), nausea/vomiting, headache, CNS depression, renal failure, severe acidosis, and blindness are all signs and symptoms of methyl alcohol poisoning.

   Management: Confirm the ABCs, 100% oxygen, monitor ECG, and establish an IV. Vomiting should be induced if patient is alert. Hospital treatment may include administration of one ounce of 80 proof whiskey (ethanol) every hour (IV or oral), which inhibits methanol metabolism.

4. Cyanide—Cyanide can be ingested in the form of fruit pits (laetrile), inhaled in the form of hydrogen cyanide (a byproduct of some types of combustion and fumigants), or absorbed through the skin. Cyanide inhibits the cellular use of oxygen and causes anoxia. In sufficient quantities, cyanide exposure may cause fatal respiratory arrest.

   Signs and Symptoms: Tachycardia, vomiting, coma, seizures, and a progression from early rapid or deep breathing with dyspnea to slow, gasping respirations are all signs and symptoms of cyanide poisoning.

   Management: Confirm the ABCs, high-flow oxygen, assisted ventilations, and use of a cyanide kit. If a cyanide kit is not available, break ampules of amyl nitrate into a sponge and hold over the patient's nose for 20-30 seconds of every minute. Establish an IV (TKO) and monitor the ECG.

   Note: Some patients contaminated with cyanide have spread dangerous amounts of the agent to their rescuers. Consider a known cyanide poisoning as a HAZARDOUS MATERIALS INCIDENT and utilize caution and personal protection.

5. Food Poisoning—Poisoning caused by bacteria contained in food is often due to inadequate refrigeration or improper food preparation and handling.

   Signs and Symptoms: Nausea and vomiting, abdominal cramping, diarrhea, dehydration, and problems with the respiratory system are all signs and symptoms. Some of the bacteria involved are:

   a. Staphylococcus (produces toxins);

   b. Clostridium (forms spores); and

   c. Salmonella (often see in poultry).

   Botulism is the most severe form of food poisoning, resulting in a significant (30% or more) mortality rate. Botulism can cause respiratory paralysis. (Example: improperly canned green beans.)

   Management: Confirm the ABCs, oxygen, assisted ventilations, if needed, and control of dehydration with IV fluids. Most cases of food poisoning are minor, often going undetected or interpreted as the flu.

6. Poisonous Plants—A wide variety of common household and garden plants are poisonous if ingested, with widely varying toxic effects and symptomotology.

   Management: Management usually includes the inducement of vomiting, identification of the plant (bring a sample to the hospital), and general care guidelines for ingested poisons.

Inhaled Poisons Inhaled poisons enter the body through the respiratory system, usually as toxic gases. Some examples of toxic gases would include:

1. Carbon Monoxide (CO)—A colorless, odorless gas produced during the incomplete burning of organic fuels, most commonly from automobiles and various types of home heaters. Half of adult suicides are a result of carbon monoxide poisoning. CO is 200 times more likely to bind to hemoglobin than oxygen, and is very difficult to remove once bonded. Less oxygen can be transported to the cells, resulting in cellular hypoxia.

    Signs and Symptoms: These are directly related to the duration and concentration of exposure, beginning with headache and nausea, and progressing to vomiting, rapid breathing, tachycardia, confusion and a roaring sensation in the ears. Sustained exposure will result in cyanosis, loss of consciousness, dilated pupils, seizures, coma and eventually death. At some point reversal becomes impossible due to the difficulty in removing the CO from hemoglobin, unless immediate access to an appropriate hyperbaric chamber is gained. Changing pressures is the only rapid way to free the hemoglobin of the carbon monoxide to make room for oxygen. A cherry-red skin color is sometimes seen with CO poisoning, but usually not until death or late exposure.

    Management: Removal from the source of CO, 100% oxygen, ventilatory assistance, monitoring ECG, an IV of D5W and treatment for shock.

2. Freon—Used primarily as a refrigerant and aerosol propellant, freon is inhaled by some as an intoxicant. Freon levels may quickly become toxic.

    Signs and Symptoms: Freon affects the heart and its electrical system, primarily in the form of dysrythmias.

    Management: Removal from the source, 100% oxygen, an IV of D5W (unless in shock, where LR would be more appropriate), ECG monitoring and medication as needed to control dysrhythmias.

3. Ammonia—Ammonia becomes a highly caustic alkaline compound when combined with water in the tissues.

    Signs and Symptoms: Watering and irritation of the eyes, nausea and vomiting, diarrhea, abdominal pain and irritation of the airways with coughing, choking and respiratory collapse.

Management: Management requires removal from the source—IF THE RESCUER IS PROTECTED FROM INHALATION OF THE AMMONIA, 100% oxygen and ventilatory assistance as needed. Severe cases may require the use of endotracheal intubation.

4. Chlorinated Hydrocarbons (example: Carbon Tetrachloride)—These may cause damage as a result of high doses or cumulative low doses, affecting the central nervous system (CNS), liver, and kidneys.

   Signs and Symptoms of Acute Exposure: Headache, mental confusion, irritation of the mucous membranes in the respiratory tract, nausea and vomiting.

   Management: Removal from the source of the poisoning—IF IT CAN BE ACCOMPLISHED WITHOUT ENDANGERING THE RESCUER, removing all contaminated clothing, careful airway maintenance (suction or intubation as needed) and 100% high-flow oxygen.

5. Methyl Chloride—A colorless, combustible gas which smells like ether and can be absorbed through the respiratory tract *and* the skin.

   Signs and Symptoms of Acute Exposure: Confusion, drowsiness, nausea, vomiting, seizures, and coma.

   Management: SAFE EXTRICATION AND REMOVAL OF THE VICTIM FROM THE SOURCE OF GAS, removal of contaminated clothing, careful airway maintenance (intubation may be necessary) and high-flow 100% oxygen. Special care must be taken to avoid sparks, open flames or the use of electrical equipment in the area during extrication.

Injected Poisons Injected poisons may be managed generally as any poisoning, with the added danger of possible anaphylactic reactions. Specific types of poisonings include:

1. Insect Stings—

   a. *Bees, hornets, wasps and yellow-jackets*—Effects are caused by injection of toxin through the sting. A significant number of deaths occur each year as a direct result of anaphylactic reactions from these insect stings.

   Signs and Symptoms: Localized pain, swelling, redness and occasional allergic reactions of varying degrees.

   Management: Carefully remove any visible stingers (without squeezing the venom sac), utilize ice or cold applications and treat any allergic reactions (epinephrine and benedryl may be needed) that may occur.

b. *Spider Bites*—Only two of the many spiders found in the United States are dangerous to man—the brown recluse spider and the female black widow spider.

   (1) Brown Recluse—Brown color, it has a band of darker color extending back from the eyes in the shape of a violin. Its venom is necrotoxic, causing necrosis by activating clotting mechanisms to form microthrombotic aggregates which plug arterioles and venules. This spider's bite is initially painless, but within 2-8 hours severe pain develops, the area becomes reddened and a blister forms. If untreated, this necrotic lesion increases in size and eventually can become an open ulcer several centimeters in diameter. Death is rare, but a few cases have been reported in the first 48 hours.

   Signs and Symptoms: Fever, chills, weakness, nausea, vomiting, joint pain, skin rash, and delirium are all symptoms. Intravascular clotting can occur, precipitating myocardial infarction or pulmonary emboli.

   Management: Confirm the ABCs, ice packs, and treat symptoms as they develop. The hospital may consider whole blood replacement to combat the clotting and pain medication. THERE IS NO ANTIVENIN TO THE BROWN RECLUSE, but antibodies to the venom can develop after surviving a bite.

   (2) Black Widow—Jet black, it has orange or red spots on its belly in the shape of an hourglass. The victim will usually feel a sharp pin-prick sensation when bitten, followed by a dull, numbing-type pain. The black widow's venom is neurotoxic, with a 5% or less fatality rate in those whose bites have been reported, and one can develop antibodies to the venom after surviving a bite. About 500 bites are reported each year. Generally, those at risk are the very young and the very old.

   Signs and Symptoms: The bite site may reveal tiny red fang marks, local swelling, mild pain, and blanching. If the bite occurred in the lower extremities, local pain will be followed by pain and rigidity of the abdominal muscles. If the bite is on an upper extremity, the pain and rigidity will be felt in the chest, back, and shoulder. In any case, all major muscles groups will eventually be involved, increasing in intensity for 12-48 hours before gradually subsiding. There may be nausea, vomiting, sweating, salivation, cramping, tremors, fever, hypertension, and possibly seizures and paralysis.

Management: Confirm the ABCs, complete rest, ice packs to bite site, consider 5-10 mg of Valium in the prehospital phase if muscle spasms are severe. ANTIVENIN IS AVAILABLE.

c. Scorpion Stings—When provoked, scorpions retaliate with the stinger located at the end of their tail. The sting of most scorpions will be uncomfortable, but not fatal. The exception is the Arizona scorpion.

Signs and Symptoms: Generally victims will experience immediate sharp pain at the site of injection, which will progress to numbness. The vast majority of scorpion stings will only involve pain and restlessness, but the sting of the Arizona scorpion may cause systemic effects that can be fatal. They might include restlessness, drooling, slurred speech, muscle twitching, abdominal pain and cramps, nausea, vomiting, seizures, dilated pupils, respiratory failure, and circulatory failure.

Management: Confirm the ABCs, constricting band above the sting, ice packs. Do not use analgesics—they seem to intensify the symptoms.

2. Snakebites—Out of about 6,000 reported bites about 20 deaths per year are attributed to snakebites. Of the 2,500 species of snakes, only about 200 are dangerous. The pit vipers and the coral snake are the only poisonous snakes indigenous to the United States.

a. *Pit Vipers*—Characterized by a deep pit (sensory organ) on either side of the nostrils below the eyes and long, erictile fangs. Their bodies are thick with broad, flat, almost triangular heads, and their length ranges from 3-8 feet (even longer). Pit viper envenomation is significant in about 70-80% of bites and is generally more serious in children. Their venom has a combination of effects that involve the heart, blood, clotting, and the nervous system.

Signs and Symptoms: Immediate severe pain at injection site, fang marks, swelling, discoloration, weakness, dizziness or faintness, sweating and/or chills, nausea, vomiting, tachycardia, hypotension, and shallow respirations that may progress to respiratory failure are the most common symptoms.

Management: Management includes removal from further danger IF THIS CAN BE DONE SAFELY, confirm the ABCs, supportive care as needed, cleanse wound, constricting band above injury site to slow venom absorption, immobilization of the injured body part, IV of LR (in uninvolved extremity). DO NOT APPLY ICE, COLD PACKS, OR FREON SPRAYS. DO NOT MAKE IN-CISIONS IN THE WOUND—the benefits of incision are minimal and the risks are great. Incising is acceptable under limited circumstances—if approved by protocols. ANTIVENIN IS AVAILABLE.

(1) Rattlesnakes—Inflict about 60% of bites reported, and are native to every state but Maine. They are shy, will flee if given a chance, but will bite when provoked or when surprised. The characteristic warning rattle is provided by the tip of the tail.

(2) Copperhead—Slightly more aggressive than the rattlesnake, but will still leave you alone if not provoked. The copperhead has no warning rattle and is usually well-camouflaged in its environment. Death is rare from copperhead bites.

(3) Cottonmouth (water moccasin)—An aggressive snake, the cottonmouth will actually detour toward you in some circumstances, especially on the water, where it most likely encountered. It gets its name from the cottony white of its inner mouth when poised to strike.

b. *Coral Snake*—Found primarily in Florida, the mid-southern, western, and southwestern states, the coral snake is about 10 to 18 inches in length and inflict only 2% of all reported bites. Its venom is essentially neurotoxic with central and peripheral activity—much more toxic than the pit viper's venom—IF IT IS INJECTED. Only a third of coral snake bites inject significant amounts of venom, while a third of the bites result in no envenomation.

Identification: The coral snake has a black nose and red and yellow adjacent bands (perhaps even red and white). If the snake has adjacent red and black bands, it is not poisonous and not a coral snake. "Red on yellow will kill a fellow", "red on black—venom lack."

Signs and Symptoms: The bite causes little pain or swelling and may be inconspicuous. In fact, there may be no real signs or symptoms for up to 12 hours. Ptosis (drooping of the eyelids) or occulomotor palsy may be the first signs of serious poisoning. Other symptoms that may occur include salivation, difficulty in swallowing, slurred speech, euphoria, confusion, sweating, nausea, vomiting, abdominal pain, dyspnea, loss of consciousness and seizures. Paralysis will progress and, if untreated, death will ensue from respiratory and cardiac failure. Most symptoms present within 1-7 hours or may be delayed up to 18 hours, but then occur quickly.

Management: Confirm the ABCs, 100% oxygen, and supportive care as needed, cleanse wound, constricting band above the bite, immobilize affected body part, complete rest, IV of LR. DO NOT APPLY ICE, COLD PACKS OR FREON SPRAY. DO NOT MAKE INCISIONS THROUGH THE WOUND. Antivenin is available and ALL VICTIMS BITTEN BY A CORAL SNAKE SHOULD RECEIVE THIS ANTIVENIN.

c. *Marine Animal Injections*—Jellyfish, sea urchins, stingrays and coral are just a few of the marine animals that can deliver toxic injections to humans.

Signs and Symptoms: Signs and symptoms vary of course, from creature to creature, but there are some general effects:

Locally = Intense pain and swelling.

Systemic = Nausea, vomiting, weakness, tachycardia, dyspnea, syncope, hypotension, dysrhythmias and possible anaphylaxis.

Management: Confirm the ABCs, oxygen and supportive care as needed, constricting band above wound if on an extremity and administer analgesics for pain. Some poisons injected by marine animals can be easily detoxified. Here are some examples:

(1) Jellyfish, coral, and anemones inject little spines or stingers. These spines can be removed manually or be inactivated by isopropyl alcohol. Baking soda paste over the site will neutralize the venom.

(2) Sea urchin and stingrays inject a venom that can be detoxified by immersion in hot water (110-115 degree Fahrenheit).

Absorbed Poisons These types of poisons make their way into body systems by absorption through the skin and mucous membranes after surface contact. These agents include:

James H. Taylor

1. Organophosphates—Chemicals utilized in insecticides and chemical weapons which are extremely toxic and may be fatal without prompt treatment.

   Signs and Symptoms: Signs and symptoms may include salivation, nausea, vomiting, diarrhea, sweating, bradycardia, hypotension, blurred vision, constricted pupils, abdominal pain, seizures, and coma.

   Management: Management should include removal of the victim from exposure (IF THIS CAN BE DONE SAFELY BY THE RESCUER), suction of large amounts of bronchial secretions and careful airway maintenance, flushing with large amounts of water, removal of contaminated clothing, repeated flushing with water, an IV of LR, ECG monitoring, and administration of atropine (2 mg IV push, repeated every 3-8 minutes as necessary). Treatment is directed toward increasing the pulse rate and reducing secretions.

2. Cyanide—SAME AS FOR INGESTED CYANIDE.

Drug Overdose

Drug overdose (OD) occurs when toxic effects occur from a larger than normal dose of a drug. Causes of such an overdose might include:

Accidental overdose;

Changes in drug strength;

Polydrug abuse (using multiple drugs);

Miscalculation; and

Suicide attempts.

The importance of a good history should be emphasized, though it is often difficult to obtain in the case of overdose. A knowledge of street drugs, slang terms for drugs and a non-judgmental demeanor will go far in helping elicit reliable overdose histories. We will briefly examine overdose with different groups of drugs:

Narcotic Overdose Narcotic overdoses include the use of heroin, morphine, demerol, codeine, methadone, Darvon, percodan, and Dilaudid.

Signs and Symptoms of Intoxication (general): Euphoria, "nodding", nausea, and pinpoint pupils (except with Demerol or combinations).

Signs and Symptoms of Overdose: Respiratory depression, apnea, CNS depression, stupor, coma, hypotension or profound shock.

Management: Confirm the ABCs, 100% oxygen, draw blood, IV of D5W, give 50 cc of D50W, give Narcan 2.0 mg IV, IM or SQ to reverse the effects of the narcotic. Darvon overdose may require more Narcan. Be prepared to restrain patient upon improvement in LOC.

Sedative Overdose (Hypnotics) Valium and Librium (benzodiazepines), and phenobarbitol, amobarbitol, and secobarbital (barbiturates) are some of the drug names in this category.

Signs and Symptoms of Overdose: Constricted pupils initially—but later pupils become fixed and dilated (even without brain damage), respiratory depression, hypotension (possibly progressing to shock) and a tendency toward easy development of hypothermia.

Management: Confirm the ABCs, 100% oxygen, draw blood, and an IV of D5W. If unconscious, give 50 cc of D50W, if no result follow with 0.08-2.0 mg of Narcan IV. Consider ipecac to induce vomiting.

Stimulant Overdose Amphetamines (Benzadrene, Desadrine, and Metaamphetamine) Stimulants (caffeine), and Cocaine are some of the drug names in this category. Cocaine has become a major drug of abuse in the United States, derived from coca leaves cultivated in Peru, Bolivia, and Columbia, especially since the development of "crack" cocaine.

Signs and Symptoms of Intoxication: Euphoria, excitement, decrease in need for sleep, decrease in appetite and increase in BP and pulse.

Signs and Symptoms of Overdose: Nausea, vomiting, chills, sweating, fever, dilated pupils, increased metabolic rate, tachycardia, hypertension, irritability, hallucination, seizures, cardiac dysrhythmias—even a form of violent paranoid psychosis can occur.

Management: Confirm the ABCs, monitor ECG, if ingestion is relatively recent and patient does not seem stimulated, consider ipecac for emesis. Be very cautious with these patients and ensure your personal safety.

Phencyclidine (PCP) Overdose: PCP is an illegally produced drug of abuse, which is snorted, ingested, smoked with marijuana or injected IV.

Signs and Symptoms: *Low doses* (patient still conscious) produce slowness and dullness, incoordination, disorientation, violent or bizarre behavior, increase in physical strength, delusional behavior and an insensitivity to pain. *High doses* (acute) produce CNS depression, sweating, salivation, hypertension, tachycardia, fever, convulsions, increase rate of respirations and coma.

Management: Confirm the ABCs, monitor ECG, consider ipecac if recent, keep quiet and calm as possible, treat the symptom (valium for seizures), restrain or prepare to restrain.

Tricyclic Antidepressants (TCA) Elavil and Tofranil are some of the "mood-elevating" drugs in this category. TCAs are prescribed primarily for depression and some types of psychological dysfunction. Almost invariably, these drugs are involved in suicide attempts by these same individuals.

Signs and Symptoms: Tachycardia, fever, restlessness, and anxiety will be seen initially, then seizures, dysrhythmias and coma. Additionally, the QRS complex may widen significantly during tricyclic overdoses.

Management: Confirm the ABCs, oxygen and supportive care as needed, monitor ECG, IV of D5W, ipecac to induce emesis IF COMPLETELY ALERT, IV of D5W, consider administering sodium bicarbonate to alkalyze blood—a specific treatment for tricyclic overdose—if allowed by local protocols.

Hallucinogens Overdose LSD, psilocybin, mescaline, peyote, and morning glory seeds are some of the substances in this category.

Signs and Symptoms: Hallucinations, distortion of sensory perception, nausea, vomiting and some anxiety reactions—but generally no major medical problems. Psychological reactions may lead to bizarre behavior.

Management: Confirm the ABCs, check for injuries that may not be apparent, find a secure quiet environment in which to "talk-down" the patient—or transport to a facility that can provide this kind of care.

Aspirin Overdose (salicylic acid) Aspirin, in tablet form, is the most common analgesic medication in the world, but aspirin is also an ingredient of many other preparations, especially cold remedies. Its primary use is for the control of pain. Most aspirin overdoses are a result of suicide attempts, accidental ingestion by children, or chronic ingestion by those dependent upon its properties. Overdose causes acute acidosis, while long-term use may cause bleeding ulcers and kidney failure.

Signs and Symptoms of Overdose: Faintness, visual disturbances, nausea, vomiting, gastrointestinal bleeding, fever, dehydration, rapid breathing and acidosis. In more advanced cases there is severe acidosis, seizures, delirium and coma (death if untreated).

Management: Confirm the ABCs, oxygen, and supportive care as needed, ipecac to induce emesis if alert, IV of NS or LR, monitor ECG and consider sodium bicarbonate to combat the metabolic acidosis—if protocols permit.

Acetaminophen Overdose Tylenol, Datril, and Tempra are just a few of the many forms and labels of acetaminophen in this category. Acetaminophen is a common over-the-counter analgesic medication manufactured as tablets, capsules, gelcaps, liquids, and so on, and is found as an ingredient in many other preparations, especially cold remedies. ACETAMINOPHEN IS A DANGEROUS DRUG WHEN OVERINGESTED. As few as 30 standard strength (325 mg) tablets will be toxic in the average adult, and 140 mg/kg is toxic in the average child. The danger of the acetaminophen overdose is two-fold:

1. Many people refer to tylenol and aspirin as the same thing, and may confuse the two when giving a history—with tragic results.
2. Some patient may survive the first phase of overdose and improve. They think the crisis has passed, do not seek medical help, and when more serious symptoms return—irreversible damage has occurred, perhaps even leading to inevitable death.

Signs and Symptoms of Overdose: Lethargy, loss of appetite, sweating, nausea, vomiting, abdominal pain and coma. If death occurs, the cause is liver toxicity and failure. After the first 24 hours, the signs of liver damage begin to appear. (the abdominal pain, later jaundice and coma)

Management: Confirm the ABCs, oxygen, and supportive care as needed, ipecac to induce emesis (if indicated), monitor ECG, IV of D5W. Do not give activated charcoal at the same time as N-ACETYLCYSTEINE, an antidote sometimes given in the emergency department, as it will absorb the antidote. Separate the administrations by at least one hour.

Drug Abuse

Though most drugs are used for medical reasons, some are used almost exclusively for their effects on mood, behavior or both. Drug abuse has been defined as:

The use of prescription drugs for non-prescribed purposes, or the use of drugs which have no prescribed medical uses.

Consider the following terms:

1. *Drug Dependency*—Patterns of drug use that are harmful (whether legal or not) and result in an unreasonable dependence (physical or psychological) upon a drug or drugs.
2. *Psychological Dependence* (habituation)—A situation in which the effects produced by a drug are necessary to maintain a person's feeling of well-being.
3. *Physical Dependence*—When regular repetitious use of a drug is required to prevent withdrawal symptoms.
4. *Tolerance*—Progressive lessening of a drug's effect after repeated doses. Growing doses are then necessary to maintain the desired effect.
5. *Compulsive Drug Use*—An unreasonable or uncontrollable compulsion to obtain and use a drug or drugs (heavy smokers, alcoholics, heavy caffeine users).
6. *Withdrawal*—A cluster of symptoms provoked by the abrupt discontinuation of a drug to which the person has become addicted. Withdrawal can be mild or severe—even fatal.

COMMON DRUGS OF ABUSE AND DEPENDENCE would include:

Alcohol	Barbiturates
Narcotics	Amphetamines
Marijuana	Cocaine
PCP	Hallucinogens
Sedatives	Tricyclics
Hypnotics	Stimulants

Remember, paramedic drug kits can be a target for desperate addicts, and drugs can play a part in many disease processes, as well as trauma. Think of drugs as a possibility whenever confronted with seizures, bizarre or changed behavior, stupor, and coma.

Alcohol

Alcohol is the most commonly used drug in the United States. The distinction between casual use, abuse, and alcoholism is sometimes a very cloudy one, especially when many alcoholics deny their addiction. As with any other drug dependency, withdrawal, and tolerance occur in alcoholism. In fact, some alcoholics substitute barbiturates if denied alcohol. Any field paramedic who has worked for a week or more has probably encountered one or more intoxicated individuals as patients, family, bystanders, witnesses, or road obstructions. *More than half of all traffic fatalities involve alcohol.* A huge amount of money is spent treating alcoholics, a portion of our economy depends upon the sale and promotion of alcoholic beverages, and alcohol is the most widely experienced drug among all ages of the population—beginning with grade school.

Effects of Alcohol One of the effects of alcohol demonstrates one its attractions to the general public—the breakdown of inhibitions and stresses with mild dosages. Unfortunately, this is just about the stage that alcohol begins impairing skilled functions like DRIVING AN AUTOMOBILE. Alcohol is a CNS depressant. In large doses it causes respiratory depression, decreased level of consciousness and decreased protective reflexes—a combination that can end in death.

Profile of an Alcoholic The alcoholic develops patterns of use/abuse that parallel other drug addictions such as tolerance, dependence, and withdrawal. Other patterns may fit into a history of alcoholism as well:

1. Drinking early in the day.
2. Drinking alone or in secret.
3. Periodic binges, where the drinker continues drinking for several days or weeks.
4. Partial or total memory loss for periods of heavy drinking.
5. Unexplained history of regular GI problems, especially bleeding.
6. Denial of any inference of a "drinking problem."
7. Cigarette burns on clothing—from falling asleep with a cigarette.
8. Chronically flushed face and palms, or tremors.
9. Odor of ETOH on breath at inappropriate times—early in the morning, while at work, after lunch breaks, or trips to the bathroom. . .

Medical Consequences of Chronic Alcohol Ingestion Frequent alcohol use over a long period of time takes its toll in medical consequences. Some of these might include:

1. Poor nutrition.
2. Cirrhosis of the liver and alcoholic hepatitis.
3. Loss of sensation in the hands or feet.
4. Pancreatitis.
5. Poor balance and coordination.
6. Upper GI tract bleeding (sometimes fatal).
7. Hypoglycemia.
8. Subdural hematoma or fractures from frequent falls.
9. Loss of recent memory.

Withdrawal Syndrome Occurs several hours after sudden abstinence and lasts for five to seven days.

Signs and Symptoms: Tremoring hands, tongue, and eyelids; nausea, vomiting and weakness; hypertension, sweating, rapid pulse, and anxiety; depression and irritability; orthostatic hypotension, brief hallucinations and difficulty sleeping.

Delirium Tremens (DTs): Usually develops on the second or third day of withdrawal. There is a decreased level of consciousness in which the patient hallucinates and misinterprets nearby events, may become agitated or excited easily, sweats heavily, trembles excessively, may talk or yell incoherently, or may be totally quiet and seem paranoid (rare).

Seizures: Seizures sometimes develop, usually within the first 24-36 hours of abstinence and may require Valium for control. Seizures or DTs are associated with significant mortality.

Methanol Poisoning (Ethylene Glycol) When alcoholics can't afford or have no access to alcoholic beverages, they have been known to drink "squeeze", sterno, wood alcohol (all forms of methanol), or antifreeze (ethylene glycol), any of which may cause blindness or death. See previous discussion on ingested poisons.

Management of the Alcohol Overdose Confirm the ABCs, supportive care as needed, ipecac to induce emesis (if indicated), Valium for seizures, and consider administration of D50W and/or thiamine—if allowed in local protocols.

Summary

Managing toxicological emergencies and substance abuse demands a great deal of the paramedic. Good base knowledge, common sense, skill, judgment and the right equipment enables paramedics to begin definitive treatment for these problems in the field (in many cases).

SELF-TEST

Chapter 21

1. 70% of the poisonings reported in the United States each year occur in the following age group:

   a. under 5   d. 36-55

   b. 5-21   e. 56-75

   c. 21-35   f. over 75

   ANSWER: a. under 5-years old

2. When assessing a suspected poisoning victim, it is important to identify possible agents involved. Name at least three ways this might be done.

   ANSWER: a. scene evaluation (medicine containers, paraphernalia, bottles, odors, and so on)

   b. patient or family information

   c. law enforcement or rescue personnel

   d. bystanders or witnesses

   e. samples of substance and/or vomitus

3. Activated charcoal is very useful in absorbing and binding poisons, but it may also neutralize a first-line medication often given to patients who have ingested poisons. What is this medication?

   ANSWER: Ipecac

4. Prevention of absorption is a major component of care in overdoses and other poisonings. Name at least three of the methods used.

   ANSWER: a. syrup of Ipecac

             b. gastric lavage

             c. activated charcoal

             d. dilution

5. Victims who have inhaled a poison present several problems for rescuers. Assuming that the rescuer is protected with appropriate gear, what should immediately be done upon reaching this kind of victim.

   ANSWER: Remove the victim from the source of the poison.

6. Is inducement of vomiting recommended in the patient who has ingested a strong acid or alkali?

   ANSWER: No. These are tricky situations requiring special care based upon the amount and type of product involved.

7. Name an antidote to methyl alcohol (wood alcohol, methanol, sterno).

   ANSWER: ethyl alcohol (such as 80-proof whiskey)

8. TRUE or FALSE. Known cyanide poisonings should be considered a hazardous materials incident—utilizing caution and personal protection.

   ANSWER: TRUE

9. Many cases of food poisoning are thought to be flu. The most severe form of food poisoning is called _____ .

   ANSWER: botulism

10. Carbon monoxide is _____ times more likely to bind to hemoglobin than is _____ , and is very difficult to remove once bonded.

    ANSWER: 200, oxygen

11. An important aspect of treatment for inhaled poisons is:

    a. removal from the source

    b. administration of oxygen

    c. monitoring the ECG

    d. all of the above

    ANSWER: d. all of the above

12. TRUE or FALSE. The sting of most scorpions is fatal.

    ANSWER: FALSE

13. Assuming significant envenomation, which of the following snakes is most deadly?

    a. rattlesnake

    b. coral snake

    c. copperhead

    d. cottonmouth

    ANSWER: b. coral snake

14. What medication is useful in treating organophosphate poisonings?

    ANSWER: atropine

15. What is the most useful medication for treating narcotic overdose?

    ANSWER: narcan

16. TRUE or FALSE. Low doses of PCP may cause an increase in physical strength, insensitivity to pain, incoordination, disorientation and violent or bizarre behavior.

    ANSWER: TRUE

17. Overdose of aspirin causes acute _____ , while long-term use may cause bleeding ulcers and kidney failure.

    ANSWER: acidosis

18. Acetaminophen overdose can cause _____ damage severe enough to be irreversible or fatal.

    ANSWER: liver

19. A cluster of symptoms provoked by the abrupt discontinuation of an addicted drug is called _____ .

    ANSWER: withdrawal

20. The most commonly abused drug in the United States is _____ .

    ANSWER: alcohol

21. TRUE or FALSE. Over half of all traffic fatalities involve alcohol use.

    ANSWER: TRUE

22. The following signs may indicate a pattern of alcoholism:

    a. drinking early in the day

    b. chronically flushed face and palms, or tremors

   c. unexplained history of regular GI problems, especially bleeding

   d. cigarette burns on clothing

   e. all of the above

ANSWER: e. all of the above

23. TRUE or FALSE. Delirium tremens (DTs) brought on by withdrawal from alcohol are extremely uncomfortable but not fatal.

ANSWER: FALSE—DT's have a significant mortality rate

CHAPTER 22

Infectious Diseases

Management of infectious diseases is handled primarily within the hospital setting. Prehospital assessment and management focuses on the recognition of possible infectious diseases, safety of responding personnel, supportive patient care, preventing cross-contamination, and cleaning/disinfecting of emergency equipment. Briefly, we will review the immune system and some specific infectious diseases.

Definitions

Virus—A minute organism (and a parasite) dependent on nutrients inside cells for metabolic and reproductive needs.

Bacteria—Any micro-organism of the class schizomycetes. Bacteria are either spherical (or ovoid), rod-shaped or spiral, they vary in size and may produce poisonous substances called toxins.

Fungus:

1. Sponge-like growth on the body that resembles fungi.

2. A vegetable cellular organism that subsists on organic matter.

Antigen—Macromolecules located at the surface of microorganisms that, when introduced into the body, cause a response.

Antibody—Considered immunoglobulins, these native proteins are produced in the body to counter specific antigens.

Interstitial Fluid—Fluid that fills the space between cells.

Extracellular Fluid—Composed of interstitial fluid and blood.

Lymph—Clear, watery, nutrient fluid found in lymphatic vessels.

Immune System

The immune system is the body's chief defense against bacteria and virus. It's primary components are:

1. *Lymphocytes* (main cells).
2. *Antibodies*—Normally present in the body, these proteins are called immunoglobulins. They will bind to foreign antigens to cause an antigen-antibody complex.
3. *Leukocytes* (white blood cells)—Mobile units of the body's protective system. White blood cells are rapidly transported to areas of serious inflammation to defend against infectious germs.

Lymphatic System

The lymphatic system is a specialized component of the circulatory system. Lymph is a clear, watery fluid (derived generally from blood, tissue fluid and lymph nodes) that moves around the body as part of the natural defense system. Lymph and interstitial fluid are similar to blood plasma, but lower in concentration of proteins.

Infectious Diseases

Infectious diseases are caused by an organism, such as a virus, bacteria or fungus, such as pneumonia, peritonitis, and meningitis.

Methods of Transmission:

1. *Direct contact* (physical touching).
2. *Indirect contact* (contact with contaminated materials).
3. *Droplets* (inhalation of airborne droplets from respiratory tract).

4. *Injection:*
   a. Bite (of an insect, animal—even a human).
   b. Puncture (contaminated needle, glass).
5. *Transfusion* (of contaminated blood products).

"Most-at-Risk" for Prehospital Personnel

Despite all the concern by prehospital providers about the possibility of contracting AIDS, the diseases with which we are most-at-risk would include:

Hepatitis Hepatitis is an inflammatory condition caused by toxins, drugs, metabolic hypersensitivity, and immune mechanisms. It causes fever, weakness, loss of appetite, nausea, abdominal pain, jaundice, dark-colored urine and light-colored stools.

Incubation Period:

Hepatitis A (viral, most common) = 25-40 days.
Hepatitis B (serum hepatitis) = 42-160 days.

Transmission: Through the blood, urine, and stool of infected patients.
Protection: Gloves, bag, and label linens and all blood specimens.

Tuberculosis Tuberculosis is an infectious disease that causes cough, fever, night sweats, weight loss, fatigue, and hemoptysis.
Incubation Period: 4-12 weeks.
Transmission: Droplets from the respiratory tract, sneezing, coughing.
Protection: Mask, fresh air, avoid contact with sputum, avoid prolonged patient contact.

Meningitis This is an inflammation of the membranes of the brain/spinal cord, caused by bacteria, viruses, or other invading organisms. It causes fever, headache, nausea and vomiting, stiff neck, and rash.
Incubation period: 2-10 days, depending on strain.
Transmission: Direct contact with respiratory discharges.
Protection: Wear a protective mask and have patient wear a mask.

Sexually Transmitted Diseases

Sexually transmitted diseases usually present little hazard for the emergency medical team. Common sense precautions should be taken (as outlined).

Syphilis This is an infectious chronic venereal disease. It causes lesions in the genital area, lymph node enlargement, inflammation of the mouth, headaches, fever, and a variety CNS and cardiovascular signs.
Transmission: Direct sexual contact, contact with contaminated material.
Protection: Avoid contact.

Gonorrhea This is a contagious inflammation of the genital mucous membranes. It causes these signs and symptoms:
Males: Yellow discharge from penis and painful urination.
Females: Urethral or vaginal discharge, painful or frequent urination, lower abdominal pain/tenderness or pelvic inflammatory disease (PID), *OR*, MAY BE ASYMPTOMATIC.
Transmission: Direct sexual contact.
Protection: Avoid contact.

Herpes (genital) These are uncomfortable weeping lesions with associated symptoms that occur on the genitals, buttocks, and thighs.
Transmission: Direct contact with lesions (sexual or skin-to-lesion). CANNOT be transmitted by toilet seats, pools, hot tubs, or sheets.
Protection: Gloves, handwashing, avoid direct contact.

Acquired Immune Deficiency Syndrome (AIDS) AIDS involves the loss of the body's ability to defend itself against invading organisms. It causes weight loss, profuse night sweats, red/purple skin lesions, and respiratory diseases (such as pneumonia).
Incubation Period: 2 months to 2 years (approximately).
Transmission: Through blood, semen, bodily secretions, and sexual contact.
Protection: Use gloves when handling blood or body fluids and handwashing after rendering care. Bag and label contaminated linens and equipment.

Childhood Diseases

Measles This is a virus that causes fever and red blotchy rash (usually starting on the face) that spreads to the rest of the body.

Incubation Period: 8-13 days.

Transmission: Droplet or direct contact with secretions.

Protection: Gloves and mask (when in close contact with secretions), measles vaccine.

Mumps This is a virus that causes fever, swelling and tenderness of salivary glands, and inflammation of testes in adult males.

Incubation Period: 12-26 days.

Transmission: Direct contact with saliva of infected person.

Protection: Gloves, handwashing, mumps vaccine.

Chickenpox This is a virus that causes fever and whole-body skin eruptions.

Incubation Period: 10-21 days.

Transmission: Droplet secretions (from infected person's respiratory tract).

Protection: Gloves and mask, chickenpox vaccine (VZIG).

Decontamination

Personal:

1. Handwashing with appropriate cleanser/disinfectants.
2. Removal of contaminated clothing and proper tagging, cleaning, or disposal.

Vehicle:

1. While wearing gloves, clean up blood with disposable linens and bleach (1:10 diluted solution).
2. Disinfectant/antibacterial aerosol of interior (if indicated).
3. Air-out vehicle with doors and windows open at least 5 minutes daily.

Equipment:

1. Dispose of used needles and syringes properly (from your "sharps" container).
2. For general cleaning, use 1:10 dilution of bleach and water or properly researched industrial cleaner.
   a. Respiratory equipment should be disposed of or taken apart, cleaned (and sterilized if appropriate) and air-dried.
   b. Suction equipment should be cleaned (bottle) and air-dried, disposed of, or bagged for incineration.

Summary

The key to proper assessment and handling of patients with infectious diseases is a combination of common sense, an understanding of the immune system and disease symptoms and a little bit of hard work keeping vehicles and equipment free from contamination. Whenever there is a chance of encountering body fluids and/or secretions, *glove up* and have a mask handy.

SELF-TEST

Chapter 22

1. What is the primary focus of prehospital management of infectious diseases?
   ANSWER: a. recognition of possible infectious disease
   b. safety of rescue personnel
   c. supportive patient care
2. Name at least three of the methods of transmission of infectious diseases.
   ANSWER: direct contact, indirect contact, droplets, injection, and transfusion
3. Which serious infectious disease are prehospital care providers most at risk to contract?
   ANSWER: hepatitis

4. Name one way to minimize the chances of contracting meningitis from a patient?

   ANSWER: wear a mask (meningitis is spread by direct contact with respiratory discharge)

5. Which sexually transmitted disease may be asymptomatic in females?

   ANSWER: gonorrhea

6. Why is AIDS (Acquired Immune Deficiency Syndrome) so severe?

   ANSWER: AIDS victims lose their ability to defend against invading organisms.

7. How is the HIV/AIDS virus transmitted?

   ANSWER: blood, semen, bodily secretions and sexual contact

8. What is the best way to prepare a disinfectant solution (using bleach) for ambulance decontamination?

   ANSWER: 1:10 diluted solution (one part bleach to 10 parts water)

The Environment

Thermoregulation

The body requires effective internal temperature regulation to maintain the narrow temperature range necessary for efficient cellular metabolism. The hypothalmus is the regulation-control mechanism.

Heat gain is due to:

1. Metabolism.
2. Environmental factors:
    a. Air temperature;
    b. High relative humidity (sweat doesn't evaporate at > 75% humidity);
    c. Infrared radiation.

Heat loss occurs by:

1. Radiation;
2. Conduction;

3. Convection;
4. Evaporation; and
5. Respiration.

Compensatory Mechanisms are in place to resist extreme fluctuations:

1. High body temperature triggers:
   a. Peripheral vasodilation;
   b. Sweating;
   c. Increase in cardiac output;
   d. Increase in respiratory rate; and
   e. Increase in metabolic rate and heat production.
2. Low body temperature triggers:
   a. Peripheral constriction;
   b. Shivering (to raise metabolic rate);
   c. Increase in metabolic rate and heat production.

Hyperthermia

Heat Cramps These are caused by excessive sweating and loss of sodium, secondary to high external temperatures (and/or vigorous exercise). Victims will complain of cramps in finger, arms, legs, and abdominal muscles. They will be alert and appear hot and sweaty with an elevated pulse, normal BP and normal temperature.

Prehospital Management

1. Move to a cooler environment. Place at rest.
2. Increase intake of sodium and fluids (consider diluted Gatorade/ equivalent).
3. If extremely nauseated, consider replenishing fluids intravenously.

Heat Exhaustion This is caused by excessive sweating, loss of fluid and sodium, secondary to high external temperatures (and/or vigorous exercise). Victims complain of weakness, dizziness, nausea, syncope, and thirst. They may appear pale or ashen, anxious or apathetic, and will be profusely sweaty. Vital signs may be normal or respirations and BP could be elevated or depressed, pulse elevated and core temperature normal to slightly high (1-2 degrees). A few patients will have higher temperatures (up to 104).

Prehospital Management

1. Move to a cooler environment. Place at rest.
2. Increase intake of sodium and fluids (consider diluted Gatorade/ equivalent).
3. If extremely nauseated, consider replenishing fluid intravenously.
4. If LOC is diminished, consider IV fluid replenishment and transport to hospital for evaluation and further treatment. Patients experiencing heat exhaustion are dehydrated, and may progress to heat stroke if their condition is not recognized and quickly treated.

Heat Stroke This results from ineffective cooling through sweating (in high-temperature, high-humidity environments) causing body core temperature to rise and metabolism to increase. Generalized vasodilation (one body response to heat gain) decreases cardiac output, while fluid and electrolyte losses decrease blood volume. The result—cardiovascular collapse. Victims will appear hot and flushed, and as the condition *worsens* the level of consciousness will diminish (eventually to coma), marked hypotension ensues (hypovolemic shock), sweating may disappear, rapid pulse will slow to bradycardia, early rapid breathing becomes slow and core temperature may be as high as 106 degrees. Untreated, heat stroke results in death.

Prehospital Management

1. Move to a cooler environment and cool patient immediately, by whatever means are at hand. Wet towels or sheets and fans work well—air conditioning at maximum in ambulance.
2. Administer oxygen.
3. IVs (two are appropriate) of LR or NS, wide open. Heat stroke victims are severely dehydrated (hypovolemic shock) and need fluid replacement.
4. Monitor ECG and transport quickly (vasopressors are contraindicated).

Hypothermia

Hypothermia develops when the rate of heat loss to the external environment exceeds the rate of heat production in the body. As body core temperature *begins* to drop, regulatory systems in the body trigger:

1. Shivering (heat generation through muscular activity).
2. Peripheral vasoconstriction (shunting blood away from the skin).

If the core temperature *continues* to drop, the basal metabolic rate increases to compensate with more heat production from body reserves. This kind of compensation may not be adequate, and in any case cannot last long. If the core temperature falls below about 95 °F, the regulatory system begins to fail. Ventilations decrease, anoxia further slows the metabolism and the core temperature spirals downward. When it reaches about 84 °F, regulatory mechanisms fail entirely and the heart is in trouble. Patients may exhibit atrial fibrillation, respiratory arrest—even ventricular fibrillation. Without oxygen for metabolism, the core temperature dives. Lower limits of survival are not clearly defined (some say about 75 °F), but individual cases of survival have been recorded with core temperatures as low as 50 °F with long-term (60 minutes) cardiac arrest before resuscitation. It is a fact that the brain of a hypothermic victim can tolerate much longer periods without perfusion than is considered ordinary at normal body temperatures. In other words—

HYPOTHERMIC VICTIMS WHO APPEAR COMPLETELY DEAD MAY STILL BE VIABLE!

Mild Hypothermia These patients present with core body temperatures of 90-95 °F. They will probably exhibit fatigue and/or mental confusion, have cold skin and be shivering.

Prehospital Management

1. Handle patient gently.
2. Remove to warmer environment (remove wet clothing, cover with blankets, crank up the heater in the ambulance).
3. Add heat to head, neck, chest, and groin.
4. Administer warm fluids with lots of sugar orally (after shivering stops and rewarming begins to take effect). ETOH is not appropriate.

Severe Hypothermia These patients present with core body temperatures below 90 °F. They will be lethargic, stuporous, or comatose with cold skin, possibly unobtainable blood pressure, slow respirations, bradycardia (pulse may not be easily felt, and heart sounds may be inaudible) and pupils that do not react to light. Some may appear dead.

Prehospital Management (with vital signs)

1. Handle patient very, very gently.
2. Avoid the use of airway adjuncts to maintain the airway when possible.
3. If you must ventilate artificially, keep the rate slow (8-10), and DO NOT hyperventilate.
4. Remove to warmer environment (cut away wet clothing, insulate with blankets, (keep ambulance at 68-72°). Do *not* try to re-warm the extremities!
5. Add heat to head, neck, chest, and groin.
6. Nothing by mouth.
7. Avoid using supplemental oxygen unless it is heated to > 99 °F.
8. IV of D5W (75 cc/hr).
9. Monitor ECG and DO NOT administer medications (they will accumulate until rewarming occurs, *then* exert a combined effect).

Prehospital Management (without vital signs)

1. Handle gently and remove to warmer environment.
2. Assess pulse and respirations for 1-2 minutes.
3. If positive there is not pulse or respirations, begin CPR.
4. Monitor ECG—if V-FIB is present, defibrillate ONCE at 400 Joules.
5. Measure core temperature (special low-reading rectal thermometer).
6. Repeat defibrillation attempt ONLY if core temperature is at least 85 °F.
7. If defibrillation is successful, administer lidocaine (1 mg/kg IV, followed by half that dose in 15 minutes).
8. Warm oxygen and intubation ARE appropriate for the *pulseless* hypothermic victim.

9. PASG (pneumatic anti-shock garment) may be used for hypovolemia.
10. Rewarming should not be attempted UNLESS you are > 15 minutes away from a medical facility. Consult your local protocols.

Remember—
THE HYPOTHERMIC PATIENT IS NOT DEAD UNTIL HE IS WARM AND DEAD!

Frostbite

Frostbite is local cooling that occurs when parts of the body are exposed to prolonged or intense cold. After vasoconstriction in the affected body part, ice crystals form in the extra and intracellular fluid and cause structural tissue damage. When thawed, circulation is impaired, edema forms, tissues become ischemic and necrosis may or may not result. Affected body parts initially become reddened (and painful), then mottled white or gray (and numb) as cooling continues, and finally white or gray with full freezing. They will feel cold and hard, lack sensation and probably lack function.

Prehospital Management

1. Gently remove any covering from the affected area.
2. Gradual rewarming IF there is no chance that the part may be refrozen.
    a. Immerse in warm (100-105 °F) water.
    b. Or place affected part against other warm parts of the body (such as a frostbitten hand placed in the armpit).
3. Cover thawed part with loosely applied dry sterile dressings and elevate.
4. DO NOT:
    a. Massage frozen part;
    b. Rub with snow;
    c. Slap, bear, or bear weight on the affected part;
    d. Puncture or drain blebs.

Near-drowning

Death by drowning claims about 8,000 persons annually in the United States (2nd leading cause of death in those aged 4-44). Approximately 80,000 others are considered "near-drowning" victims, by virtue of having escaped the ultimate fate. Most victims are male (85%), most (2/3) do *not* know how to swim, and in nearly half of adult victims, alcohol (ETOH) intoxication was a factor.

Sequence of Events As drowning victims submerge and panic, they gasp and swallow water. Some of the water makes it past the epiglottis, causing laryngospasm and functional airway obstruction (asphyxia) and unconsciousness. Reflex swallowing of more water often causes gastic distention (increasing the possibility of vomiting and aspiration). If the victim is not soon rescued, the laryngospasms relax and water is allowed into the lungs (in 10% of cases, the laryngospasm maintains and the lungs remain dry). Several factors determine the continued pathophysiology at this point:

1. *Fresh-water Drowning:*
   a. Water passes quickly from the alveoli into the pulmonary capillaries (fresh-water is of lower solute concentration than blood—remember that in osmosis, water passes from areas of lower concentration across semi-permeable membranes to areas of higher concentration). This tends to dilute the blood and its chemistry significantly.
   b. Surfactant (a chemical that helps keep alveoli from collapsing) is decreased, making ventilation difficult and decreasing the ability to exchange oxygen and CO_2.
2. *Salt-water Drowning*—Fluid from the pulmonary capillaries passes into the alveoli (attracted by the heavy solute concentration of sodium in salt-water that has passed into the lungs), causing massive pulmonary edema.
3. *Cold-water Drowning*—Cold water (water less than 70°F) can mean a real break for both rescuer and victim because:
   a. *Cerebral Hypothermia*—Delays the damage caused by cerebral hypoxia.
   b. *Mammalian Diving Reflex*—If present, kicks the metabolism into low gear, causing profound bradycardia, dramatically slowed

respirations and profound peripheral vasoconstriction (shunting the blood around the central core).

Note: Many victims of cold-water drowning have been resuscitated with little or no permanent deficits after long periods (up to an hour) of submersion.

So remember—

> *DO NOT HESITATE TO RESUSCITATE AFTER LONG PERIODS OF SUBMERSION IN COLD WATER!*

Prehospital Management

1. Do not become an additional victim! Throw a line, throw something that will float (preferably with line attached), remove by boat or call for specialized personnel. Swimming for a still-struggling victim is the *last* alternative, and then only for an experienced trained swimmer.

2. Remove victim from the water (if there is suspicion of spinal injury, quickly slide a backboard under them first). If there will be a delay, begin resuscitation while victim is still in the water (if this can be done without danger to rescuers).

3. Begin CPR. DON'T TRY TO PUMP WATER OUT OF THE LINGS— HEIMLICH MANEUVER IS CONTRAINDICATED. Follow resuscitation routine as indicated in ACLS or local protocols. *If you suspect severe hypothermia,* follow the guidelines given earlier in this chapter under—

> *SEVERE HYPOTHERMIA (WITHOUT VITAL SIGNS)*

Note: There is no difference in treatment between salt-water or fresh-water drownings.

Nuclear Radiation

Ionizing Radiation This is the type of radiation that disrupts atoms into their charged particles which can be very detrimental to body tissues. Ionizing radiation can be divided into four types:

1. *Alpha Particles*—Large, low-energy positively-charged particles that can only penetrate skin a few cells deep. They can be stopped by

clothing, paper—even a few inches of air. Alpha particles *can* be harmful if inhaled or ingested in sufficient quantities.

2. *Beta Particles* (electrons)—Negatively-charged particles that are faster and have slightly more penetrating energy than alpha particles. Beta particles *can* be harmful if inhaled or ingested in sufficient quantities.

3. *Gamma Rays* (and X-rays)—Made of energy, not particles, gamma rays are highly penetrating and can cause direct damage to body tissues. Gamma rays can penetrate the whole body—only thick shielding materials such as lead, thick concrete and lots of earth can stop their penetration.

4. *Neutrons*—High-energy particles that can penetrate several inches of tissue and cause direct tissue damage. Neutron exposure in the field would be very rare—normally they are present only near the core of a nuclear reactor.

Measurement Radiation is measured in Roentgens, Rads, and Rems.

Sources of Background Radiation Radiation is generated by natural sources (cosmic radiation, terrestrial radionucleides, elements in human tissues) and man-made sources (medical, atomic energy industries, laboratories, consumer products, radioactive fallout).

Damage from Ionizing Radiation Ionizing radiation damages genetic material, impairing cellular reproduction and seriously affecting tissues that rapidly reproduce. Damage can be categorized as:

1. *Long-Term*—Cumulative damage over a lifetime:
   a. Decrease in the number of white cells;
   b. Impaired reproduction (sterility, genetic defects in offspring);
   c. Bone damage;
   d. Increase in incidence of cancer.
2. *Short-Term*—Based on amount of dose—the greater the *volume of body exposure* and *dose,* the greater the damage.
   a. *Acute Radiation Syndrome* (based on whole body exposures):
      1. 150 rads = Usually asymptomatic.
      2. 400 rads = Transient nausea and vomiting.
         = Mild decrease in number of white cells.

3. 500-600 rads = Severe blood disorders.

   = Gastrointestinal (GI) damage.

   = 50% mortality within 30 days.

4. 600-1500 rads = Accelerated GI and blood disorders.

   = Death within 2 weeks.

5. 2000 or more rads = Severe CNS effects.

   = Death within a few hours.

Prehospital Management   Normal principles of emergency care still apply, but attention must be paid to the source of exposure and extent of patient contamination.

1. *Externally radiated patient*—Presents no danger to paramedics, and requires normal care for injuries OTHER than radiation.

2. *Internally radiated patient*—Ingestion or inhalation of radioactive material presents no danger to paramedics. Normal care procedures should be used, but these additional precautions are in order:

   a. Collect body wastes.

   b. Use airway adjuncts if artificial ventilation is required.

   c. If radiation was inhaled, collect sample (swab of nasal passage).

3. *Externally contaminated patient*—May have contacted liquids, dirt particles or radioactive smoke particles. Normal emergency care procedures may be used, but decontamination of patient is required, as is decontamination of paramedic (after rendering of emergency care).

4. *Patient with open, contaminated wounds*—Normal emergency care procedures may be utilized, taking care not to cross-contaminate wounds.

Summary

Radiation exposures, usually from accidents while transporting wastes or radioactive materials, are no longer something to worry about in the future. Calm, informed rescuers can do their jobs effectively if they know the hazards and take appropriate precautions. Your best protections from exposure to harmful ionizing radiation are:

1. *Time*—Limiting duration of exposure (work in shifts).
2. *Distance*—Putting distance between you, your patient and the source of radiation (double your distance—you get only 1/4 the exposure, triple your distance—you get only 1/9 the exposure).
3. *Shielding*—Utilizing natural shielding from the radiation source whenever possible (filtration masks, complete clothing cover—tape up seams and cuffs).
4. *Common Sense*—Approach from upwind, don't contaminate co-workers and hospital personnel by poor precautions and pre-plan for trouble.

SELF-TEST

Chapter 23

1. The _____ is responsible for regulating the body's internal temperature.
   ANSWER: hypothalmus
2. Name at least three ways that the body loses heat.
   ANSWER: radiation, conduction, convection, evaporation, and respiration
3. Differentiate between heat exhaustion and heat stroke.
   ANSWER: a. Heat exhaustion is caused by excessive sweating that produces a fluid and sodium loss. Signs and symptoms include profuse sweating, weakness, dizziness, thirst and possibly syncope.
   b. Heat stroke is caused by ineffective cooling through sweating. Signs and symptoms include, very hot dry skin, elevated body temperature, hypotension and eventually coma. Can be fatal.
4. When are severely hypothermic patients considered dead?
   ANSWER: When they are warm and dead.
5. What happens to water in the alveoli when resuscitating a fresh-water drowning victim?
   ANSWER: It passes quickly into the pulmonary circulation, as the higher solute concentration of the blood osmotically draws the water across the capillary membranes into the bloodstream.

6. Why do salt-water drowning victims usually have massive pulmonary edema?

ANSWER: Salt-water in the alveoli is of a higher solute concentration than the blood, thus osmotically drawing fluid from the bloodstream across capillary membranes into the alveoli.

7. Cold-water drowning victims are likely to survive long periods of submersion without significant brain damage. Name at least one of the mechanisms responsible for this phenomena?

ANSWER: cerebral hypothermia and/or the "mammalian diving reflex"

8. What form of ionizing radiation can penetrate the entire body and cause direct damage to body tissues?

ANSWER: gamma rays

_____

The Geriatric Patient

Every year, a greater percentage of our population passes the age of 65, and the number is sure to rise. In 1900, the average life expectancy was about 48 and only 4% of the population was 65 or older. In 1985, the average life expectancy was about 75 years and over 12% of the population was 65 or older, an increase in life expectancy of about 56%. A large percentage of ambulance transports involve the geriatric patient. The elderly have their own special set of problems that must be considered when rendering emergency care—especially when trying to make an accurate assessment of illness or injury. They, like children, are especially vulnerable to both physical and psychological abuse by family, criminals, and care-givers. This chapter tries to outline the principal problems involved when treating the "older" patient.

Definitions

Syncope—A brief loss of consciousness caused by temporary reduction in blood flow to the brain (from a variety of causes).

Vertigo—A dizzy sensation that mimics movement, usually a "spinning" of the world around you.

Delirium—A mental disturbance marked by hallucination, excitement and restlessness, usually lasting only a short period of time.

Dementia—A severe emotionally disturbed state, which is often characterized by irrational behavior.

Chronic Senile Dementia—A loss of mental faculties caused by the aging process.

Organic Brain Syndrome—Neurological disease process that causes disruptive and irrational behavior.

Alzheimer's Disease—A degenerative brain disorder that can strike early in the aging process, causing a progressive loss of brain function and a marked decrease in the ability of a person to care for himself.

Stroke (CVA)—Cerebrovascular accident. Usually a blood vessel in the brain ruptures or becomes obstructed by clot or embolus, depriving an area of the brain of oxygenated blood. May cause necrosis of brain tissue.

TIA (Transient Ischemic Attack)—Temporary reduction in blood flow to the brain that mimics a stroke. However, the effects of a TIA dissipate within a few minutes to a few hours (if effects last > 24 hours, it is not a TIA).

Carcinoma—Cancer.

Aging of Body Organs and Systems

As the body ages, it suffers a decline in the function of organ systems—usually a predictable decline.

Respiratory System At about age 30, degenerative changes begin to occur in the respiratory system, and after age 60 these changes progress rapidly. At age 80, there is a:

1. 50% decrease in vital capacity;
2. 60% decrease in breathing capacity; and
3. 30% reduction in pulmonary blood flow.

Cardiovascular System By age 65:

1. Stroke volume declines (as does the force of contractions);
2. Degenerative changes slow conduction pathways;

3. The left ventricle loses 25% of function (hypertrophy); and

4. Progressive atherosclerosis increases peripheral vascular resistance (causing hypertension) and decreases the ability of the arteries to dilate and constrict.

Renal System The bladder is reduced to half its size, and filtration and reabsorption by the kidneys can be inhibited by these degenerative changes:

1. Renal blood flow is reduced by 50%;

2. The number of functioning neurons is reduced by 30-40%.

Nervous System Brain weight actually declines as we age (6-7%) and some cortical areas of the brain lose as many as 45% of their brain cells. Some elderly subjects experience a change in how the brain processes pain, thus it is difficult to assess their problems and level of discomfort. There may be an absence of pain in situations that should normally elicit pain. Changes include:

1. Decreased cerebral blood flow—usually due to increased resistance (caused by atherosclerosis). This can result in a variety of symptoms, including confusion, amnesia, anxiety, altered sleep patterns, and so forth.

2. 15% reduction in nerve conduction velocity.

Musculoskeletal System These include changes in posture, bone deterioration, reduction in joint flexibility. These are just some changes due to aging. Also:

1. Decrease in height of 2-3 inches due to narrowing of vertebral disks;

2. Decrease in total skeletal muscle weight;

3. Widening and weakening of certain bones (become porous and brittle).

Gastrointestinal (GI) System Structural changes occur with age in the GI tract, and digestion can be a real problem due to the following:

1. The volume of saliva available decreases by 30%;

2. Gastric secretions diminish by 80% (1/5 of what it was when young);

3. Esophageal motility (the ease of moving food down the esophagus from the pharynx to the stomach) decreases.

General Changes Some other general physiologic changes include:

1. A decrease in total body water;
2. A decrease of 15-30% in total body fat;
3. Progressive loss of ability to bounce back as quickly from illness or injury (a loss in the adjustment capacity of homeostatic systems);
4. The total number of body cells decreases by 30% by age 65, but there is no evidence of a decline in metabolic activity.

Assessment of Geriatric Patients

Factors that complicate clinical evaluation are:

1. It is extremely difficult to separating the effects of aging from the effects of disease. These factors contribute:
   a. Chief complaint may be trivial and misleading;
   b. Patient may fail to report important symptoms;
   c. EMT may fail to note important symptoms.
2. Multiple disease processes often exist, confusing the clinical picture:
   a. Chronic problems may make assessment for acute problems difficult;
   b. Symptoms of chronic illness may be confused with symptoms of acute illness (or injury).
3. Aging affects our body and mind's response to illness or injury:
   a. Pain may be diminished or absent, thus the patient and/or the EMT may severely underestimate the severity of the condition.
   b. Temperature regulating mechanisms don't function as well:
      (1) There may be minimal or absent fever with a severe infection;
      (2) The elderly are very prone to environmental thermal syndromes.
   c. Social and emotional factors may have greater impact on health than in any other age group.

4. Communication problems may be present:
   a. Diminished sight (glaucoma, cataracts, blindness);
   b. Diminished hearing (deafness, poor hearing aids);
   c. Diminished mental faculties (not necessarily intelligence);
   d. Depression (often mistaken as dementia or organic brain syndrome).

History Taking This can be very difficult, even in the non-emergency.
1. Common complaints of the geriatric patient:
   a. Fatigue and weakness;
   b. Dizziness/vertigo/syncope;
   c. Falls;
   d. Headache;
   e. Insomnia and altered sleeping patterns;
   f. Dysphagia (difficulty in expressing oneself);
   g. Loss of appetite (usually a strong instinct);
   h. Inability to void the bladder;
   i. Constipation/diarrhea.
2. Probing for significant symptoms, a chief complaint may be trivial and a patient may not volunteer significant information.
3. Dealing with communication problems in history taking:
   a. Diminished sight:
      (1) Increased anxiety in those with sight reduction—due to an inability to exert control over their situation, compounded by their inability to see their surroundings;
      (2) Speak to the patient calmly;
      (3) Position yourself so patient can best see you.
   b. Diminished hearing or deafness:
      (1) This can make obtaining a history virtually impossible if patient cannot hear questions or lip read;
      (2) Don't assume patient is deaf without inquiring (be polite);
      (3) Don't shout—it distorts sound if patient has some hearing (and doesn't help if patient is deaf);
      (4) Write short notes, if possible;

      (5) If patient can lip read, speak slowly and directly towards the patient;

      (6) Whenever possible, verify history with reliable friend or relative, or seek assistance from these individuals to communicate with the patient.

  c. Diminished mental status (NOT intelligence, which does not fade):

      (1) Patient is often confused and unable to remember detail.

      (2) Noise of radios, ECG sounds, strange voices—all add to the confusion for elderly patients who summon you. Try to cut down on the radio noise and/or explain clearly and carefully what's going down.

      (3) Both senility and acute organic brain syndrome may present in a similar manner: delirium, confusion, distractibility, excitement, restlessness, or hostility.

      (4) Attempt to determine if patient's mental status represents a significant change from normal (most important).

      (5) Alcoholism is more common in elderly than is generally realized—an intoxicated patient may further hamper attempts at taking a good history.

  d. Depression:

      (1) Very common in the elderly, especially those in nursing homes. It may mimic senility or organic brain syndrome.

      (2) Often inhibits patient cooperation.

      (3) A depressed patient may be malnourished, dehydrated, overdosed, contemplating suicide, or simply imagining physical ailments for attention.

      (4) Question carefully regarding drug ingestion and the presence of suicidal thoughts—suicide is the fourth leading cause of death among the elderly in the United States.

4. Past medical history:

  a. It may be complicated—try to determine what is significant.

  b. Obtaining medication history is very important:

      (1) Geriatric patients are usually on multiple drugs.

      (2) Medication errors and noncompliance are common.

      (3) Find all drugs and take to hospital with patient (or make a really good list).

(4) Try to establish old versus current drugs—including over-the-counter medications.

5. Information from the environment:
    a. Attempt to verify patient history with reliable family/neighbors (this is less offensive if done out of patient's presence).
    b. Observe the surroundings for indication of patient's ability to care for himself (note subjective findings on run report).
    c. Observe for evidence of drug/alcohol ingestion.
    d. Look for medic alert tags, Vial of Life (in the refrigerator), and so on.
    e. Observe for signs of violence/abuse (report if found).

Physical exam considerations in geriatric patients are:

1. Patients tire easily.
2. Layers of clothing may hamper or discourage proper examination.
3. Explain actions clearly before initiating patient exam in patient with diminished sight.
4. Patient may minimize or deny symptoms due to fear of being bedridden, institutionalized, or losing self-sufficiency—you may need to dig.
5. Peripheral pulses may be difficult to evaluate.
6. Chronic versus acute problems—you must differentiate.
    a. Elderly may have nonpathological rales.
    b. Loss of skin elasticity and mouth breathing may give false appearance of dehydration.
    c. Dependent edema may be secondary to varicose veins and inactivity/position versus congestive heart failure (CHF).
7. Experience and practice are the greatest allies in trying to differentiate between acute and chronic physical findings.

Pathophysiology and Management

Trauma

1. Biologically, geriatric patients are more at risk from trauma, especially falls.

2. Contributing factors:

   a. Slower reflexes;

   b. Failing eyesight and hearing;

   c. Arthritis;

   d. Blood vessels are less elastic, and very subject to tearing;

   e. Tissues and bones are more fragile.

3. The elderly are at high risk for trauma from criminal assault by the "low-lifes" of our society. They are easy prey and can be intimidated out of money, social security checks, and so on. Many of these assaults go unreported.

4. Head injury:

   a. More prone to head injury, even from relatively minor trauma.

   b. There is a difference in proportion between brain and skull.

   c. Signs of brain compression may develop more slowly, sometimes over days and weeks—patient may have forgotten he was injured.

5. C-spine injury is often associated with cervical spondylosis:

   a. The elderly often have a significant degree of this disease.

   b. Arthritic changes of the spine gradually compress existing nerve roots to arms or even spinal cord.

   c. If injury occurs to cervical spine, spinal cord is more likely to be injured.

   d. Sudden neck movement, even without fracture, may cause spinal cord injury—and the patient may have less than usual amount of pain in absence of fracture.

6. Trauma management considerations:

   a. *Cardiovascular system:*

      (1) Consider MIs (recent or past) as a possible cause of cardiac dysrhythmias.

      (2) The heart may be less able to adjust rate and stroke volume to combat hypovolemia.

      (3) The body may require higher arterial pressures to perfuse critical organs (due to increased peripheral vascular resistance caused by atherosclerosis hypertension).

      (4) Because of the decrease in the elderly heart's ability to compensate for hypovolemia, you must monitor IV infusions carefully.

(5) Trauma may alter cardiovascular system response to medications.

b. *Respiratory system:*

(1) Physical changes due to aging are responsible for decreasing chest cage movement and vital capacity, therefore the capacity to compensate for injuries to the chest are reduced.

(2) All organs have less tolerance to anoxia and hypoxia.

(3) COPD is common, therefore airway and management and ventilation must be carefully performed (positive pressure easily damages or ruptures the alveoli of these patients).

c. *Renal system:*

(1) The ability of the kidneys to maintain adequate acid-base balance *and* compensate for fluid changes (such as hypovolemia) is decreased.

(2) If the patient has pre-existing renal disease, this decrease in ability to compensate (during trauma) is markedly worse.

(3) The decrease in compensatory function also places the patient at risk for fluid overload during resuscitation therapy. Observe carefully for the development of rales and pulmonary edema.

7. Immobilization—Positioning, immobilization, and packaging of the elderly trauma patient may be an adventure in ingenuity. Physical deformities and other special conditions unique to the individual elderly patient often demand modifications of the usual techniques to accomplish the same objectives of immobilization. (Stretching certain elderly patients out flat on their back on a rigid spineboard would almost break them in half.) Strategic application of padding to support the patient anatomically, and perhaps transporting on their side may be necessary. Paramedics are expected to improvise to accomplish treatment objectives, but if you do—DOCUMENT THE REASON FOR THE VARIATION IN USUAL TECHNIQUE.

Respiratory Distress Respiratory distress can be caused by a variety of factors:

1. Pulmonary embolism;

2. Silent MI (heart attack without pain)—dyspnea may be primary symptom;

3. Pulmonary edema;

4. Asthma/COPD;
5. Respiratory infections;
6. Cancer.

Management is the same for all age groups.

Cardiovascular Conditions This is very common in geriatric patients due to a long duration of atherosclerosis. You may see:

1. Syncope (common, orthostatic, vasovagal, or cardiac);
2. Myocardial infarction (MI);
3. Stroke (CVA);
4. Congestive heart failure (CHF);
5. Dysrhythmias;
6. Aortic dissection;
7. Abdominal aortic aneurysm;
8. Peripheral arterial and venous conditions.

Management is the same for all ages.

Neurologic Disorders Geriatric patients suffer a myriad of neurological disorders, many of which can be linked to atherosclerosis and cardiovascular problems. They are:

1. Coma;
2. Stroke;
3. Seizures;
4. Dizziness; and
5. Senile dementia.

Management is similar for all age groups.

Psychiatric Disorders These are very common in the elderly. Though they suffer more dementia and depression, there is less schizophrenia and alcoholism. Psychiatric disorders common to the elderly can be classified as follows:

1. Organic brain syndrome;
2. Affective disorders (especially depression);

3. Neurotic disorders (anxiety, phobia, hypochondriasis);

4. Personality disorders;

5. Paranoid disorders;

6. Alcoholism;

7. Suicides.

Management is similar for all age groups.

Environmental Emergencies Constant high or low temperatures are tolerated poorly by the elderly.

1. Predisposing factors for hypothermia:
   a. Accidental exposure is not uncommon in the elderly;
   b. Some drugs taken regularly interfere with heat production;
   c. CNS disorders;
   d. Endocrine disorders;
   e. Chronic illness, reduction in movement;
   f. Low and/or fixed incomes—probably the most common factor.
2. Predisposing factors for hyperthermia:
   a. Decrease in the function of the thermoregulatory center;
   b. Some drugs taken regularly interfere with sweating (and cooling);
   c. Low and/or fixed incomes—again the most common factor. They may not be able to afford air conditioning or fans.

Gastrointestinal (GI) Disorders GI bleeds are the most common problem in elderly patients (both upper and lower GI tract). Some causes are:

1. Peptic ulcers and gastritis;

2. Esophageal varices;

3. Diverticulitis;

4. Tumors; and

5. Ischemic colitis.

Signs of Significant Blood Loss:

1. "Coffee grounds" or blood in emesis or stool;

2. Orthostatic hypotension;

3. Pulse > 100 at rest (unless on beta blockers);

4. Confusion, restlessness, fatigue.

Prehospital Management:

1. Airway maintenance and high-flow oxygen therapy;

2. Shock trousers (if indicated);

3. Begin rapid transport;

4. Large-bore IVs of LR or NS enroute (two are appropriate, if there's time).

Pharmacology

1. Factors contributing to adverse drug reactions:
   a. Drug interactions are common. Many elderly patients have lots of prescriptions and over-the-counter drugs (25% of all sold). Often, taking several of these medications will cause adverse reactions, which are more difficult to detect in the aged.
   b. The aging process affects the absorption, distribution, metabolism and excretion of drugs. For example, if renal function is impaired, excretion of a drug may be difficult and a cumulative effect of the drug may be seen as blood levels increase.

2. Drug-induced illnesses are common (30% of hospital admissions).

3. Drugs that commonly cause toxicity in elderly include:
   a. Digitalis—leading cause (Lanoxin, Digoxin).
   b. Antiparkinsonian drugs.
   c. Diuretics (Lasix, Hydradiuril).
   d. Anticoagulants (Coumadin, Warfarin).
   e. Lidocaine.
   f. Quinidine.
   g. Propranolol (Inderal).
   h. Theophylline (Theo-Dur).
   i. Narcotic analgesics (Darvon, Percodan, Demerol).
   j. Acetaminophen (very dangerous if overdosed).
   k. Sedatives and hypnotic drugs.
   l. Phenothiazines.
   m. Tricyclic antidepressants (Elevil).

Geriatric Abuse/Neglect

Abuse and/or neglect is a syndrome in which elderly persons have received serious physical (or psychological) injury from their children or their care providers.

Profile of Potential Abused/Neglected Elderly The average age is 80. They usually suffer from chronic multiple health disorders (CHF, cancer, incontinence, heart disease, Alzheimers, and so on).

Signs and Symptoms Unexplained trauma is the primary finding. A high index of suspicion is needed to adequately "key-in" on geriatric abuse.

Profile of Potential Geriatric Abuser The abuser may be sleep-deprived (newborns and geriatrics have strange sleeping patterns). They usually show a high level of stress (a geriatric patient at home keeps stress levels high—nowhere to go to relax). They may have marital problems (often complicated by caring for the geriatric). They may have work-related problems (which can complicate the stress of caring for geriatric patient at home).

Obtain a Complete Patient and Family History Particularly note any suspicious inconsistencies. Just as you are obligated to report child abuse, you should pass any reasonable suspicions regarding geriatric abuse/neglect on to the patient's physician or the appropriate person/agency.

Summary

The increasing numbers of our population over the age of 65 pose problems for society and health care professionals, both now and in the future. When to intercede in the degenerative process, whether to view quality of life from a functional or clinical frame of reference, how to differentiate between chronic and acute problems—all these are considerations when dealing with the geriatric patient. It is important for paramedics to make their assessment in a systematic manner, communicate constantly and effectively, obtain a good history and use common sense in treating the geriatric patient.

SELF-TEST

Chapter 24

1. A loss of mental faculties caused by the aging process is referred to as _____ _____ .

   ANSWER: senile dementia

2. Name several factors that may complicate a clinical evaluation of the geriatric patient?

   ANSWER: a. separating the effects of aging from the effects of disease

   b. multiple disease processes

   c. responses to illness or injury are affected by age

   d. communication difficulties

3. A temporary reduction in blood flow to the brain that mimics a stroke is called a _____ _____ _____ .

   ANSWER: transient ischemic attack (TIA)

4. A degenerative brain disorder that can strike early in the aging process, causing a progressive loss of brain function and a marked decrease in the ability of a person to care for oneself is called _____ _____ .

   ANSWER: Alzheimer's Disease

5. Define geriatric abuse/neglect.

   ANSWER: A syndrome in which elderly persons have received serious physical (or psychological) injury from their children or their care providers.

6. Why are geriatric patients more at risk from trauma (especially falls)?

   ANSWER: a. slower reflexes

   b. failing eyesight and hearing

   c. arthritis

   d. blood vessels are less elastic and tear easily

   e. tissues and bones are more fragile

7. Why are the elderly more at risk for hypothermia?

   ANSWER: a. low and fixed incomes (proper heat may not be affordable)

      b. endocrine and CNS disorders

      c. accidental exposure is common

      d. some drugs taken regularly interfere with heat production

      e. chronic illness may cause a reduction in movement

8. Gastrointestinal (GI) bleeding is a common cause of problems in the geriatric patient. Name at least two signs of a GI bleed.

    ANSWER: a. "coffee grounds" or blood in emesis or stool

           b. orthostatic hypotension

           c. pulse > 100 at rest

           d. confusion, restlessness, fatigue

CHAPTER 25

Pediatrics

Children are not small adults—they have needs and problems specific to their own age group. Paramedics are generally more comfortable providing advanced care to adults, yet children and infants require swift intervention with aggressive advanced treatment when their systems have been stretched past compensation. The reserves adults call upon when compromised are yet to be developed in the pediatric patient and recognition of respiratory distress, compensation and decompensation (respiratory failure) is critical. Correction of respiratory failure is the name of the game, followed closely by correction of volume depletion—cardiac components (unlike the adult) are rare and nearly always secondary to respiratory or volemic insufficiency. This chapter briefly reviews specific pediatric problems, their management and special treatment techniques.

Few calls evoke quite the same feeling in paramedics as those involving a known pediatric emergency. Enroute to the scene after hearing "child hit by a car", "baby not breathing", or "woman having a baby", there is a heightened sense of awareness as you anticipate needed equipment, hope for a visible vein, and wish you had studied your pediatric drug dosages better. Training in special techniques, appropriate-sized equipment, a good pediatric knowledge base, and solid experience are your best weapons against pediatric emergencies. We urge you to attend specialized courses in Pediatric Advanced Life Support (PALS) and Pediatric Trauma.

Specific Medical Problems

Sudden Infant Death Syndrome (SIDS) SIDS refers to the sudden death of an infant or young child which is unexpected by history and in which a thorough postmortem exam fails to reveal an adequate cause of death. Generally, SIDS deaths occurs during sleep and are commonly called crib deaths.

Statistics

1. SIDS is the leading cause of death in the United States in children from one week to one year of age (approximately 10,000 per year).
2. Ninety percent of deaths occur between 1-6 months (peak incidence—2-4 months).
3. Frequency—2 deaths per 1,000 live births.
4. Occurs more often in:
   a. Winter months;
   b. Males (60%);
   c. Young mothers;
   d. Low birth weight babies;
   e. Families from lower socioeconomic groups; and
   f. Babies with urinary tract infections (URIs).

SIDS is *not* caused by external suffocation, aspiration of vomitus, child abuse, heredity, or allergy to cow's milk. Many theories are being pursued, but the cause is still unknown.

Prehospital Management

1. Vigorous resuscitation attempts (even when death is obvious);
2. Unconditional parental support;
3. Good care will include understanding the grief process that parents experience (denial, anger, depression, blame, and acceptance).

Child Abuse/Neglect Consider the possibility of abuse in a child that presents with an injury that *does not fit* with the cause of injury given. Learn to recognize the injuries commonly suffered by abused children:

1. *Pattern injuries*—handprints, cord and belt tattoos, finger bruise marks.
2. *Burns*—immersion burns (scalds of the buttocks/lower extremities, "stocking" burns), cigarette burns, palm burns.
3. *Fractures*—spiral fractures from twisting of extremities, skull fractures, "nursemaids elbow", multiple fractures.
4. *Soft tissue injuries*—multiple bruising and abrasions (especially about the trunk and buttocks), injuries about the mouth (from being force-fed with a bottle).
5. *Head injuries*—the "shaken child syndrome."

Learn to recognize suspicious situations and behavioral responses:

1. Poorly nourished or poorly cared-for children.
2. Parents who exhibit indifference to treatment, prognosis, and child, in general.
3. Apathetic child that does not cry despite injuries or a child who does not turn to parents for support or comfort.
4. Child whose injury occurred several days before medical assistance was sought.
5. Frequent visits to the emergency room for related complaints.
6. Child who constantly appears on the alert for danger.

Prehospital Management

1. Treatment of the presenting injuries.
2. Accurate documentation of care-giver statements (especially about mechanism of injury).
3. Careful injury description.
4. Alerting the physician who will be evaluating the child to your suspicions. In most states, you must report your suspicions of child abuse/neglect to a designated authority or agency.

Seizures Seizures in children are not uncommon and can be due to a wide variety of causes such as fever (most common), head trauma, hypoxia, hypoglycemia, infections (meningitis, and so on), toxic ingestions and exposure, epilepsy, tumors, electrolyte imbalance, and CNS malfunction. History is all-important here.

Febrile Seizures These seizures occur most commonly between 6 months and 6 years of age and usually last 1-2 minutes. If longer than 2 minutes, it may be from a different cause. Suspect a febrile seizure with a temperature of 103°F, but remember that some children are prone to seizures at much lower temps. Five percent of high fevers result in seizure.

Prehospital Management

1. Maintain airway and position on side (away from potential injury).
2. Administer oxygen.
3. Remove clothing.
4. Sponge bath with tepid water.
5. Consider acetaminophen/aspirin for fever reduction.
6. If condition is non-acute, check with child's pediatrician—he can advise you as to the need for transport. If you are unable to contact the pediatrician, advise transport and follow parental decision.

Status Epilepticus This is a prolonged seizure or multiple seizures without a lucid interval between seizures. This is a true emergency, as repeated seizures sap the reserves of children quickly.

Prehospital Management

1. Maintain airway and position on side (away from potential injury).
2. Administer high-flow oxygen.
3. IV of D5LR or D5NS (TKO) (if not available, use LR or NS and consider glucose administration based on dextrostick or medical control direction).
4. Valium, slow IV push:
   a. 30 days-5 years = 0.2-0.5 mg slowly IV every 2-5 minutes up to maximum of 2.5 mg.
   b. 5 year or older = 1 mg every 2-5 minutes to a maximum of 5 mg.
5. Draw a blood tube and measure blood glucose (if possible). If results

suggest significant low blood sugar, give 0.5-1.0 gm/kg IV of 25% solution (mix one part saline or water with one part D50W).

6. Monitor ECG and vitals signs carefully during transport.

Dehydration Children can dehydrate very quickly. Fluid loss may be due to fever, diarrhea, vomiting, burns, or environmental factors. Taking a good history can clue you in to suspect dehydration, as well as a careful physical examination.

Signs and Symptoms

1. Weakness, lethargy, possible decreased LOC (or even coma).
2. Poor skin turgor ("tenting" when you pinch the skin), dry skin and mucous membranes.
3. Recent weight loss ($<$ 4% = mild, 5-9% = hospitalization, $>$ 9% = severe, with significant mortality).
4. Concentrated urine.
5. Dull eyes (may be sunken-looking).
6. Depressed anterior fontanelle in infants.
7. Weakness, irritability, may have a pinched anxious expression.
8. Cherry red lips or ashen gray color

Prehospital Management

1. Maintain airway.
2. Monitor vital signs.
3. IV of D5LR or D5NS, if shocky (LR or NS if you don't carry the other).
4. Smooth transport to hospital.

Infectious Problems

Meningitis Meningitis is a bacterial, fungal, or viral infection of the tissues covering the brain and spinal cord. Infants and children are at higher risk than adults. These kids may have been ill for one or several days, with fever, and perhaps an ear or respiratory infection (usually 4 days after exposure). The infection is spread by droplets—especially when in closed spaces.

Signs and Symptoms

1. High fever.
2. Stiff neck (hallmark of meningitis).
3. Lethargic and/or irritable.
4. Severe headache.
5. Vomiting.
6. Blotchy red/bluish rash.

Prehospital Management

1. Airway maintenance and supportive care as needed.
2. Smooth transport.

Septicemia More commonly seen in children than adults, septicemia is a generalized infection of the bloodstream. The child has usually been ill for several days before evaluation.

Signs and Symptoms

1. Fever.
2. Lethargic and/or irritable.
3. Possibility of shock symptoms.

Prehospital Management

1. Airway maintenance and supportive care.
2. Smooth transport.
3. Consider IV of D5LR or D5NS enroute, if shocky (profound shock would merit pediatric shock trousers prior to transport and IV).

Reyes Syndrome First recognized as a disease in 1963, Reyes Syndrome attacks the brain and causes increasing intercranial pressure. Most patients die of cerebral complications.

Statistics

1. Usually occurs in younger children (peak incidence—5-15 years).
2. More cases in the fall and winter—clusters of cases during influenza B epidemics.

3. Many victims have history of recent upper respiratory infection (URI).
4. Ten to 20% if victims are in latter stages of chickenpox when struck.

Signs and Symptoms

1. Sudden onset of vomiting in the early stages.
2. Irrational behavior.
3. Hyperexcitability, restlessness and convulsions.
4. Progressive stupor.
5. Coma—may demonstrate decerebrate or decorticate posturing.
6. Rapid, deep, possibly irregular respirations.
7. Dilated, sluggishly reactive pupils.
8. Other signs of increased intercranial pressure.
9. Late stages may include respiratory failure, acute pancreatitis, and cardiac arrhythmias.

Prehospital Management

1. Airway maintenance and high-flow oxygen therapy.
2. Support ventilations as needed.
3. Rapid transport to the appropriate facility.

Respiratory Emergencies

Obstructed Airway American Heart Association standards for infant and child obstructed airways are recommended. In complete obstruction, quick action is needed to prevent brain damage from hypoxia. In infants, back blows and chest thrusts are recommended, while abdominal thrusts (6-10) are recommended in the child.

Bronchiolitis This is a viral infection of the bronchioles in children under 2 years, characterized by prominent expiratory wheezing (the same symptoms as asthma), respiratory distress, and possibly accompanying rales. There may be a family history of asthma/allergies or a patient allergy history.

Prehospital Management

1. Airway maintenance and humidified oxygen therapy (by mask).
2. Ventilations assisted as needed.
3. Semi-sitting position.
4. Consider epinephrine (1:1,000). Sub-Q if bronchospasms are severe.
5. Consider racemic epinephrine.
6. Smooth transport.

Croup (Laryngotracheal Bronchitis) This is a viral infection of the upper airway that causes edema beneath the glottis, progressively narrowing the airway and producing a barking sound when patient coughs. Croup is generally seen in kids between 6 months and 4 years, often after a cold or infection, and is usually more pronounced at night.

Signs and Symptoms

1. Hoarse high-pitched stridor/"seal bark."
2. Nasal flaring, tracheal tugging, and retractions.
3. Restlessness, tachycardia, and cyanosis in more severe cases.
4. Patient will refuse to lie down.

Prehospital Management

1. Airway maintenance and humidified oxygen therapy (by mask).
2. Place in position of comfort.
3. Consider racemic epinephrine (1:1,000).
4. Smooth transport.
5. DO NOT examine the throat!

Epiglottitis This is a bacterial infection that causes the epiglottis to swell and turn cherry red, occurring most often in children of 2 months to 4 years. Epiglottitis has the dangerous potential to cause complete airway obstruction. The onset is usually rapid.

Signs and Symptoms

1. High fever (that develops quickly).
2. Drooling.

3. Pain on swallowing—refuses to swallow.

4. Respiratory distress—may be shallow with retraction and stridor.

5. Anxiety.

6. Child will "look" extremely ill.

Prehospital Management

1. Airway by positioning and humidified oxygen therapy. If patient won't tolerate mask—don't push it. Keep the child as calm as possible. If you can figure a way to provide supplemental oxygen, do it (try "blow-by" administration).

2. Position of comfort—may be held by parent if that seems calming.

3. Rapid, smooth transport (keep intubation equipment close at hand, but do not intubate unless there is a complete obstruction).

4. In the case of complete obstruction, vigorous bag-valve ventilation with a good mask seal (may require two people) can force air past the swelling in about 50% of cases (assuming intubation is unsuccessful).

5. Consider transtracheal ventilation as alternative, if necessary.

Note: Never try to examine the patient's throat if you remotely suspect epiglottitis. Keep them quiet and unagitated.

Asthma This is characterized by respiratory difficulty produced by spasm and constriction of bronchi with edema and congestion of the bronchial linings (including hypersecretion of mucous plugs). Exhalation becomes progressively more difficult as "air trapping" occurs in the lower airways and the chest becomes hyperinflated. As acidosis increases, broncho-constriction increases—a vicious circle. When taking a history, be sure and determine:

1. How long wheezing has been present.

2. Recent fluid intake.

3. Presence of any recent infections.

4. Current medications—especially any administered in last 2 hours.

5. Any allergies to drugs, food or environmental elements.

6. If hospitalization has ever been necessary to control asthma.

Signs and Symptoms

1. Wheezing, rales, rhonchi and/or difficulty in exhalation.
2. Use of accessory muscles in respiration (often "barking" expulsions of breath in attempt to clear airways).
3. Sleepy or stuporous.
4. Cyanosis.
5. Hyperinflation of the chest.
6. Vital signs—fast pulse, rapid or labored breathing, elevated BP.

Prehospital Management

1. Airway maintenance and humidified high-flow oxygen therapy (by mask or "blow-by").
2. IV of NS or LR, if easily accomplished—consider intraosseous infusion if patient is significantly compromised. (Don't delay!)
3. Consider racemic epinephrine (if your protocols address nebulized drug therapy).
4. Consider epinephrine (1:1,000) .01 mg/kg (sub-Q) up to 3 mg. (In rare circumstances, physician may direct you to repeat the dose.)
5. If epinephrine is ineffective, consider aminophylline 2–4 mg/kg in 10 ml of NS LR (given over at least 15 minutes) while enroute to hospital.
6. Monitor vital signs carefully during smooth transport.

> *Note:* Find out what medications may have been used before your arrival. Epinephrine may be contraindicated in the presence of high doses of bronchodilators.

Respiratory Failure Respiratory failure is one of the major causes (and most frequent) of cardiopulmonary failure (shock syndrome is the other).

Respiratory Rates

1. Infants = 40 (normal)
2. 1-year old = 24 (normal)
3. 18-year old = 18 (normal)
4. Tachypnea = It may be the first and earliest sign of respiratory stress (or it may be benign).

5. Bradypnea = An ominous sign—it indicates fatigue (most common), hypothermia, or CNS problems.

Signs and Symptoms of Respiratory Distress

1. Nasal flaring.
2. Subcostal retractions.
3. Intercostal retractions.
4. Supracostal retractions.
5. Head-bobbing = Impending respiratory failure—BAD sign.
6. Stridor = Upper airway problem.
7. Prolonged expiration = Bronchial and bronchiolar destruction.
8. Grunting = Alveolar collapse, pneumonia, pulmonary edema, atelectasis, or ARDS.
9. See-saw respirations = upper airway problems or alveolar collapse.
10. Cyanosis = Very late finding, differentiate from peripheral shock.
11. Altered states of consciousness = May not exhibit many of the other signs because of fatigue.

Prehospital Management

1. *Airway positioning*—If cervical spine is suspect, use neutral position with jaw thrust. When extending (never hyperextend in infants)—you can occlude trachea. Use oropharyngeal or nasopharyngeal airway to keep tongue from obstructing airway. If appropriate, head elevation helps.
2. *Administer supplemental oxygen*—Use nasal cannula, oxygen hood (if < 1), pediatric oxygen mask, partial rebreathing mask, non-rebreathing mask or face tent. Use oxygen connecting tube when utilizing adjuncts. Children not tolerating these may benefit from "blow-by" oxygen.
3. *Ventilate if necessary*—Use mouth-to-mouth, mouth-to-nose, mouth-to-mask, bag-valve-mask, or bag-valve with endotracheal tube. When using all but the endotracheal tube, consider cricoid pressure to occlude esophagus and minimize gastric distention.

Trauma

Trauma is the untreated disease of children.

Statistics

1. Trauma is the leading cause of death among children over the age of one year (25,000 pediatric trauma deaths annually in the United States).
2. Seventy percent of accidents in the preschool age occur in and around the home.
3. The most common causes of traumatic deaths are from:
    a. Motor vehicle accidents (most often when unrestrained);
    b. Fires; and
    c. Falls.

Children are definitely not "little adults" when it comes to trauma. They are capable of extreme vasoconstriction—to the point that you may not see signs of hypotension until the child has lost a major portion of his blood volume. Hemorrhage of a few hundred mls may cause shock, and the signs of hypovolemic shock in children are very subtle. Children may lose 25% of their blood volume before developing measurable hypotension—thus blood pressure may be maintained until just before complete cardiovascular collapse.

Signs and Symptoms of Traumatic Shock

1. Rapid pulse and breathing.
2. Apathy and listlessness.
3. Cold, pale, perhaps mottled skin.
4. Increase in capillary refill time:
    a. < 2 seconds = normal;
    b. 2-4 seconds = delayed;
    c. > 4 seconds = absent (or profoundly delayed).
5. Collapsed neck and peripheral veins.
6. Little or no urinary output.
7. Increasing abdominal girth.

Prehospital Management

1. Airway maintenance and supplemental high-flow oxygen.

2. Pediatric PASG (if > 40 lbs)—remember, use of PASG in children is controversial.

3. IV of LR. 20 ml/kg bolus—may repeat twice if no improvement in:
   a. Heart rate;
   b. Skin color;
   c. Capillary refill;
   d. Level of consciousness;
   e. Blood pressure (not reliable).

4. Rapid transport to an appropriate facility.

Note: DO NOT DELAY TRANSPORT to start IVs—do them enroute, and if difficulty is encountered with peripheral veins or none are clearly available, go directly to the intraosseous technique.

Special Pediatric Techniques

Cardiopulmonary Resuscitation (CPR) American Heart Association's current standards for infant and child are recommended as performance standards.

Defibrillation The dosage is 2 joules/kg. If unsuccessful, the dose may be doubled (to 4 joules/kg). If still unsuccessful, correct hypoxia and acid base. Use pediatric paddles if at all possible, but if you are stuck with adult paddles on a small infant, use an anterior/posterior placement.

Endotracheal Intubation This must be preceded by ventilation with 100% oxygen via bag-valve mask (BVM). You can estimate tube size by matching the size of the patient's little finger or using this formula:

(16 + patient's age) divided by 4 = endotracheal tube size.

Endotracheal tubes used in children less than 8 years old (approximately 5-6 mm) do not need distal cuffs—the cricoid region is narrower in infants and young children and provides an adequate seal for the tube without trauma.

Intravenous Techniques The method of IV placement you use will depend upon the situation, the suitability of your patient, your level of skill, and your confidence in the various techniques. Use a microdrip administration set unless going for rapid volume expansion.

1. *Peripheral Vein*—Generally considered as first choice for IV site.
2. *Intraosseous*—In kids under 5, use after peripheral attempt or for rapid access in life-threatening emergencies.
3. *External Jugular Vein*—Use it if you can see it, but only after trying peripheral access or in life-threatening situations. If child is under 5, use intraosseous method instead.
4. *Femoral Vein*—Use if peripheral, intraosseous and external jugular are unavailable. Be sure to puncture medial to the femoral artery just below the inguinal ligament.
5. *Endotracheal Tube*—Can serve as a temporary alternate for intravenous cannulation in an arrest or other serious event. Epinephrine, atropine, lidocaine and nalaxone can be administered through the tube.

PASG (Shock Trousers) Use of the pneumatic anti-shock garment in children is controversial. If used, the patient should weigh at least 40 lbs (18 kg), and the trousers should be especially designed as *pediatric* PASG. *DO NOT* USE ONE LEG OF ADULT PASG in any attempt to improvise.

Pediatric Drug Dosages

In prehospital care, drug administration is usually secondary to correction of respiratory and hypovolemic components. We recommend that you keep a pediatric drug and dosage chart on the wall of the ambulance and with your resuscitation equipment, easily accessible—don't depend on memorization of pediatric dosages, which are usually weight-dependent. When given, the drugs most commonly ordered will be epinephrine, atropine and dextrose. The following is a list of prehospital drugs with corresponding pediatric dosages for your reference:

Aminophylline: 5 mg/kg, diluted with 50-100 cc D5W over 15 minutes.

Atropine: .01-.03 mg/kg IV slow push or down ET (diluted).

Benadryl: 2 mg/kg IV slowly.

Decadron: .25 mg/kg IV.

Dextrose: .5-1 gm/kg IV push. (25% solution). If you have D50W, dilute it 1:1 with D5W or sterile water.

Dopamine: 5-20 mg/kg/min IV drip (6 mg × wt (kg) in 100 ml D5W or LR).

Epinephrine: .1 cc/kg IV push of 1:10,000 or down ET.

Isuprel: .05-1.5 mg/kg/min IV drip (.6 mg × wt (kg) in 100 ml D5W or LR).

Morphine: .1-.2 mg/kg IV or IM.

Sodium Bicarbonate: 1-2 mEq/kg IV push (dilute in neonates).

Narcan: .4-.8 mg IV or IM (may increase as needed).

Valium: .2-.3 mg/kg IV slow push.

Average Weight and Vital Signs

Age	Wt(kg)	Pulse	BP	Resp(awake)	ET-Tube
Newborn	1	160	60/40	64	2.5 mm
Newborn	3	160	65/40	64	3.0 mm
1 month	4	160	65/40	64	3.5 mm
6 months	7	160	70/45	64	3.5 mm
1 year	10	160	80/50	35	4.0 mm
2-3 years	12-14	140	84/55	30	4.5 mm
4-5 years	16-18	120	90/60	26	6.0 mm
6-8 years	20-26	120	95/60	23	6.5 mm
10-12 years	32-42	120	100/65	21	7.0 mm
> 14 years	> 50	100	110/70	18	7.5-8.5 mm

Formulas (Rapid Approximations Only)

Blood Pressure:

(2 × age in years) + 80 = Systole (minimum normal)
2/3 of systole = Diastole

ET Tube: Age + 16 (divided by 4) = Tube Size

Weight: (2 × age in years) + 8 = Weight in kg

Urine Output: 1 cc/kg/hr = Minimum normal urinary output

Summary

Pediatric emergencies offer a real challenge to field paramedics. The development of a broad base knowledge about pediatric problems and treatment priorities is essential to adequate emergency treatment. Most life-threatening problems in kids are respiratory or hypovolemic in nature, seldom requiring prehospital medication. Early application of oxygen, effective ventilation, aggressive fluid replacement and timely transport to an appropriate hospital are the key components to providing good emergency prehospital pediatric care.

SELF-TEST

Chapter 25

1. What is the leading cause of death in children between the age of 1 week and 1 year of age?

   ANSWER: SIDS (sudden infant death syndrome).

2. What is the cause of SIDS?

   ANSWER: the cause is unknown

3. What is a key in recognizing the possibility of child abuse?

   ANSWER: A child presenting with an injury that *does not fit* with the cause of injury given.

4. The most common cause of seizures in children is _____ .

   ANSWER: fever

5. Status epilepticus in children is life-threatening and may require use of the drug _____ to control the seizures.

   ANSWER: valium

6. A bacterial, fungal or viral infection of the tissues covering the brain and spinal cord is called _____ .

   ANSWER: meningitis

7. Which childhood infection of the upper airway progressively narrows the airway and produces a barking sound when the patient coughs?

   ANSWER: croup (laryngotracheal bronchitis)

8. A generalized infection of the bloodstream is called _____ .

ANSWER: septicemia

9. Which childhood infection has a rapid onset, causes the epiglottis to swell and turn cherry-red, makes swallowing painful, causes excessive drooling and has the dangerous potential to cause a complete airway obstruction.

ANSWER: epiglottitis

10. Which childhood infection of the lower airways is characterized by prominent expiratory wheezing?

ANSWER: bronchiolitis

11. What is the major cause (and most frequent) of cardiopulmonary failure in children?

ANSWER: respiratory failure

12. Name at least three of the signs and symptoms of respiratory distress.

ANSWER: a. nasal flaring

　　　　　　b. retractions and/or the use of accessory muscles

　　　　　　c. head-bobbing (warns of impending respiratory failure)

　　　　　　d. stridor (signals an upper airway problem)

　　　　　　e. prolonged expiration

　　　　　　f. grunting

　　　　　　g. see-saw respirations

　　　　　　h. cyanosis (very late finding)

　　　　　　i. altered states of consciousness

13. The most common cause of pediatric trauma deaths is _____ _____ _____ .

ANSWER: motor vehicle accidents (MVA's)

14. Children may lose 25% of their blood volume before developing measurable _____ .

ANSWER: hypotension

15. What are the parameters for normal, delayed and absent (profoundly delayed) capillary refill (CR)?

ANSWER: normal = < 2 seconds

　　　　　　delayed = 2-4 seconds

　　　　　　absent = > 4 seconds

16. List at least three signs or symptoms of traumatic shock in children?

ANSWER: a. rapid pulse and breathing

b. apathy and listlessness—if not unconscious

c. cold, pale, perhaps mottled skin

d. increase in capillary refill time

e. little or no urinary output

f. increasing abdominal girth

17. What is the pediatric dose for defibrillation?

ANSWER: 2 joules/kg initially—if unsuccessful, double to 4 joules/kg

18. Name at least one way to estimate endotracheal tube size in children.

ANSWER: a. match the tube size to the patient's little finger

b. use the formula $\dfrac{16 + \text{age}}{4}$ = ET tube size

19. Name at least three techniques for gaining intravascular access for medications or fluid in children.

ANSWER: a. peripheral vein

b. intraosseous (in kids under 5, use after peripheral attempt *or immediately* in life-threatening situations where confidence is low for hitting a peripheral vein—go by protocols)

c. external jugular vein

d. femoral vein

e. endotracheal tube (may be used as temporary alternate for some IV medications, but not for fluid replacement)

20. TRUE or FALSE. Early application of oxygen, effective ventilation, aggressive fluid replacement and timely transport to an appropriate hospital are the key components to providing good emergency prehospital pediatric care.

ANSWER: TRUE

OB-GYN/Neonatal

This chapter will briefly review the female reproductive system, pertinent definitions, gynecologic dysfunction, obstetrical complications, normal and abnormal birth, specific treatments for all, and care for the neonate. Our focus is necessarily limited, but should provide the paramedic with adequate review of the material.

Definitions

Ovulation—The growth and discharge of an unfertilized egg, usually coincidental with the menstrual period.

Fertilization—The fusion of sperm and egg within the fallopian tube, where the egg remains for three days.

Implantation—When the fertilized egg attaches to the lining of the uterus (after coming from the fallopian tube).

Amniotic Sac and Fluid—The bag (of thin membrane) that contains the fetus and waterlike fluid to protect the fetus—approximately 1,000 cc at term.

Menstrual Cycle—This usually occurs in a 28-day cycle after initial onset of puberty (at age 12-14). The body readies for possible fertilization of eggs, and if fertilization does not occur, the extra cells and blood (uterine lining) that had been retained are excreted.

Menopause—Permanent cessation of ovarian function and menstrual activity.

Antepartum—Before delivery.

Postpartum—The maternal period following childbirth.

Prenatal—Before birth.

Natal—Connected with birth.

Gravida—The number of pregnancies a woman has had.

Primigravida—A woman who is pregnant for the first time.

Multigravida—A woman who has been pregnant several times.

Para—The number of pregnancies that have produced an infant of viable age.

Primipara—A woman who has given birth to her first child.

Multipara—A woman who has borne several or many children.
  EXAMPLE: A woman has been pregnant three times and has two
              live children is "gravida 3—para 2."

Effacement—The thinning and shortening of the cervix in the latter stage of pregnancy as the fetus moves down the birth canal.

Cervical Dilitation—Stretching of the opening of the cervix to accommodate birth of the fetus.

Crowning—Phase in the second stage of labor when a large part of the top of the fetal head becomes visible in the vaginal opening.

Presenting Part—The part of the infant that is first visible during birth (or that part that presents first at the os of the cervix).

Trimester—Approximately three months.

Meconium—Thick green fluid sometimes present in the amniotic fluid of the fetus at birth—extremely dangerous if inhaled with first breaths.

Structures

Ovaries—These organs secrete estrogen and produce eggs. There are two, located on each side of the uterus.

Fallopian Tubes—Muscular tubes that extend from each ovary to the uterus, through which eggs travel for possible fertilization.

FIGURE 26.1.

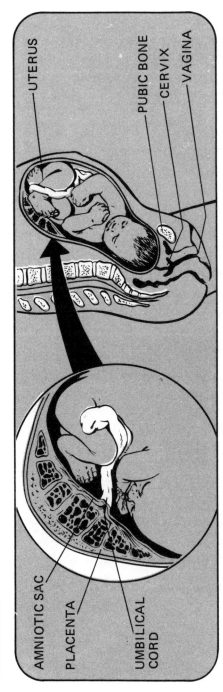

UTERUS

PUBIC BONE

CERVIX

VAGINA

AMNIOTIC SAC

PLACENTA

UMBILICAL CORD

Uterus—A muscular organ that protects the fetus while it grows and matures inside the body. The uterus normally lies within the pelvic girdle, but grows upward and outward as fetus develops.

Placenta (afterbirth)—A vascular organ attached to the wall of the uterus that supplies oxygen and nutrients to the fetus (through the umbilical cord).

Umbilical Cord—A flexible structure that connects placenta with fetus (containing two arteries and one vein).

Cervix—The lower portion (narrowing) of the uterus.

Vagina—Extends from the uterus to the birth canal (vulva).

Vulva—External genitalia.

Labia—The folds of skin and mucous membrane that comprise the labia.

Perineum—The area between the genitalia and the anus.

Endometrium—The inner layer (mucous membrane) of the uterus.

Gynecological Emergencies

Pelvic Inflammatory Disease (PID) This is an infection of the uterus, ovaries, fallopian tubes, or adjacent structures. These patients may have a history of erratic menstrual periods, recent painful sexual intercourse, and onsets of pain just after menses.

Signs and Symptoms

1. Generalized pain in the lower abdominal quadrants, more severe upon palpation, near the menstrual period (may radiate to right shoulder).
2. Possible fever, chills, rapid pulse, nausea and vomiting, or vaginal discharge.
3. Tense abdomen with rebound tenderness.

Prehospital Management

1. Smooth transport.
2. Position patient how she is most comfortable.

Vaginal Bleeding (Due to Trauma) This can be caused by foreign body insertion, straddle injuries, blows to the perineum, lacerations to genitalia, sexual assault, and abortion attempts. Usually involves soft tissue.

Prehospital Management

1. If bleeding is external—use direct pressure.
2. If bleeding is internal:
   a. Do *not* pack vagina with dressings.
   b. IV of LR.
   c. PASG if indicated.
   d. Monitor vital signs carefully for signs of hypovolemia.

Spontaneous Abortion This is the termination of a pregnancy (usually prior to the 12th week) before the fetus has attained viability.

Signs and Symptoms

1. Abdominal pain and cramping (may be mild to severe).
2. Vaginal passage of blood and tissue.
3. Sometimes evidence of infection.

Prehospital Management

1. Oxygen.
2. Trendelenberg position.
3. Large bore IV of NS or LR.
4. Shock trousers, if indicated.
5. Smooth transport, rapid if hypotensive.

Ectopic Pregnancy Pregnancy that ensues when a fertilized egg impants anywhere other than the uterus (1 out of 200). Usually, that place will be a fallopian tube (because that's where the egg is fertilized), after an egg does *not* make it down the tube to be implanted in the uterine wall. As the egg grows, the tube stretches and eventually ruptures, bleeding profusely. If the fallopian tube ruptures within its own intima, the blood will follow the tube to the uterus and present as severe vaginal bleeding. If the tube ruptures externally, dumping blood into the abdominal cavity, it presents as abdominal pain (perhaps with fever and spotting). In either case, the problem quickly becomes one of hypovolemic shock, and can be fatal.

Signs and Symptoms of Rupture (or Near Rupture)

1. Lower abdominal pain (may have rebound tenderness).
2. Significant history (symptoms of early pregnancy, skipped period[s], previous ectopic pregnancy, previous pelvic infection, intermittent spotting).
3. Possible severe vaginal bleeding (but may only be spotting).
4. Signs of hypovolemic shock (pale, cold clammy skin, rapid thready pulse, and eventually hypotension and decreased LOC).

Prehospital Management

1. High index of suspicion.
2. Airway and high-flow oxygen therapy.
3. Shock trousers.
4. Begin rapid transport to hospital/operating room.
5. Large-bore IVs of LR, wide open (two, if there is time), while enroute.
6. Monitor vital signs and ECG carefully enroute.

Complications of Pregnancy

Abruptio Placenta This refers to the premature separation of the placenta from the uterus, causing serious bleeding. Some causes would include trauma, hypertension, preeclampsia, multiple pregnancies, or short umbilical cord.

Signs and Symptoms

1. Acute onset of *severe* abdominal pain.
2. Vaginal bleeding.
3. Tender abdomen.

Prehospital Management

1. Airway and high-flow oxygen therapy.
2. Shock trousers, if indicated (leave abdomen section uninflated).
3. Begin rapid transport to hospital/operating room.

4. Large bore IV of NS or LR (while enroute).

5. Monitor vital signs closely.

Placenta Previa This refers to implantation of the placenta in the lower uterus, over the internal cervical os. This location completely or partially blocks the route for normal delivery of the fetus (requiring a cesarean section) and causes bleeding late in pregnancy when the cervix begins to change shape. These patients are generally multigravida and often have a history of early bleeding in their pregnancy.

Note: Any painless bleeding late in pregnancy should be considered placenta previa until proven otherwise.

Signs and Symptoms

1. Profuse painless bleeding (often associated with uterine contractions).

2. Uterus soft on palpation with no tenderness.

Prehospital Management

1. Airway and high-flow oxygen therapy.

2. Shock trousers, if indicated.

3. Begin rapid transport to hospital/operating room.

4. Large-bore IV of LR (while enroute).

5. Monitor vital signs carefully for signs of hypovolemia while continuing rapid transport.

Preeclampsia Preeclampsia is a disorder exclusive to late pregnancy or soon after birth, characterized chiefly by hypertension and edema. It can progress to eclampsia.

Prehospital Management

1. Secure patient in a dark, quiet environment.

2. Position on side.

3. IV of NS or LR (TKO).

4. Smooth transport.

Eclampsia (Toxemia) This is a serious toxic condition occurring in late pregnancy or soon after birth that presents itself with seizures, hypertension, edema, and coma (5-15% mortality—second leading cause of maternal death).

Prehospital Management

1. Airway and oxygen therapy.
2. IV of NS or LR (TKO).
3. Consider IV Valium if still seizing (Diazepam 2-10 mg.).
4. Smooth transport to the hospital.

Uterine Rupture Characterized by sudden severe abdominal pain, a ruptured uterus will cause significant internal bleeding (external hemorrhage may not be severe, masking significant internal losses) and can quickly result in profound shock. There may be a history of trauma, previous cesarean section, prolonged labor, or abnormal fetal presentation.

Prehospital Management

1. Airway and high-flow oxygen therapy.
2. Shock trousers, if indicated (legs only).
3. Begin transport immediately.
4. Large-bore IV(s) of LR, wide open (two, if there's time), while enroute.
5. Rapid transport to appropriate hospital/operating room.

Postpartum Hemorrhage This type of hemorrhage would involve more than 500 cc (rough estimate) of bleeding following a birth, often after a prolonged delivery, delivery of large or multiple infants, or in concert with some other complication. Severe postpartum hemorrhage is not uncommon and can result from a variety of causes such as:

1. Poor uterine tone.
2. Clotting disorders.
3. Failure of the uterus to return to normal size following delivery.
4. Retention of placental parts.
5. Cervical or vaginal tears.

Prehospital Management

1. Airway and high-flow oxygen therapy.
2. Shock trousers, if indicated.

3. Begin rapid transport to hospital/operating room.

4. Large-bore IV(s) of LR, wide open (two, if enough time enroute).

5. Consider Oxytocin (10-20 units in 1,000 LR at 20-30 drops per minute, titrated to severity of hemorrhage or uterine response).

Note: It may be helpful to put baby to the breast (which may stimulate uterine contractions) and/or to massage the uterus externally—see your local protocols. *Never* pack vagina, and *never* attempt to force placental delivery.

Supine Hypotensive Syndrome This may occur in the late stages of pregnancy when the abdominal mass is large. When the mother is supine, the large abdominal mass compresses the inferior vena cava, reducing venous return and thus reducing cardiac output. (This syndrome may be more likely in the patient with marginal blood volume.)

Prehospital Management If volume depletion is *not* present—place patient in left lateral recumbant position. (This position takes the pressure off the vena cava.) If volume depletion *seems likely*:

1. Airway and high-flow oxygen.

2. Shock trousers, if indicated (legs only).

3. Begin transport.

4. Large-bore IV(s) of LR, wide open (two, if enough time enroute).

5. Monitor vital signs and ECG carefully.

Note: It is good practice to transport any near-term patient with the abdominal mass shifted slightly to the left, either manually, by positioning, or by tilting a spineboard to the left with some kind of cribbing underneath (towel, blanket, small cat).

Delivery

Though we assume the presence of an obstetrical kit, it must be remembered that you may be called upon to deliver infants without specialized equipment. You can improvise for the essentials—shoelace for clamping umbilical cord, newspaper to wrap baby, turkey baster for suction, and so on.

Stages of Labor In a normal delivery there are three stages of labor:

1. *First*—From the onset of regular contractions to complete dilitation of the cervix.
2. *Second*—From full dilitation of the cervix to delivery of the baby.
3. *Third*—From delivery of the baby to delivery of the placenta.

Decision to Transport Whether to begin transport or stay and prepare for on-site delivery depends upon the imminence of delivery. This is affected by several factors:

1. The number of pregnancies (labor tends to shorten progressively).
2. The frequency of hard contractions—traditionally, contractions less than two minutes apart mean delivery should be soon.
3. The mother's urgent need to push.
4. Crowning (the ultimate sign of imminent delivery).
5. Abnormal presentations (may require immediate transport in mid-birth).

Management of Normal Delivery Assuming that the immediate area for delivery has been made as clean as possible, and that time allowed some kind of clean or sterile draping of the mother and delivery area, these are the usual steps in the managing the normal delivery:

1. Oxygen therapy for the mother throughout.
2. Large-bore IV placement as a precaution (if time permits).
3. Put on sterile gloves (or clean hands thoroughly).
4. Coach mother's breathing—coordinate pushing with contractions and urge controlled panting when pain or pressure seems unbearable.
5. When head begins to appear (crowning), place fingers gently on the fetal head to prevent an "explosive" delivery.
6. If the amniotic sac still covers the head as it delivers, quickly tear the membrane with your fingers and allow the amniotic fluid to escape.
7. If, as the head delivers, the umbilical cord is wrapped around the baby's neck, slip it over the head (if there is enough slack). If it's tight around baby's neck, clamp the cord in 2 places and cut carefully between the clamps.

8. Suction the infant's nose and mouth as soon as they are accessible.

9. Support the head as it rotates and support the shoulders as they deliver.

10. Once the baby has been delivered, keep it at or above the level of the vagina. This prevents fluctuations in blood supply to the infant.

11. Clamp the umbilical cord twice (at least 4 inches from the baby) and cut between the clamps.

12. Suction infant again, wipe dry, check the cord, wrap baby in dry blanket, towels, and so on and lay on side with the head slightly lower to aid drainage. Aluminum foil works well to maintain the infant's body heat, a *critical* step. Babies can't easily regulate or maintain body heat.

13. Note the time of the birth.

14. If you have time, take an APGAR score at one minute after birth, and again at five minutes for comparison.

15. Deliver placenta if it comes while you're still on the scene, but *don't delay transport* for delivery of the placenta. If you do deliver it, save it and bring it with the mother.

16. If bleeding seems excessive, massage the uterus externally.

17. Manage any perineal tears with direct pressure.

18. Be vigilant in observing the mother for signs of bleeding or shock (check vital signs frequently).

19. Keep communicating with the mother throughout, as her normal apprehension is heightened by the worry of an out-of-hospital delivery. She is your best asset in assisting with the delivery.

Breech Presentation This situation exists when the baby presents itself with its feet or buttocks. Delivery is best done in the hospital, but if field delivery is unavoidable, it often can be successful.

Prehospital Management

1. Make sure you administer high-flow oxygen to the mother.
2. Allow the body to be delivered with contractions only. DO NOT ENCOURAGE MOTHER TO PUSH.
3. Support the body once the arms are delivered.
4. Gentle traction may be applied once the head is past the pubis, until the mouth appears.

FIGURE 26.2.

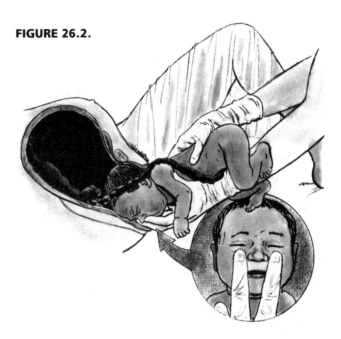

5. If the head has not delivered and spontaneous breathing attempts begin, place a gloved hand in vagina, form a V with the fingers on either side of the baby's nose and push the vaginal wall away from the face. Maintain this position and transport rapidly. Delivery may or may not complete enroute.

Arm or Leg Presentation Sometimes one leg or one arm may be the presenting part. Do not pull, and do not push back into birth canal.

Prehospital Management

1. Stop, reassure mother, and load immediately (if not already enroute).

FIGURE 26.3.

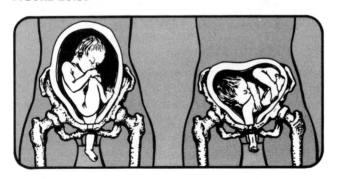

2. Rapid transport to the hospital/operating room (with high-flow oxygen, of course). Immediate cesarean section is required.

Prolapsed Cord This condition exists when the umbilical cord is compressed between the presenting part and the pelvis, shutting off fetal circulation. The cord may present first, followed by part of the infant's body.

FIGURE 26.4.

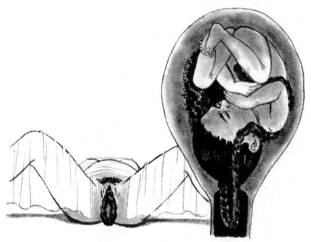

- Elevate hips, administer oxygen and keep warm
- Keep baby's head away from cord
- Do not attempt to push cord back
- Wrap cord in sterile moist towel
- Transport mother to hospital, continuing pressure on baby's head

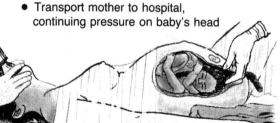

Prehospital Management

1. If the umbilical cord can be seen or felt in vagina, insert 2 fingers to remove pressure against the cord if possible. Check for pulsations in the cord.
2. Place mother in Trendelenburg position, or "knee-to-chest" of possible.
3. High-flow oxygen therapy.
4. Immediate rapid transport.

Multiple Births Most mothers having multiple births will be aware of the fact or possibility and can tell you—especially if you *ask*! This can still be a surprise, however, and you must be ready. The biggest tipoff is when the abdomen remains large after delivery of the first baby and contractions continue.

FIGURE 26.5.

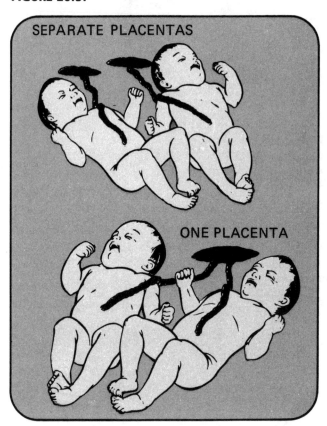

Prehospital Management

1. There may or may not be more than one placenta, so tie the cord of the first baby at the first opportunity.
2. Pay very special attention to keeping these babies warm—they will usually be very small and very vulnerable to heat loss. Don't forget the aluminum foil for maintaining heat.

Neonatal Care

Gentle stimulation after birth (rubbing the back) will generally get things started off well. Avoid spanking or vigorous rubbing. The biggest prehospital problem with the neonate is keeping him warm, so use common sense and avoid unnecessary heat loss. (And don't forget the foil or special neonatal wrap.)

Prehospital Assessment

1. Vital signs:
   a. 150-180 at birth, slows to 130-140 per minute after.
   b. If pulse is < 100, begin resuscitation to combat asphyxia.
   c. Crying indicates good respiratory effort.
   d. Respiratory rate should be 40-60 per minute.
2. APGAR score at one minute and five minutes. This is a tool to help identify those infants who may need more than routine care.

Premature Infants These are babies born before the 38th week of pregnancy. They are usually significantly smaller and are really at risk for:

1. Hypothermia.
2. Volume depletion.
3. Respiratory problems.
4. Cardiovascular problems (caused by hypoxia).

Prehospital Management

1. KEEP WARM. Use dry towels, aluminum foil, "silver swaddlers", your shirt, whatever it takes to maintain the little one's body heat.

FIGURE 26.6.

Sign	0	1	2	Score	
				1 min	*5 min*
Heart Rate	absent	below 100	over 100		
Respiration (effort)	absent	slow and irregular	normal; crying		
Muscle Tone	limp	some flexion—extremities	active; good motion in extremities		
Irritability	no response	crying; some motion	crying; vigorous		
Skin Color	bluish or paleness	pink or typical newborn color; hands and feet are blue	pink or typical newborn color; entire body		
			TOTAL SCORE		

2. Monitor the airway closely and suction as needed. Infants are obligatory nose-breathers, so keep that nose clear.

3. Check and prevent bleeding from the cut umbilical cord.

4. Keep clean and as free from germs and dirt as possible.

Meconium Staining A potentially serious complication, meconium staining (thick green fluid in the amniotic fluid or covering infant) requires quick decisive action by paramedics. If inhaled, meconium may cause severe lung inflammation, hypoxia, even brain damage. Some infants may already have some in their lungs. This must be removed from the airway before the first breath is taken.

Prehospital Management

1. Vigorous suctioning before the first breath.

2. If possible, after initial suctioning with an ear-bulb syringe, quickly intubate infant and perform trachal suction. Avoid stimulation of the baby until this is done.

3. Report the meconium staining to the physician assuming care.

Note: The presence of meconium may indicate fetal distress, possible due to placental insufficiency or obstruction of the cord.

Resuscitation Resuscitation of infants is directed primarily toward *ventilation* and *oxygenation,* as hypoxia is the usual culprit in the distressed neonate. You can pretty much forget the IVs and cardiac care. Oxygen toxicity is not a problem in the prehospital setting, so *do not* withhold. If the infant is pale or cyanotic, give oxygen until pink. You can use oxygen tubing or a mask, run at 4-5 L/min. and hold near face. If you must provide ventilatory assistance, use infant-size bag-valve mask (or mouth-to-mouth-and-nose if BVM is not available) with supplemental oxygen. Watch for lung rise and fall—DO NOT OVERINFLATE. You may intubate with endotracheal tube if you are confident in your training. Remember to ventilate at 30-40/minute and follow current American Heart Association (AHA) guidelines if performing CPR.

Summary

It is vital that paramedics have an understanding of the general nature and specific treatment of obstetrical and gynecological emergencies. Further, management of normal and abnormal births will sometimes be necessary, and should therefore be thoroughly understood. Recognition of hemorrhage and/or shock in the OB/GYN patient and maintenance of warmth and ventilation in the neonate are the most important lessons in this chapter.

SELF-TEST

Chapter 26

1. The stretching of the opening of the cervix to accommodate the birth of the fetus is called _____ _____ .

   ANSWER: cervical dilitation

2. The thick green fluid sometimes present in the amniotic fluid of the fetus at birth is called _____ .

   ANSWER: meconium

3. The muscular organ that protects a fetus while it grows and matures is called the _____ .

   ANSWER: uterus

4. The _____ is a vascular organ attached to wall of the uterus that supplies oxygen and nutrients to the fetus through the

   _____ _____ .

   ANSWER: placenta, umbilical cord

5. _____ is the phase in a normal birth when a large part of the top of the fetal head is visible in the vaginal opening.

   ANSWER: Crowning

6. _____ is the technical term that refers to the number of pregnancies a woman has had.

   ANSWER: Gravida

7. The area between the genitalia and the anus that sometimes tears during delivery is called the _____ .

   ANSWER: perineum

8. The growth and discharge of an unfertilized egg (usually coincidental with the menstrual period) is called _____ .

   ANSWER: ovulation

9. In most ectopic pregnancies, a fertilized egg implants somewhere in the _____ _____ instead of the uterus. Eventually, rupture occurs, often resulting in profound _____ .

ANSWER: fallopian tube, shock (hypovolemic)

10. Termination of a pregnancy (usually before the 12th week) by the body before the fetus has attained viability is called _____ _____ .

ANSWER: spontaneous abortion

11. Hypertension and edema late in pregnancy (or soon after birth) may be indicative of _____ .

ANSWER: preeclampsia

12. Premature separation of the placenta from the uterus is called _____ _____ .

ANSWER: abruptio placenta

13. Any woman who has skipped a period, has lower abdominal pain and bleeding (or spotting) should be suspected of having an _____ _____ until proven differently.

ANSWER: ectopic pregnancy

14. The "pregnancy hormone" secreted by the ovaries is called _____ .

ANSWER: estrogen

15. Any profuse painless bleeding late in pregnancy should be assumed to be _____ _____ until proven otherwise.

ANSWER: placenta previa

16. If preeclampsia goes undiagnosed (and untreated), it may progress to a more serious toxic condition called _____ .

ANSWER: eclampsia (toxemia)

17. *More than* 500 cc of bleeding following birth is often referred to as _____ _____ .

ANSWER: postpartum hemorrhage

18. Explain "supine hypotensive syndrome".

ANSWER: While supine, the pregnant patient's large abdominal mass may compress the inferior vena cava, significantly reducing venous return and cardiac output.

19. Infants are considered to be premature when delivered before the _____ week of pregnancy.

ANSWER: 38th

20. Name some of the factors that affect the decision to transport a mother in active labor.

ANSWER: a. number of previous pregnancies

b. frequency of hard contractions

c. the mother's urgent need to push

d. crowning (the ultimate sign of imminent delivery)

e. abnormal presentations

21. TRUE or FALSE. A breech presentation cannot be successfully delivered in the prehospital environment.

ANSWER: FALSE—breech presentations are often successfully accomplished outside of the hospital.

22. If the umbilical cord is wrapped around the infant's neck as the head delivers, what should be done?

ANSWER: a. Slip the cord over the head if there is enough slack.

b. If the cord is wrapped tightly around the baby's neck, clamp the cord in two places and cut carefully between the clamps.

23. What condition exists when the umbilical cord is the presenting part.

ANSWER: prolapsed cord

24. TRUE or FALSE. An arm or leg presentation or prolapsed cord must be transported to the hospital for an emergency cesarean section.

ANSWER: TRUE

25. Ideally, an APGAR score should be taken at one minute and five minutes after birth. What do the letters in A-P-G-A-R stand for?

ANSWER: A = appearance

P = pulse

G = grimace

A = activity

R = respiratory effort

26. If there appears to be meconium staining as the baby is born, what should be accomplished *before* the first breath is taken by the infant?

ANSWER: suctioning (preferably tracheal)

27. TRUE or FALSE. Resuscitation of infants is directed primarily toward *ventilation* and *oxygenation*.

ANSWER: TRUE

28. What is the most important thing you can do for a newborn (once that adequate breathing has been established) in the prehospital arena?

ANSWER: Keep the newborn *WARM.*

Behavioral Emergencies

Paramedics are at a disadvantage when confronted with behavioral and psychiatric emergencies. Our training (like most other uniformed personnel on the streets) has been directed in other critical areas, with little time spent in understanding and managing the patient in behavioral crisis. Most of our learning has been "on the job", and errors we might have made had immediate consequences. Local protocols (if available) seldom deal with these patients, and if they do it's generally a "hands off" policy—don't do anything without the police, don't deal with behavior presentations, just wrap em' in Kerlix when the police say "bring your gurney, boys." That's not a very realistic policy for a great many situations. Safety of the paramedic is the TOP PRIORITY, absolutely true—but there is a time to pull back and call in the troops and there is a time to take charge and provide stability for the patient in crisis—and education and experience are the key.

Some paramedics have a natural tendency to avoid behavioral situations, often believing that intervention on the streets does little to affect patient outcome. An uncertainty in how to handle behavior/psychiatric situations is normal. This chapter reminds you that you can make a significant difference in patient/situation outcomes, that there is a systematic organized approach to evaluation, and that not only is safe intervention usually possible—it may be essential to keep the crisis from becoming worse.

Definitions

Anxiety—Often caused by a feeling of helplessness or loss of control, especially in those whose self-esteem depends upon being active, independent, and aggressive.

Regression—A return to an earlier, more primitive mode of behavior—often a return to being child-like and depending upon others for direction, usually as a response to stress.

Confusion—A response, often due to illness or injury, in which the subject is disoriented (very common in the elderly).

Anger—A response to discomfort or limitation of function that may be inappropriately directed toward the rescuer.

Catatonia—Periods of physical rigidity, stupor, non-communication—a total separation of subject from interacting with surroundings.

Conversion Reaction—A subconscious conversion of anxiety into bodily dysfunction, such as being unable to hear, see, or move an extremity.

Fear—A response of anticipation. Perhaps related to anxiety in facing pain, disability, the unknown, economic difficulties, emotions—even death.

Denial—An attempt to ignore a problem because of the anxiety it causes.

Depression—Sadness, feelings of dejection, melancholy, and a decrease in functional activity. The subject may not want to do anything, may not want to move, answer questions or cooperate, and may even experience insomnia and weight loss. Depression can be situational, pathological, or part of a grief reaction to a sense of loss.

Suicide—Willful act intended to bring an end to one's own life.

Paranoia—Mental disorder characterized by distrust, seclusion, abnormal suspicions of persecution "they're out to get me. . ." and delusions.

Facilitation—Reinforcing and encouraging continued patient communication by small positive responses, such as nodding the head, saying "I see. . ." or "go on. . .". It can also be used to direct conversation back to a pertinent topic—"so you say you wanted to just go to sleep?. . ."

Confrontation—Technique of pointing out to a patient significant points in conversation or behavior of which he may not have been aware.

Open-ended Questions—A leading question that urges the subject to talk—"How is this making you feel? . . ."

Phobia—An unfounded, exaggerated dread or fear.

Withdrawal—Refusal to deal with a situation or a reality.

Understanding Behavioral Emergencies

Behavioral Emergencies Defined Behavioral emergencies are defined as a change in a person caused by intrapsychic, environmental, situational, or organic alterations resulting in behavior that cannot be tolerated by the person or others and requires immediate attention.

Intrapsychic Causes Behavioral changes that come from within can be expressed in a wide range of behaviors, whether due to an acute situation or underlying mental disorder. Some of these include;

1. Depression;
2. Withdrawal;
3. Catatonic state;
4. Violence;
5. Suicidal acts;
6. Homicidal acts;
7. Paranoid behavior;
8. Phobia;
9. Conversion hysteria; and
10. Disorientation/disorganization.

Interpersonal/Environmental Causes Sometimes the abnormal behavior is a reaction to external events or overwhelming incidents such as:

1. Death of a loved one;
2. Rape;

3. Natural disaster (tornado, flood, earthquake, hurricane);
4. Man-made disaster (war, explosions, industrial catastrophes);
5. Career change;
6. Loss of a job;
7. Marital stress or divorce;
8. Physical/psychological abuse; and
9. Personal economic disaster.

Changes in behavior can often be linked to a specific incident or series of incidents.

Organic Causes Disruption of the physical or biochemical state can cause significant changes in behavior. Possible causes would include:

1. Drugs (wide range of causal agents and responses);
2. Alcohol (CNS depressant, complication of underlying behavior);
3. Trauma (head injury, hypoxia);
4. Illness (diabetes, electrolyte imbalance);
5. Dementia (organic brain syndrome)—changes in behavior due to the aging process affecting the brain.

Scene Evaluation

Due to the nature of the profession, emergency providers are constantly at risk for injury. Evaluation of the scene for possible dangers is the initial top priority responsibility—no matter what the situation. *A dead paramedic is an ineffective paramedic!* The following potentially hazardous situations are obviously beyond the scope of the typical field paramedic, unless specifically cross-trained or in prearranged concert with appropriate backup:

1. Patients with weapons;
2. Riot scenes;
3. Fire scenes;
4. Hostage situations;
5. Hazardous materials potential.

If the scene is judged sufficiently safe for entry, enter and look carefully for clues that may aid in patient care or evaluation:

1. Evidence of violence;
2. Evidence of substance abuse;
3. Evidence of suicidal attempt.

Obtaining a History

Your initial course of action will be to perform a primary survey to identify life-threatening conditions. If you are able to complete the primary survey, you can begin to get a more complete picture of the situation while finishing your secondary survey, utilizing your own observations and patient history obtained from family, friends, bystanders and first responders. These points may be important:

1. What (if known) triggered the behavioral crisis that resulted in emergency care being summoned.
2. Current life situation—married with ten kids, going to school, working in vaudeville, takes drugs regularly, and so on.
3. Medical and behavioral/mental history (both recent and past).
4. Physical signs/symptoms.
5. Behavior that resulted in help being summoned (also current behavior).

Guidelines for Managing Interview You may want to separate the patient from the immediate environment (if inflammatory) or from persons involved who continue to interact with the patient and keep things riled up. These points may be helpful in interviewing the patient:

1. Encourage the person to sit, relax and speak freely.
2. When the person begins to speak, interrupt as little as possible.
3. If the person stops talking and begins to cry, don't start talking or change the subject, just let it happen. Also, long periods of silence are okay, just remain attentive.
4. Facilitate the conversation by nodding your head and "I see. . ." or "so then?. . .".

5. If you must ask questions to keep things moving, avoid "yes or no" questions.

6. If the situation seems like total chaos to the patient, try to build a structure and communicate confidence in yourself, honesty, firmness and reasonableness on important issues.

7. Position yourself in non-intimidating manner, don't try and outyell the patient, and don't touch the patient unless he indicates this is allowable—if it is allowable, it is important to touch.

Psychiatric Disorders

Depression Depression may have internal (frozen anger, guilt) or external (grief, situational) causes.

Symptoms The patient may exhibit some of the following:

1. Persistent pessimism—"things will never get better. . . ."
2. Tendency to cry easily.
3. Feelings of hopelessness, worthlessness and isolation.
4. Withdrawal from social relationships.
5. Agitation and hyperactivity *OR* slowness and lethargy.

Suicide Some primary motivations for suicide may be:

1. Feelings of hopelessness, and a loss of ability to communicate effectively.
2. Wavering decisions whether to live or die (a strong human instinct is to live—this can be used in managing patient).
3. Manipulation of personal relationships—attempting to arouse sympathy or anxiety in others.

Assessment of Suicide Potential—Risk Factors
Sex:

1. Men are more successful at committing suicide than women.
2. Men use more violent means (guns, knives, ropes) than women (pills, carbon monoxide).

The Suicide Plan:

1. How lethal is the method selected?
2. How available is the method selected?
3. How specific is the plan? (The more specific, the greater the threat.)
4. Have there been prior attempts?

Stress Stress increases the likelihood of suicidal behavior and should be evaluated from the patient's point of view. If the stress level is high, than the risk of suicidal behavior is higher. If stress is low, so is the risk of suicide. If the stress level is low, but the symptoms pointing to probable suicidal behavior are high, than the facts are incomplete or the patient is unstable.

Symptoms:

1. Depression (see previous heading).
2. Agitation (feelings of anger, revenge, tension, guilt).
3. Agitation is more likely if the patient is alcoholic, addicted to drugs, or in a psychotic state.
4. Disorganization—in both activity and thought processes.

Prehospital Management

1. Access to patient (may have to have proper personnel break in if threat has been made but no contact established).
2. If patient turns out to be armed, they may be homicidal as well as suicidal. Leave immediately—stay away until police indicate the scene is safe.
3. Emergency care for illness or injury is first priority.
4. Brief assessment interview, search of scene for clues, history from relatives, friends, bystanders or first responders.
5. Every attempted suicide should be evaluated by a physician. This often involves the help and authority of the police.

Rage, Hostility, Violent Behavior Basically, this is the disruptive patient. Behavior is probably a symptom of an underlying problem (such as illness, head injury, feelings of helplessness or loss of control) and not necessarily a psychiatric problem.

Prehospital Management

1. Once the scene is safe, isolate the subject (if possible) and let him know what he can expect from you—and what you expect from him.
2. If he is angry (and you are protected), investigate the source of the anger.
3. Tell him your primary concern is to help him and keep the peace.
4. Tell the subject what you need him to do, and allow him a chance to comply voluntarily.
5. Follow through with what you say—do not make idle threats.
6. If patient refuses to comply, restraint may be required and police involvement becomes mandatory. Utilize soft restraints whenever possible.

Paranoid Reactions Acute anxiety usually precipitates the emergency of paranoid behavior. This behavior often presents as a conviction that the subject is being persecuted or plotted against. Check the validity of the patient claims, if possible. An objective person's observations sometimes reassure the patient. Paranoid reactions can occur suddenly, with some warning, or very gradually over a long period of time.

Prehospital Management

1. Clearly identify yourself and your reason for being there.
2. Be civil, business-like, or neutral. Do not be overly friendly or very warm, as you might be with most patients—this can be taken as an attempt to get close to the patient in order to "get" them.
3. Never respond to the patient's anger.
4. Don't talk behind the patient's back, or in whispers.
5. Don't lie to the patient, use tact and firmness in advocating a professional evaluation.

Hysterical Conversion Reaction This is a situation in which stress or anxiety is psychologically transformed into physical symptoms such as psychic blindness, deafness, or paralysis.

Prehospital Management Don't try to convince the patient that he is imagining the symptoms, but treat the signs and symptoms as if they were real. Be sure to inform the receiving facility or staff of the possibility that the patient may be experiencing a conversion reaction.

The Disorganized/Disoriented Patient Uncontrolled and disconnected thoughts characterize a disorganized patient, as well as incoherent or rambling speech. He may be wandering aimlessly, or be dressed inappropriately. A disoriented patient does not know where he is, what day it is—perhaps not even his own name. Some causes of disorientation include head injury, drug ingestion and metabolic disorders.

Prehospital Management

1. With *disorganized* patients, try to provide some structure. Explain who you are, what you are trying to do and what his role is as the patient.
2. With *disoriented* patients, orient them to time, place and person. Be patient, because you may have to repeat the information several times. This is a relatively common condition in the elderly, and it may be complicated at times by regression.

General Management and Intervention

1. Assess the risk to your own safety. If in doubt, hang back until the scene is secure. A dead or injured paramedic is an ineffective paramedic.
2. Maintain a professional attitude. Most of the time, it is appropriate to be warm, sensitive and compassionate.
3. Take command of the situation, calmly, and be reassuring when possible.
4. Practice good scene management. This may mean separating patient from others closely related to the situation, removing unnecessary bystanders and/or physically changing location from scenes of stressful events.
5. Make an attempt to establish some kind of rapport before performing physical examinations.
6. When dealing with emotionally disturbed patients:
   a. Intervene only to the degree that you feel fully capable. Be aware of your professional limitations as well.
   b. Communicate to the patient the importance of seeking professional help when unable to deal effectively with a problem alone.
   c. Don't overreact to behavior or emotional attacks.
   d. Assess patient needs and try to meet them.

7. Paramedics are not equipped to deal effectively with many behavioral/psychological disorders. Learn to recognize early when intervention must be accomplished by appropriate facilities and personnel and find a legal way to get the patient there. Maintain a good rapport with the police.

8. Know your local mental health resources and how to access them at any time.

9. Remember that detailed repetitive explanations may be required for some anxious or confused patients.

Controlling Violent Behavior If, for whatever reason, a paramedic finds himself in the middle of a violent situation, he should remember several points:

1. Protecting himself from harm is appropriate. So is running away.

2. When forced to restrain a patient, use only the amount of force required to accomplish the restraint.

3. Don't get separated from your partner. You are each other's backup until more help can arrive.

4. Utilize standard restraining techniques (practice these) and practice self-control.

Transporting Resistive Patients When authorized to transport the resistive patient, remember these points.

1. When possible, place the patient prone or laterally recumbant.

2. It is always safer to use restraints—but it's a judgment call.

3. Know what kind of method you will use to strap the patient to the stretcher. Keep the stretcher in its lowest position (for stability) and allow for good maintenance of the airway.

4. When appropriate, request that police personnel ride with you. (Be ready to insist.)

5. Once applied, do not remove restraints until there are enough personnel present to maintain control.

Summary

Patients in behavioral or psychiatric crisis are a challenge to the paramedic, and one in which we are not generally well-prepared to handle.

Management often depends upon experience and judgement. Top priority while handling these calls is for the paramedic's own safety. Emergency care remains the same for these patients as for any other, but other intervention will depend greatly upon the kind of rapport you can establish in a brief period of time. Enlist the aid of the police whenever necessary, stay within your legal bounds (don't transport against a patient's will unless legally authorized to do so), protect yourself and protect the best interests of your patient.

SELF-TEST

Chapter 27

1. Sadness, feelings of dejection, pessimism, isolation, agitation, hyperactivity or slowness, melancholy and a decrease in functional activity are some possible symptoms of _____ .

   ANSWER: depression

2. List some of the primary motivations for suicide.

   ANSWER: hopelessness, ambivalence, depression, anxiety, and so on.

3. Define paranoia.

   ANSWER: A mental disorder characterized by distrust, seclusion and abnormal suspicions or convictions that one is being persecuted or plotted against.

4. When stress or anxiety is transformed into physical symptoms (such as paralysis, deafness or blindness) the result is called a _____ _____ .

   ANSWER: conversion reaction

5. An unfounded, exaggerated fear or dread is called a _____ . Give some examples of these kind of fears.

   ANSWER: phobia

   Examples: fear of confined spaces, fear of water, fear of open spaces, fear of writing checks, fear of flying, fear of heights, fear of depths

6. When a subject becomes totally separated from interacting with surroundings, this is called _____ .

   ANSWER: catatonia (catatonic state)

7. Name some potentially hazardous situations that may be beyond the scope of the typical field paramedic (unless specifically cross-trained or in prearranged concert with appropriate backup).

ANSWER: a. patients with weapons
            b. riot scenes
            c. fire scenes
            d. hostage situations
            e. hazardous materials potential
            f. combatibe patients

8. TRUE or FALSE. Transporting a patient against his or her will legally requires the consent of the spouse or immediate family.

ANSWER: FALSE

ACLS Algorithms

The American Heart Association provides a course in Advanced Cardiac Life Support (ACLS) that has set a standard for prehospital emergency cardiac care. The algorithms (recommended care guidelines) currently approved by the AHA are included in this appendix. This includes the use of an additional algorithm dealing with the use of Automated External Defibrillators (AEDs).

FIGURE 1. Ventricular fibrillation (and pulseless ventricular tachycardia).[a] This sequence was developed to assist in teaching how to treat a broad range of patients with ventricular fibrillation (VF) or pulseless ventricular tachycardia (VT). Some patients may require care not specified herein. This algorithm should not be construed as prohibiting such flexibility. Flow of algorithm presumes that VF is continuing. CPR indicates cardiopulmonary resuscitation.

[a]Pulseless VT should be treated identically to VF.

[b]Check pulse and rhythm after each shock. If VF recurs after transiently converting (rather than persists without ever converting), use whatever energy level has previously been successful for defibrillation.

[c]Epinephrine should be repeated every five minutes.

[d]Intubation is preferable. If it can be accompanied simultaneously with other techniques, then the earlier the better. However, defibrillation and epinephrine are more important initially if the patient can be ventilated without intubation.

[e]Some may prefer repeated doses of lidocaine, which may be given in 0.5-mg/kg boluses every eight minutes to a total dose of 3 mg/kg.

[f]Value of sodium bicarbonate is questionable during cardiac arrest, and it is not recommended for routine cardiac arrest sequence. Consideration of its use in a dose of 1 mEq/kg is appropriate at this point. Half of original dose may be repeated every ten minutes if it is used.

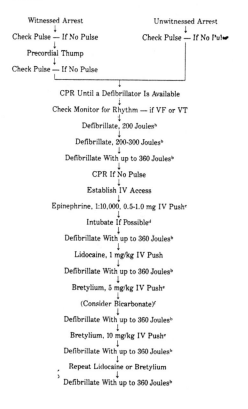

FIGURE 2. Asystole (cardiac standstill). This sequence was developed to assist in teaching how to treat a broad range of patients with asystole. Some patients may require care not specified herein. This algorithm should not be construed to prohibit such flexibility. Flow of algorithm presumes asystole is continuing. VF indicates ventricular fibrillation; IV, intravenous.

[a]Asystole should be confirmed in two leads.

[b]Epinephrine should be repeated every five minutes.

[c]Intubation is preferable; if it can be accomplished simultaneously with other techniques, then the earlier the better. However, cardiopulmonary resuscitation (CPR) and use of epinephrine are more important initially if patient can be ventilated without intubation. (Endotracheal epinephrine may be used.)

[d]Value of sodium bicarbonate is questionable during cardiac arrest, and it is not recommended for the routine cardiac arrest sequence. Consideration of its use in a dose of 1 mEq/kg is appropriate at this point. Half of original dose may be repeated every ten minutes if it is used.

If Rhythm Is Unclear and Possibly Ventricular Fibrillation, Defibrillate as for VF. If Asystole is Present[a]

↓

Continue CPR

↓

Establish IV Access

↓

Epinephrine, 1:10,000, 0.5 - 1.0 mg IV Push[b]

↓

Intubate When Possible[c]

↓

Atropine, 1.0 mg IV Push (Repeated in 5 min)

↓

(Consider Bicarbonate)[d]

↓

Consider Pacing

FIGURE 3. Electromechanical dissociation. This sequence was developed to assist in teaching how to treat a broad range of patients with electromechanical dissociation. Some patients may require care not specified herein. This algorithm should not be construed to prohibit such flexibility. Flow of algorithm presumes that electromechanical dissociation is continuing. CPR indicates cardiopulmonary resuscitation; IV, intravenous.

[a]Epinephrine should be repeated every five minutes.

[b]Intubation is preferable. If it can be accomplished simultaneously with other techniques, then the earlier the better. However, epinephrine is more important initially if the patient can be ventilated without intubation.

[c]Value of sodium bicarbonate is questionable during cardiac arrest, and it is not recommended for routine cardiac arrest sequence. Consideration of its use in a dose of 1 mEq/kg is appropriate at this point. Half of original dose may be repeated every ten minutes if it is used.

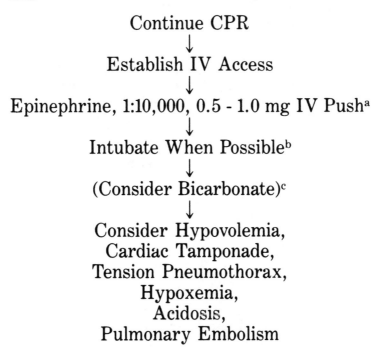

Continue CPR
↓
Establish IV Access
↓
Epinephrine, 1:10,000, 0.5 - 1.0 mg IV Push[a]
↓
Intubate When Possible[b]
↓
(Consider Bicarbonate)[c]
↓
Consider Hypovolemia,
Cardiac Tamponade,
Tension Pneumothorax,
Hypoxemia,
Acidosis,
Pulmonary Embolism

FIGURE 4. Sustained ventricular tachycardia (VT). This sequence was developed to assist in teaching how to treat a broad range of patients with sustained VT. Some patients may require care not specified herein. This algorithm should not be construed as prohibiting such flexibility. Flow of algorithm presumes that VT is continuing. VF indicates ventricular fibrillation.

[a]If patient becomes unstable (see footnote b for definition) at any time, move to "Unstable" arm of algorithm.

[b]Unstable indicates symptoms (e.g., chest pain or dyspnea), hypotension (systolic blood pressure <90 mm Hg), congestive heart failure, ischemia, or infarction.

[c]Sedation should be considered for all patients, including those defined in footnote b as unstable, except those who are hemodynamically unstable (e.g., hypotensive, in pulmonary edema, or unconscious).

[d]If hypotension, pulmonary edema, or unconsciousness is present, unsynchronized cardioversion should be done to avoid delay associated with synchronization.

[e]In the absence of hypotension, pulmonary edema, or unconsciousness, a precordial thump may be employed prior to cardioversion.

[f]Once VT has resolved, begin intravenous (IV) infusion of antiarrhythmic agent that has aided resolution of VT. If hypotension, pulmonary edema, or unconsciousness is present, use lidocaine if cardioversion alone is unsuccessful, followed by bretylium. In all other patients, recommended order of therapy is lidocaine, procainamide, and then bretylium.

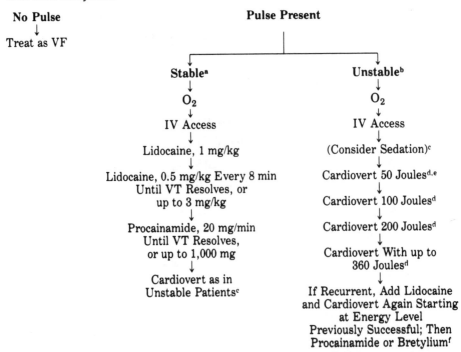

```
No Pulse                          Pulse Present
   ↓
Treat as VF                            |
                          ┌────────────┴────────────┐
                          ↓                          ↓
                       Stableᵃ                   Unstableᵇ
                          ↓                          ↓
                          O₂                         O₂
                          ↓                          ↓
                      IV Access                  IV Access
                          ↓                          ↓
                 Lidocaine, 1 mg/kg        (Consider Sedation)ᶜ
                          ↓                          ↓
          Lidocaine, 0.5 mg/kg Every 8 min   Cardiovert 50 Joulesᵈ·ᵉ
               Until VT Resolves, or                 ↓
                  up to 3 mg/kg           Cardiovert 100 Joulesᵈ
                          ↓                          ↓
            Procainamide, 20 mg/min        Cardiovert 200 Joulesᵈ
               Until VT Resolves,                    ↓
               or up to 1,000 mg          Cardiovert With up to
                          ↓                     360 Joulesᵈ
                  Cardiovert as in                   ↓
                Unstable Patientsᶜ        If Recurrent, Add Lidocaine
                                          and Cardiovert Again Starting
                                               at Energy Level
                                          Previously Successful; Then
                                          Procainamide or Bretyliumᶠ
```

FIGURE 5. Bradycardia. This sequence was developed to assist in teaching how to treat a broad range of patients with bradycardia. Some patients may require care not specified herein. This algorithm should not be construed to prohibit such flexibility. AV indicates atrioventricular.

[a]A solitary chest thump or cough may stimulate cardiac electrical activity and result in improved cardiac output and may be used at this point.

[b]Hypotension (blood pressure <90 mmHg), premature ventricular contractions, altered mental status or symptoms (e.g., chest pain or dyspnea), ischemia, or infarction.

[c]Temporizing therapy.

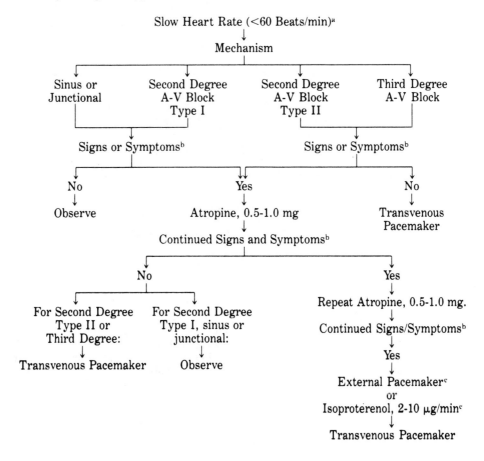

FIGURE 6. Ventricular ectopy: acute suppressive therapy. This sequence was developed to assist in teaching how to treat a broad range of patients with ventricular ectopy. Some patients may require therapy not specified herein. This algorithm should not be construed as prohibiting such flexibility.

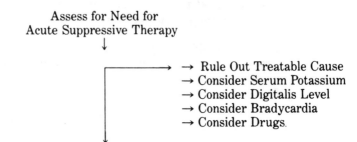

Assess for Need for
Acute Suppressive Therapy
↓

→ Rule Out Treatable Cause
→ Consider Serum Potassium
→ Consider Digitalis Level
→ Consider Bradycardia
→ Consider Drugs.

Lidocaine, 1 mg/kg
↓
If Not Suppressed,
Repeat Lidocaine, 0.5 mg/kg Every 2-10 min
Until No Ectopy, or up to 3 mg/kg Given
↓
If Not Suppressed,
Procainamide 20 mg/min
Until No Ectopy, or up to 1,000 mg Given
↓
If Not Suppressed,
and Not Contraindicated,
Bretylium, 5-10 mg/kg Over 8-10 min
↓
If Not Suppressed,
Consider Overdrive Pacing

Once Ectopy Resolved, Maintain as Follows:
    After Lidocaine, 1 mg/kg ... Lidocaine Drip, 2 mg/min
    After Lidocaine, 1-2 mg/kg ... Lidocaine Drip, 3 mg/min
    After Lidocaine, 2-3 mg/kg ... Lidocaine Drip, 4 mg/min
    After Procainamide ... Procainamide drip, 1-4 mg/min (Check Blood Level)
    After Bretylium .... Bretylium Drip, 2 mg/min

FIGURE 7. Paroxysmal supraventricular tachycardia (PSVT). This sequence was developed to assist in teaching how to treat a broad range of patients with sustained PSVT. Some patients may require care not specified herein. This algorithm should not be construed as prohibiting such flexibility. Flow of algorithm presumes PSVT is continuing.

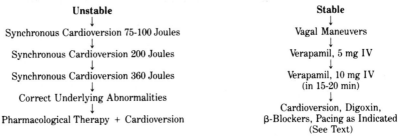

Unstable
↓
Synchronous Cardioversion 75-100 Joules
↓
Synchronous Cardioversion 200 Joules
↓
Synchronous Cardioversion 360 Joules
↓
Correct Underlying Abnormalities
↓
Pharmacological Therapy + Cardioversion

Stable
↓
Vagal Maneuvers
↓
Verapamil, 5 mg IV
↓
Verapamil, 10 mg IV
(in 15-20 min)
↓
Cardioversion, Digoxin,
β-Blockers, Pacing as Indicated
(See Text)

If conversion occurs but PSVT recurs, repeated electrical cardioversion is *not* indicated. Sedation should be used as time permits.

ACLS Algorithms

FIGURE 8. Recommended treatment algorithm for ventricular fibrillation and pulseless ventricular tachycardia when ACLS cannot be provided and an automated external defibrillator and a trained provider are present.

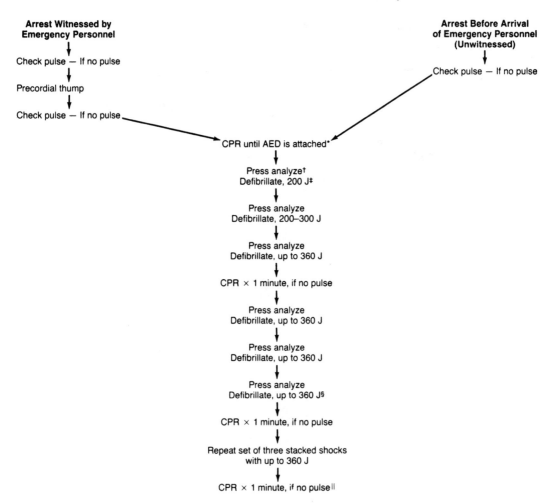

Ventricular Fibrillation and Pulseless Ventricular Tachycardia

*The single rescuer with an AED should verify unresponsiveness, open the airway (A), give two respirations (B), and check the pulse (C). If a full cardiac arrest is confirmed, the rescuer should attach the AED and proceed with the algorithm.
†If "no shock indicated" appears, check pulse, repeat 1 minute of CPR, and then reanalyze. After three "no shock indicated" messages are received, repeat analyze period every 1–2 minutes.
‡Pulse check is not required after shocks 1, 2, 4, and 5 unless the "no shock indicated" message appears.
§If ventricular fibrillation recurs after transiently converting (rather than persists without ever converting), restart the treatment algorithm from the top.
‖In the unlikely event that ventricular fibrillation persists after nine shocks, then repeat sets of three stacked shocks, with 1 minute of CPR between each set.

Bibliography

American Academy of Orthopaedic Surgeons, *Emergency Care and Transportation of the Sick and Injured* (4th ed.), Menasha, WI: George Banta Company, 1987.

American Heart Association, *Textbook of Advanced Cardiac Life Support* (2nd ed.), Dallas, TX: American Heart Association, 1987.

Campbell, M.D., John Emery, *Basic Trauma Life Support: Advanced Prehospital Care* (2nd ed.), Englewood Cliffs, N.J.: Prentice Hall, Inc., 1988.

Caroline, M.D., Nancy L., *Emergency Care in the Streets* (3rd ed.), Boston, MS: Little, Brown and Company, 1987.

Gazzaniga, Alan B., Lloyd T. Iseri, and Martin Baren, *Emergency Care: Principles and Practices for the EMT-Paramedic* (2nd ed.), Reston, VA: Reston Publishing Company, Inc., 1982.

Grant, Harvey D., Robert H. Murray, Jr., J. David Bergeron, *Emergency Care* (4th ed.), Englewood Cliffs, N.J.: Prentice-Hall, Inc., 1986.

Greenwald, Jonathan, *The Paramedic Manual*. Englewood, CO: Morton Publishing Company, 1988.

Guyton, M.D., Arthur C., *Human Physiology and Mechanisms of Disease* (4th ed.), Philadelphia, PA: W.B. Saunders Company, 1987.

Huszar, M.D., Robert J., *Emergency Cardiac Care* (2nd ed.), Bowie, MD: Robert J. Brady Company, 1982.

Pre-Hospital Trauma Life Support Committee of the National Association of Emergen-
cy Medical Technicians in Cooperation With The Committee on Trauma of The
American College of Surgeons, *Pre-Hospital Trauma Life Support.* Akron, OH:
Educational Direction, Inc., 1986.

Shade, Bruce R., Joann Grif Alspach, Michael J. Ballenger, Victor A. Morant, *Advanced
Cardiac Life Support: Certification, Preparation and Review* (2nd ed.), Englewood
Cliffs, N.J.: Prentice-Hall, Inc., 1988.

Tortora, Gerald J., *Principles of Human Anatomy* (4th ed.), New York, NY: Harper &
Row, Publishers, 1986.

Department of Transportation, *Emergency Medical Technician—Paramedic: National
Standard Curriculum.* Washington, D.C.: U.S. Government Printing Office, 1985.

Walraven, Gail, *Basic Arrhythmias* (2nd ed.), Englewood Cliffs, N.J.: Prentice-Hall, Inc.,
1986.

Index